Nursing Delegation and Management

of Patient Care

Nursing Delegation and Management

of Patient Care

THIRD
EDITION

Kathleen Motacki, MSN, BSN, RN
Clinical Professor
Nursing
Saint Peter's University
Jersey City
NJ, USA

Kathleen M. Burke, PhD, RN
Assistant Dean in Charge of Nursing
Adler Center for Nursing Excellence
Ramapo College of NJ
Mahwah
NJ, USA

ELSEVIER

Elsevier
3251 Riverport Lane
St. Louis, Missouri 63043

NURSING DELEGATION AND MANAGEMENT OF PATIENT CARE,
THIRD EDITION

ISBN: 978-0-323-62546-3

> **Notices**
>
> Knowledge and best practice in this field are constantly changing. As new research and experience broaden our understanding, changes in research methods, professional practices, or medical treatment may become necessary. Practitioners and researchers must always rely on their own experience and knowledge in evaluating and using any information, methods, compounds or experiments described herein. Because of rapid advances in the medical sciences, in particular, independent verification of diagnoses and drug dosages should be made. To the fullest extent of the law, no responsibility is assumed by Elsevier, authors, editors or contributors for any injury and/or damage to persons or property as a matter of products liability, negligence or otherwise, or from any use or operation of any methods, products, instructions, or ideas contained in the material herein.

Content Strategist: Yvonne Alexopoulos
Content Development Manager: Meghan Andress
Content Development Specialist: Kevin Travers
Publishing Services Manager: Shereen Jameel
Project Manager: Janish Paul
Design Direction: Margaret Reid

Printed in the United States of America

Last digit is the print number: 9   8   7   6   5   4   3   2   1

Working together
to grow libraries in
developing countries

www.elsevier.com • www.bookaid.org

ABOUT THE AUTHORS

KATHLEEN MOTACKI, MSN, RN, BC

A Clinical Professor at Saint Peter's University School of Nursing, Jersey City, New Jersey, Kathleen Motacki has more than 40 years of experience in nursing, 12 years as a Professor of Nursing, and currently teaches 4-year traditional nursing courses and in the RN-to-BSN program at the Jesuit College of New Jersey. Her areas of clinical and classroom expertise include pediatric nursing, leadership, and community health. She has taught pediatric NCLEX® review sessions. She holds board certification in pediatric nursing from the American Nurses Credentialing Center (ANCC). She was on the ANCC examination-standard-setting committee and on the content expert panel for the new pediatric credentialing examination. She was the lead investigator for the American Nurses Association School of Nursing Curriculum Study on Safe Patient Handling and Movement. She received the 2008 National Occupational Research Agenda (NORA) Partnering Award for the American Nurses Association Safe Patient Handling and Movement Training Program for her role in the Schools of Nursing research project. She also received the Daisy Award and the Marianne Rooney Award for nursing excellence from the New Jersey Consortium of Chapters, Sigma Theta Tau International Nursing Honor Society. She is past president of the Epsilon Rho Chapter and the Mu Theta Chapter at Large and currently serves as the Secretary for the New Jersey Consortium of Chapters, Sigma Theta Tau International Nursing Honor Society. Professor Motacki obtained her BSN and MSN in transcultural nursing administration from Kean University, Union, New Jersey. She has published a continuing nursing education series for contact hours, "Safe Patient Handling in Pediatrics," in the *Journal of Pediatric Nursing*. She has published two books with Springer Publishing: *The Illustrated Guide to Safe Patient Handling and Movement* and *The Illustrated Guide to Infection Control*. She has presented at conferences throughout the country on safe patient handling and movement, as well as on peer-reviewed nursing publications.

KATHLEEN M. BURKE, RN, PhD

Kathleen Burke presently serves as the Assistant Dean in Charge of Nursing at Ramapo College of New Jersey, the state's public liberal arts college. In this position, she is the chief administrator of a 700-student program with prelicensure and RN-to-BSN, RN-to-MSN, and DNP programs. She has been in this position since 2007. In this role she has created academic/clinical partnerships between the college and The Valley Hospital, Ridgewood, New Jersey; University of Sierra Leone in West Africa; and Kwame Nkrumah University of Science and Technology in Kumasi, Ghana. Additionally, she has served as research advisor to three large Magnet Hospitals in New Jersey and is presently working with St. Joseph's Regional Medical Center (a four-time Magnet-recognized organization). Before that, she was the Assistant Dean of the UMDNJ (the state's health sciences university) School of Nursing, in charge of the Northern Region.

She has extensive clinical nursing experience, having started as a staff nurse in the Veterans Administration system, then moving to local community hospitals and up the professional ladder to supervisory roles, Director of Performance Improvement, Director of Clinical Education, and Senior Vice President of Nursing.

Kathleen has served as a member of Quality New Jersey as an examiner, trainer, senior examiner, and Member of the Board of Judges from 1995 to 2003. She was a 10-year member of the Baldrige Board of Examiners. She has also facilitated training and served on writing panels and scorebook review panels. She has participated in and led numerous site visits at both state and national levels. She led the first of the Baldrige Collaborative Assessment Teams. She holds a Green Belt in Quality and Lean Six Sigma from Villanova University.

Kathleen is presently serving on the Board of Trustees of the New Bridge Medical Center in Paramus, New Jersey. She previously served on the Board of Trustees of The Valley Home Care System in Ridgewood, New Jersey, and on the Board of Mountainside Hospital in Glen Ridge, New Jersey. She is the sole academic representative to the New Jersey Council of Magnet

Organizations and the Northern New Jersey Council of Magnet Organizations.

She holds a Bachelor's Degree from Rutgers, The State University of New Jersey, College of Nursing. Her Master of Arts degree is from New York University, Division of Nursing, and she holds a PhD in Nursing Theory and Research from New York University. She was an AACN/Wharton Leadership Fellow in 2014. She is a member of the American Nurses Association, the National League for Nursing, New Jersey Organization of Nurse Executives, Sigma Theta Tau International, and the New Jersey Council of Magnet Organizations.

Nursing Delegation and Management of Patient Care, Third Edition, is designed to assist nursing students and novice nurses to begin developing an understanding of the myriad issues facing them as managers of care and the potential nursing leaders of tomorrow. This is only a beginning; the concepts of management and leadership are changing daily. Health care is moving at an unprecedented speed, and it is imperative that we all attempt to keep up. The important lesson here is that we as nurses need to keep current, questioning and focusing on what is "best" for our patients and practice.

There is massive information, in both the scholarly and commercial literature, that focuses on what makes a good manager or leader. It is important that nurses keep in touch with this literature, but they need to be able to differentiate between what is "best evidence" and what is best-selling fiction. As you move into practice, your professional organizations, your health care library/librarian, and your own engagement in the profession will be your best allies. Keep in touch with the current literature, and continually strive to improve the care that you deliver to patients and families. Remember: continuous improvement is continuous!

This book is divided into five sections, four of which deal with the components of the Magnet Model; the final section deals with issues of importance to new graduate nurses. The Magnet-focused sections deal with:
- Transformational leadership
- Structural empowerment
- Exemplary professional practice
- New knowledge, innovations, and improvements

The last section deals with issues of importance to newly graduated nurses.

Integrated throughout these components are the delineated areas of competence for the nurse manager (AONL). These areas of competence include:
- Financial management
- Human resource management
- Performance improvement
- Technology
- Strategic management
- Clinical practice based on current evidence

Other competencies are necessary for the art of managing health care. This is leading the people of health care. These competencies include:
- Human resource skills
- Relationship management and influencing behaviors
- Diversity
- Shared decision-making

Finally, there are competencies for creating the leader in yourself:
- Personal and professional accountability
- Career planning
- Personal journey disciplines
- Optimizing the leader within

PREFACE TO THE STUDENTS

Nursing Delegation and Management of Patient Care, Third Edition, is designed to assist you as you prepare to become the nursing leaders of tomorrow. To help you make the most of your learning experience, here are the key features that you will find in this text:
- Objectives begin each chapter and explain what students should accomplish on completion of each chapter.
- Key Terms with definitions are placed at the beginning of each chapter for quick reference.
- Summaries review key points covered in each chapter.
- Updated Clinical Corner boxes discuss topics related to practice process improvements made by nurses.
- Evidence-Based Practice boxes review current research and/or best practice.
- Each chapter ends with NCLEX® exam–style review questions.
- **NEW** to this edition: each section ends with a Next-Generation NCLEX® (NGN)–style case study.

FEATURES AND ANCILLARIES

The text is organized according to these competencies of nurse leaders and managers. Each chapter includes a Clinical Corner box written by a nurse leader who shares a current practice that is used in practice. Additionally, there is an evidence-based discussion from a current piece of literature that reviews current research and/or best practice. It is our hope that the reader gleans some ideas from these sections to spark their own practice. Each chapter concludes with some NCLEX® exam–style questions that may prove helpful in reviewing the content. **New** to this edition are Next-Generation NCLEX® (NGN)–style case studies after each of the five sections.

ANCILLARIES

Evolve Resources for Nursing Delegation and Management of Patient Care, Third Edition, are available at http://evolve.elsevier.com/Motacki/delegation/ to enhance student instruction. This online resource is organized by chapter and includes:For instructors:
- TEACH for Nurses
- Test Bank Questions

- PowerPoint Slides
- Image Collection
- Next-Generation NCLEX® (NGN)–Style Leadership and Management Case Studies
  For students:
- NCLEX® exam–style practice questions for each chapter

CONTRIBUTORS AND REVIEWERS

Josephine Bodino, DNP, MPA, RN, NEA-BC, HN-BC
Assistant Vice President, Professional Practice/PCS Finance
The Valley Hospital
Ridgewood, NJ

Laura Cima, PhD, RN, MBA, FACHE
Adjunct Faculty,
Ramapo College of New Jersey
Mahwah, NJ

Gina M. Dovi, MSN, RN, CPHON
Adjunct Faculty
Ramapo College of New Jersey
Mahwah, NJ

Kathy Faber, MSN, RN, CNL
Clinical Nurse Leader, Chair of EBP Council,
St. Joseph's Health
Paterson, NJ

Annemarie Flatekval, DNP, RN, NE-BC
Assistant Professor
Ramapo College of New Jersey
Mahwah, NJ

Donna Grotheer, MSN, RN
Epic Educator
University Hospital
Newark, NJ

Stephanie Herr, DNP, RN
Director of Organizational Education
St. Joseph's Health
Paterson, NJ

Catherine Herrmann, MSN, RN, CCRN, NE-BC
Nurse Manager III, Endoscopy Services
Hackensack University Medical Center
Hackensack, NJ

May Ann Hozak, MSN, RN, NEA-BC
Director of Cardiology
St. Joseph's Health
Paterson, NJ

Beverly S. Karas-Irwin, DNP, RN, NP-C, HNB-BC, NEA-BC
Director of Nursing and Advanced Practice
The Summit Medical Group
Summit, NJ

Judith Kutzleb, DNP, RN, CCRN, CCA, NP-C
Holy Name Medical Center
Holy Name Medical Partners
Teaneck, NJ

David Liguori, DNP, NP-C, ACHPN
Assistant Professor of Nursing
Ramapo College of New Jersey
Mahwah, NJ

Karen Madigan, MSN, RN
Hackensack University Medical Center
Hackensack, NJ

Maureen Mulligan, MSN, RN
Clinical Educator
St. Joseph's Health
Paterson, NJ

Joan Orseck, RN
Human Resources Business Partner
Holy Name Medical Center
Teaneck, NJ

Karen M. Stanley, MS, APRN, BC
Medical University Hospital Authority
Charleston, SC

Shirley Bennett Thompson, RN, BSN, BSBA, MSHA, FACHE
Shirley Bennett Thompson Consulting LLC
Jackson, FL

Melissa Tunc, DNP, RN, HN-BC, CPHQ, PMCP
Lean Six Sigma Black Belt
System Director for Quality and Performance
  Improvement
Valley Health System
Ridgewood, NJ

Maureen Washburn, RN, ND, CPHQ, FACHE
Certification and Program Development
DNV-GL-Business Assurance
Healthcare Accreditation Services
Milford, OH

**Linda Wendling, MA, MFA , English Composition
  and Writing**
Writing-Learning Theory Specialty
University of Missouri–St. Louis
St. Louis, MO

REVIEWERS

JoAnne M. Pearce, MS, RN
Assistant Professor
Nursing Department
Idaho State University, College of Technology Nursing
  Department
Pocatello, ID

**Michael Wayne Rager, PhD, DNP, MSN, FNP-BC,
  APRN, CNE**
Dean of Nursing
Daymar College
Owensboro, KY

Haywood Smith, RN, BSN, MSA, MSN/Ed, CNE
Instructor
Department of Nursing and Allied Health
Norfolk State University
Norfolk, VA

ACKNOWLEDGMENTS

The collaborative partnership with the New Jersey Council of Magnet Organizations has been an invaluable asset to the continued refinement of our understanding of current nursing practice for this text. I thank them for their commitment to sustained excellence.

CONTENTS

Transformational Leadership

SECTION OUTLINE

Transformational leaders are those who stimulate and inspire followers to achieve extraordinary outcomes and in the process develop their own leadership potential. The transformational nursing leader communicates expectations, develops leaders, and evolves the organization. (American Nurses Credentialing Center [ANCC], 2019, p. 19). They also evolve the organization through strategic planning to meet current and future needs and strategic challenges. Nursing leaders at all levels of the organization demonstrate advocacy and support on behalf of staff and patients (ANCC, 2016, 2019).

The strategic planning of the organization occurs at all levels and must align with the organizational priorities to continually improve the levels of performance across the organization. Wherever nursing is practiced, the nursing leadership must develop structures, processes, and expectations for clinical nurse input and involvement across the organization (ANCC, 2016).

This section deals with the leadership structure within health care organizations, such as the structures and processes, underlying strategic planning, regulatory environments, and financial management.

1

Leadership and Management

OBJECTIVES

- Identify the various leadership theories.
- Differentiate between leadership and management.
- Discuss the role of a manager.
- Review the different management levels in nursing.
- Identify differences between a nurse manager and a nurse executive.

- Differentiate between the various types of competencies of patient care managers.
- Compare the nursing process and the management process.
- Discuss activities used by a nurse manager to support the nursing and management processes.
- Identify the day-to-day activities of a care manager.

KEY TERMS

chief nursing executive the highest level nurse within an integrated health system, who has responsibility for all nursing practice within the system (American Organization of Nurse Leaders, 2019)

chief nursing officer the highest level nurse with ultimate responsibility for all nursing practice within the single organization (ANCC, 2019)

first-level manager manager responsible for supervising nonmanagerial personnel and day-to-day activities of specific work units

leadership ability to influence people to work toward the meeting of stated goals

management act of planning, organizing, staffing, directing, and controlling for the present; process of coordinating actions and allocating resources to achieve organizational goals

middle-level manager manager who supervises first-level managers within a specified area and is responsible for the people and activities within those areas; generally acts as liaison between first-level and upper-level management

upper-level manager top level to whom middle manager reports; primarily responsible for establishing organizational goals and strategic plans for entire division of nursing

Nursing leadership has transitioned from the silo-based oversight of only nursing to the coordination and leadership of strategic, interprofessional teams responsible for structures and processes necessary for quality patient care. Today's health care environment promotes the value of nursing across all settings in the quest to achieve the *Triple Aim*, which is effective, safe, quality care that exceeds patient/family/community expectations and is efficient to reduce the total cost across the health care continuum.

LEADERSHIP VERSUS MANAGEMENT

Just because someone is in a leadership position, it does not automatically follow that this person is a leader. Some people have false assumptions about leaders and leadership. Many people believe that the position and title are the same as true leadership. Having the title of chief nurse does not necessarily mean that the person in that position is a leader, whereas being a staff nurse does not mean that person is not a leader. New nurse managers often make the mistake of believing that along with the new title comes the mantle of leadership. Leadership takes a tremendous amount of effort, time, and energy. Leadership can be defined as the use of individual traits and personal power to influence and guide strategy development. Leaders need to "do the right thing," be future oriented, be visionary, focus on purposes, and empower others to set and achieve organizational goals. According to Porter-O'Grady and Mallach, 2015) the major tasks of the 21st century health care leader include:

- Deconstructing the barriers and structures of the 20th century
- Alerting staff about the implications of changing what they do
- Establishing safety around taking risks and experimenting
- Embracing new technologies as a way of doing work
- Reading the signposts along the road to the future
- Translating the emerging reality of health reform into language the staff can use

- Demonstrating personal engagement with health reform
- Helping others adapt to the demands of a value-driven health system
- Creating a safe milieu for the struggles and pain of changing practice and service
- Enumerating small successes as a basis for supporting staff
- Celebrating the journey and all progress made

Management is the act of planning, organizing, staffing, directing, and controlling for the present. Management can be taught, whereas leadership is usually a reflection of personal experience.

As shown in Table 1.1, leaders show the way, although managers labor to produce the day-to-day outcomes. Leaders focus on effectiveness, and managers deal with efficiencies (see Table 1.1).

TABLE 1.1 Comparison of Leadership and Management Functions

Management Produces Order and Consistency	Leadership Produces Change and Movement
• Planning and budgeting • Establishing agendas • Setting timetables • Allocating resources	• Establishing direction • Creating a vision • Clarifying the big picture • Setting strategies
• Organizing and staffing • Providing structure • Making job placements • Establishing rules and procedures	• Aligning people • Communicating goals • Seeking commitment • Building teams and coalitions
• Controlling and problem solving • Developing incentives • Generating creative solutions • Taking corrective action	• Motivating and inspiring • Inspiring and energizing • Empowering subordinates • Satisfying unmet needs

Northouse, P. (2007). *Leadership theory and practice* (p. 10). Thousand Oaks, CA: Sage Publications.

COMPARISON OF LEADERSHIP AND MANAGEMENT

A further review of leadership and management focuses on the major themes of each role (see Table 1.1). The nurse, as manager, works collaboratively to achieve the desired outcomes of quality care, fiscal responsibility, and customer satisfaction by coordinating the care of individuals, families, groups, or populations through the effective use of technology, resources, information, and systems.

THEORIES OF LEADERSHIP

There are numerous theories of leadership. How the leader approaches leadership is often very dependent on their personal experiences. Leadership also relies on the organizational structure and culture of the health care facility. Four of the more common leadership theories have evolved over time: trait theory, behavioral theory, contingency theory, and contemporary theory.

Trait Theory

Leaders are presumed to possess certain traits that are leadership specific. Leadership traits include drive, persistence, creative problem solving, initiative, self-confidence, ability to influence others, and intelligence. The thought is that these traits, when put into practice, will result in positive outcomes.

Behavioral Theory

The focus of behavioral theory is not what leaders do, but how they behave. Behaviorists characterize leaders by their style of practice:

- Autocratic leaders change behaviors within the organization through the use of coercion, authority, punishment, and power.
- Democratic leaders influence change within the organization through participation, involvement of staff in goal setting, and collaboration.
- Permissive or laissez-faire leaders assume that people are able to make their own decisions and complete their work without any facilitation of the leader.
- Bureaucratic leaders influence the behavior of the organization through organizational policies and rules.

Contingency Theory

Often leaders use different leadership styles in different situations. A leader may use an autocratic style in a disaster management situation but use a democratic style in strategic planning. This ability to adjust one's approach to the situation is called situational leadership or contingency theory.

Newer concepts of leadership are a combination of prior work in the field and include such descriptors as charismatic, connective, shared, and servant leadership. A charismatic leader has the ability to engage others because of his or her powerful personality. Connective leadership draws on the leader's ability to bring others together to effect change. Shared leadership acknowledges that no one person can accomplish the work of the organization. Self-directed work teams and shared governance epitomize this philosophy. Servant leadership puts other people and their needs before the leader's self-interest and works to build community.

Two leadership theories prevalent within health care today are transactional leadership and transformational leadership. In transactional leadership, there is an exchange between the leader and the employee. The needs of the employees are identified, and the leader provides rewards to meet those needs in exchange for performance. This type of leadership usually occurs in a hierarchical organization, that is, one in which decision making occurs at the top of the structure and is communicated to the employees. Transformational leadership is more consultative and collaborative. (Kouzes & Posner, 2017) identified five basic practices in transformational leadership:

1. Challenging the process, questioning the ways that things have always been done, and creatively thinking of new ways of doing things
2. Motivating and inspiring shared vision or bringing everyone together, moving toward the shared goal
3. Empowering others to act
4. Modeling the change
5. Praising the employee for the work done

Transformational leaders behave in ways to achieve superior results by employing one or more of the four core components of transformational leadership:

Idealized Influence (II): Leaders serve as a role model for followers. They exhibit high ethical behavior, instill pride, and gain respect and trust. Followers tend to identify with their leaders and desire to emulate them; leaders are perceived by their followers as having extraordinary capabilities, persistence, and determination.

Inspirational Motivation (IM): This is the degree to which the leader articulates a vision that is appealing, motivating, and inspiring to followers. Leaders with IM communicate optimism about future goals, provide meaning for the task at hand, and challenge followers with high standards. The visionary aspects of leadership are supported by communication skills that make the vision understandable, precise, powerful, and engaging. The followers are willing to invest more effort in their tasks because they are encouraged and optimistic about the shared vision and goals.

Intellectual Stimulation (IS): This is the degree to which leaders challenge assumptions, take risks, and stimulate and solicit followers' ideas. Transformational leaders encourage followers to be innovative and creative by questioning assumptions, by reframing problems, and by challenging them to approach old situations in new ways.

Individualized Consideration (IC): This is the degree to which the leader attends to each follower's need for achievement and growth, acts as a mentor or coach to the follower, and listens to the follower's concerns and needs. The leader provides empathy and support, keeps communication open, and places challenges before the followers. IC also encompasses the need for respect and celebrates the individual contribution that each follower makes to the team (Bass and Riggio, 2005, cited in American Nurses Credentialing Center [ANCC], 2019, p. 161).

One form of governance often used by transformational leaders is shared governance. This is a democratic, dynamic process resulting from shared decision making and accountability (Porter-O'Grady, 2001, 2003). Shared governance is a structure and process for partnership, equity, accountability, and ownership (Guanci, 2018) It is a key principle in the ANCC's Magnet Recognition Programs. ANCC shared leadership/participative decision making is a model in which nurses are formally organized to make decisions about clinical practice standards, quality improvement, staff and professional development, and research (American Nurses Credentialing Center [ANCC], 2019, p. 160).

LEADER VERSUS MANAGER

As you advance in your nursing proficiency, you will eventually take over some managerial tasks. You may even be asked to become a nurse manager. However, just because you take on some managerial tasks does not necessarily make you a nurse manager. Also, just because you are an excellent clinical nurse does not mean that you will become an excellent manager. In some organizations the only promotion opportunities occur through progression to management. If you do not see yourself in such a role, it will be important for you to work in an organization that also has promotion opportunities for nurses who remain at the bedside. The competencies of a nurse manager need to be developed, and the process of manager development occurs through education, mentorship, and professional growth. A *Transition to Practice* program supports you as you move into a management role. As discussed earlier, management is not synonymous with leadership, although management is a part of leadership.

Management and leadership are different. The distinctions between leaders and managers are as follows (Kerr, 2015):

- Leadership inspires change; management manages transformation.
- Leadership requires vision; management requires tenacity.
- Leadership requires imagination; management requires specifics.
- Leadership requires abstract thinking; management requires concrete data.
- Leadership requires the ability to articulate; management requires the ability to interpret.
- Leadership requires an aptitude to sell; management requires an aptitude to teach.
- Leadership requires an understanding of the external environment; management requires an understanding of how work gets done inside the organization.
- Leadership requires risk-taking; management requires self-discipline.
- Leadership requires confidence in the face of uncertainty; management requires commitment to completing the task at hand.
- Leadership is accountable to the entire organization; management is accountable to the team.

In addition, the leader needs to be able to operate under the evidence-based management tenets identified in the Institute of Medicine, 2004 report on work environment. These five tenets are (1) balancing efficiency and patient safety, (2) promoting trust, (3) creating and managing change, (4) implementing shared decision making around work design and flow, and (5) establishing a learning environment. Leadership is

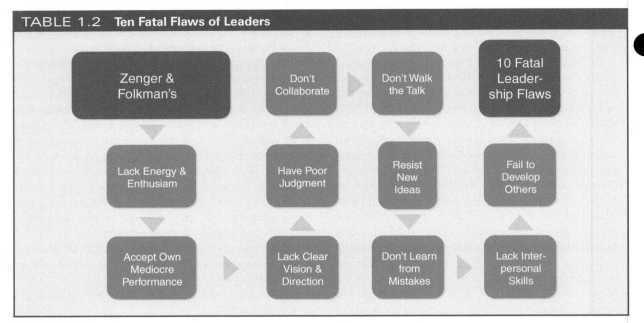

TABLE 1.2   Ten Fatal Flaws of Leaders

Zenger, J. & Folkman, J. (2009). Ten fatal flaws that derail leaders. *Harvard Business Review, 87*(6), 18. <https://hbr.org/2009/06/ten-fatal-flaws-that-derail-leaders/sb1> Accessed 24.9.19.

mission driven, whereas management is task driven. There are, however, 10 fatal leadership flaws (Table 1.2). These flaws can derail leaders and transformational leadership.

Management is a complex process of coordinating and directing the actions of others to accomplish an organization's objectives. It also involves the assignment of resources to these groups so that the objectives can be met. It is achieved through six functions: planning, staffing, organizing, directing, controlling, and decision making (Carroll, 2006).

Planning determines what needs to be done. This may refer to what needs to be done for a single shift or for a longer period, such as the year. Management planning is not the same as the strategic planning done by senior leadership. Staffing refers to the selection and assignment of specific people to accomplish the tasks (see Chapter 13 for discussion on delegation). Organizing is the process of coordinating all resources to meet the goals. It is a fluid activity requiring knowledge of the organization and people and having the ability to alter the plan, staffing, and organization if the goals are not being met. Management also includes directing deals with the skills necessary to motivate the

staff to accomplish the assigned tasks. In this function, you need to be able to provide the proper resources, set clear goals, and foster a work environment that encourages goal achievement. Controlling is accomplished through the setting of professional standards, compliance with standards of performance, and the ability to lead a staff to excellence. Finally, decision making is the result of these actions. The seven steps to decision making include: (1) identify the problem, (2) gather relevant information, (3) identify the alternatives, (4) weigh the evidence, (5) choose among alternatives, (6) take action, and (7) review your decision and evaluate the consequences.

COMPARING THE NURSING PROCESS WITH THE MANAGEMENT PROCESS

The nursing process focuses on assessing, analyzing, planning, implementing, and evaluating. The management process is used to meet patient needs in an efficient and effective manner with available resources. The management process consists of five phases: identification of needs, identification of resources, planning, organizing and direction, and controlling.

LEVELS OF MANAGEMENT

Cipriani, 2011 stated that nurse managers "at all levels work together to address emerging trends, adopt innovative ideas, and work toward the shared goals of quality, efficiency, and excellence in practice. They guide and lead frontline nurses while contributing to an organization's success." There are levels of patient care management in most institutions. The organizational structure of the organization will determine the titles and the span of authority of the various levels of patient care management (Box 1.1).

First Level

The first-level manager, also known as a front-line manager, nurse manager, or head nurse is responsible for supervising the work of nonmanagerial personnel and the day-to-day activities of a specific work unit or units (Box 1.2). This manager is responsible for the units 24/7. The first-level manager straddles the worlds of staff and upper management, ensuring a two-way flow of information (Cipriani, 2011).

Key tasks for a first-line (front-line) nurse manager may include (adapted from Cipriani, 2011):

- Preparing orientation and transition to practice schedules in collaboration with nursing education department
- Submitting time schedules for nursing shifts
- Assigning staff for patient care during shifts
- Making budget recommendations to the middle- and upper-levels of management; these budget needs are made based on unit needs and patient acuity (see Chapter 4).
- Calculating the amount of staff needed per shift, per day, and so forth. This will also include the alteration of staffing plans based on emergencies, sick calls, and changes in patient acuity
- Making daily patient rounds
- Conducting staff meetings
- Conducting employment reviews, including counseling reports and termination
- Overseeing peer evaluation
- Interviewing potential staff members (this is often done in conjunction with middle management)
- Participating in performance improvement and evidence-based practice activities; reviewing unit performance on National Database of Nursing Quality Indicators (NDNQI) outcome measures, CORE measures, National Patient Safety Goals, infection rates, and other unit-based performance indicators
- Setting goals with individual staff and for patient care areas
- Maintaining current knowledge of the profession and regulatory requirements

The scope and standards from the American Nurses Association (ANA) (2016) for nurse administration stated that to fulfill the responsibilities, the nurse manager, in collaboration with nursing personnel and members of other disciplines, has to have the following core competencies:

- Accountability and advocacy for employees
- Clinical care delivery and optimal patient outcomes
- Healthy work environments
- Legal and regulatory compliance
- Networking, partnering, and collaborating
- Patient and population health advocacy
- Safety, quality, and risk management
- Strategic, financial, and human resource management
- Assess the effect of and plan strategies to address the following issues:
  - Ethnic, cultural, and diversity changes in the population
  - Political and social influences
  - Financial and economic issues
  - Aging of society and demographic trends
  - Ethical issues related to health care

Middle Level

The middle-level manager, also known as supervisor, director, assistant director, or associate director of nursing, supervises a number of first-level managers. They are positioned on the organizational chart between the

BOX 1.1 **Three Levels of Management Are Used in Nursing**	
First	Nurse manager
Middle	Director
Upper	Executive

From Sullivan, Eleanor J., *Effective leadership & management in nursing*, 6th edition, ©2005. Reprinted by permission of Pearson Education, Inc.

BOX 1.2 Levels of Managers and Responsibilities

	Upper Level	Middle Level	First Level
Examples	Chief nursing officer Chief nursing executive	Unit supervisor Department head Director	Nurse manager Charge nurse Team leader, Primary nurse
Scope of responsibility	Look at organization as a whole and external influences	Focus on integrating unit(s) level day-to-day needs with organizational needs	Focus on day-to-day needs at unit level
Primary planning focus	Strategic planning	Combination of long- and short-range planning	Short-range operational planning
Communication flow	More often top-down but receives shared governance feedback both directly and via middle-level managers and nursing councils	Upward and downward with great centrality	More often upward; generally relies on middle-level managers to transmit communication to top-level managers

Adapted from Marquis, B., & Huston, C. (2017). *Leadership roles and management Functions in nursing* (p. 299). Wolters Kluwer: Philadelphia, PA.

nurse manager and the chief nursing officer (CNO) of the site. These managers usually are within the same specialty or the same geographic location. Specialty directors may manage all specialty care for both inpatient and outpatient experience. They may spend more time planning, evaluating, and coordinating and less time with direct patient care supervision than the first-line manager (see Box 1.2). They are responsible for the people and activities within the departments they supervise 24/7.

Key tasks that the middle-level manager may perform include (adapted from Carroll, 2006, p. 33):

- *Assessment:* Observe whether unit policies and objectives are meeting the needs of the patients and staff. Initiate changes to unit policies based on current evidence.
- *Planning:* Set short-term and long-term goals for patient care; revise as needed. Align these goals with the goals of the larger patient care services department.
- *Organization:* Put plans in action via delegation, committee work, and through shared governance processes.
- *Control:* Analyze results of action plans and evidence-based projects, make changes as necessary, facilitate the growth of staff, and communicate changes and opportunities to upper-level staff and to staff reporting to managers.

Upper Level

The upper-level manager, or the executive-level manager, is also known as the senior vice president of patient care, vice president for nursing, chief nurse executive (CNE), or CNO. Middle management reports to the vice president for nursing. ANCC defines the CNO as the highest level nurse with ultimate responsibility for all nursing practice within the organization (American Nurses Credentialing Center [ANCC], 2019, p. 146). In this time of mergers and large health care systems, there is a further division to include a CNE that is responsible for all of the nursing practice within the larger system, with site-specific CNOs reporting to the CNE in the larger table of organization.

The CNO spends the least amount of time in direct supervision. Most of the time is spent planning and working with key stakeholders to move the organization forward. According to the Magnet standards, "the CNO is a knowledgeable, transformational leader who develops a strong vision and well articulated philosophy, a professional practice model, and strategic and quality plans in leading nursing services" (American Nurses Credentialing Center [ANCC], 2019, p. 19). The CNO is responsible for influencing change beyond the scope of nursing to provide for continued excellence (American Nurses Credentialing Center [ANCC], 2019, p. 31). They are responsible for establishing organizational goals and strategic plans for the patient care department and driving leadership development and the continued path toward excellence (see Box 1.2).

Key competencies of the nurse administrator (ANA, 2016) include:

- Collection of comprehensive data and information about pertinent problems, issues, and trends
- Analysis of assessment data to identify problems, issues, and trends
- Identification of expected outcomes for the system, organizational, or population problem issue or trend
- Development of a plan that defines, articulates, and establishes strategies and alternatives to attain expected outcomes
- Implementation of the plan
- Coordination of implementation of the plan and other associated processes
- Establishment of strategies to promote health, education, and safe environment
- Provision of consultation to influence the identified plan and effect changes
- Evaluation of progress toward attainment of outcomes
- Practice ethically
- Attainment of knowledge and competence that reflects current nursing practice
- Awareness that decisions are evidence-based and research findings are translated into practice
- Contributions to quality nursing practice
- Effective communication in a variety of formats in all areas of practice
- Provision of leadership to the profession, health care industry, and society
- Collaboration with health care consumers, colleagues, community leaders, and other stakeholders to advance nursing practice and health care transformation
- Evaluation of own nursing practice to professional practice standards and guidelines, relevant statutes, rules, and relevant regulations
- Utilization of appropriate resources to plan and provide evidence-based, high-quality nursing services that are patient-centered, culturally appropriate, safe, timely, effective, and financially responsible
- Practice in an environmentally safe and healthy manner

Other managerial roles have evolved over the last few years. To assist the nurse manager or head nurse, the role of charge nurse (patient care manager) has been developed. This expanded staff nurse role grants a staff nurse managerial responsibility on a given shift. This role may be a permanent position or a rotating one. The care manager functions as a liaison between the nurse manager and the activities and staff of the off-shifts.

Key tasks that the care manager may perform include (adapted from Carroll, 2006, p. 33):

- Assist in shift coordination
- Create patient assignments for the shift
- Deal with personnel issues arising during shift (e.g., sick calls, real-time conflict management)
- Make patient care rounds during shift
- Troubleshoot problems that occur during shift
- Assist staff members with making decisions and prioritizing care
- Use resources efficiently
- Perform staff evaluations (this will depend on the organization)
- Serve as liaison between staff of off-shift and first-line management

COMPETENCIES OF PATIENT CARE MANAGERS

Patient care managers use organizational resources and routines while providing direct patient care. They need to use time productively and collaborate with the interdisciplinary work group. They use leadership characteristics to manage others within the nursing work group. More specifically, to manage patient care, entry-level nurses perform the following tasks:

- Identify organizational resources and determine when they are needed
- Work within various nursing service delivery patterns
- Use position descriptions to establish the scope and limitations of their own and other nursing work group member practices
- Manage time purposefully and productively
- Prioritize patient needs and related care
- Exhibit flexibility in providing care within available time constraints
- Show initiative, flexibility, and creativity as leadership qualities
- Think critically to make decisions required to solve patient care problems
- Collaborate with other health team members
- Resolve conflicts within the work group
- Delegate appropriately

The role of the patient care manager differs from that of the first-line manager in that the charge nurse or care manager has more limited authority and a limited span of control. The charge nurse may or may not perform staff evaluations; this will depend on the organization.

The charge nurse may have more knowledge of staff performance, especially if the position deals with the off-shifts.

Resource nurses are being used in many organizations. The role of resource nurse has developed to role model nurses in areas of clinical decision making and use of resources. The resource nurse is usually a nurse with recognized clinical expertise (clinical ladder position, certification, and experience) who is able to mentor less experienced nurses as they grow within the profession (St. Luke's Medical Center, 2015). Clinical resource nurses serve as a clinical resource for the identified unit(s). They collaborate with nurse leaders and medical and nursing staff and provide clinical support to improve patient care and patient outcomes in the unit (Quinn-O'Neil et al., 2011).

SUMMARY

The role of the manager is very different from that of the nurse. Although nurses need to have strong management skills to deliver patient care, there are additional skills and tasks that are needed to be a nurse manager at any level. Not every nurse will want to be a nurse manager, even though they manage patient care on a daily basis. As a new nurse moves into a managerial role, it is important to realize that a different set of skills and knowledge is required to advance in this role. The American Organization of Nurse Executives has many resources for these roles, and the ANCC manages the certification examinations for nurses working in nursing administration.

CLINICAL CORNER

Topic

A successful nursing future is reliant on strong nursing leadership. Health care has become more complex and challenging and requires adequately prepared nurse managers to lead the health care organizations. Nurse managers that are not provided with appropriate leadership development can result in high turnover rates for staff, and poor patient and staff satisfaction, which ultimately negatively affect the fiscal health of the organization. Therefore, leadership development is crucial for nurse manager and organizational success. However, leadership training for this position may not be satisfactory.

Literature Search

Nurse managers are crucial to the optimal functioning of health care organizations. Their responsibilities are numerous and affect not only the present but the future of the organizations as well. The development and preparation of the front-line managers, if inadequate, has far-reaching effects. Therefore, effective leadership development of nurse managers is warranted.

The effect of nurse managers on the optimal functioning of our health care organizations is well documented in the literature. Positive leadership skills enable higher patient satisfaction and reduction in the incidence of adverse outcomes Chism (2013). The current health care environment is very complex and changes rapidly. It requires effective leaders to steer through the changes effectively Rees, Glynn, Moore, Rankin, and Stevens (2014). The expectation is to still provide quality patient care in an environment with limited resources and to handle the uncertainty in health care organizations Sherrod and Harper- Harrison (2010). The nurse managers are the role models for staff Rees et al. (2014). Leadership preparation for nurse managers leads to retention of staff, decreased turnover costs, and better quality and financial outcomes for the health care organization Fennimore and Wolf (2011).

This role encompasses accountability to various stakeholders including patients, family members, staff, the interdisciplinary team, the hospital, and the entire health care organization; therefore, it would greatly benefit the health care organizations to ensure that nurse managers receive the appropriate development and support. Many nurse mangers are often promoted based on clinical expertise and they may not receive sufficient preparation and support for this essential role Zwink, et al. (2013). Even though these nurse managers have expertise at the bedside, they are novices in this new role, which requires additional support and training to acclimate to this new role. Leadership training will enable them to have the tools they need to function appropriately in this new role. Investing the time to develop nurse managers has demonstrated benefits for the short and long term Martin, McCormack, Fitzsimons, and Spirig (2012).

Nurse managers are role models for the staff. If time and resources are given to them for their development,

Continued

they will have the skills to develop their staff as well. It will enable them to be proficient in the role. Leaders must be identified, supported, and developed to enable the provision of excellence in nursing care. An important component to attaining this goal is that "informal, negative leaders be discouraged, and positive leaders, possessing the evidence-based qualities of leadership be identified and nurtured to lead the profession."(Scully, 2014)

Nurse managers that had received education and training for leadership expressed this investment in them as a positive Parry, Calarco, Hensinger, Kearly, and Shakarjian (2012). It made them feel highly valued by the organization. Respondents stated, "the opportunity to develop leadership skills, knowledge and attributes in a protected space and during a specific time was described as a privilege" (Wilson, Paterson, & Kornman, 2013, p. 60). Additionally, this will help them to develop a positive culture at the unit level and value their own staff. If they feel valued, they will want to stay, thus leading to higher staff satisfaction, higher retention rates, and higher patient satisfaction (Fennimore & Wolf, 2011; Moore, Sublett, & Leahy, 2016).

When providing training, it is important to connect the content to actual situations that the manager encounters McNamara et al. (2014). Collaborating with each other and discussing best practices as nurse managers enables this leadership development to continue and allows them to work with their peers to problem solve Mackoff, Glassman, and Budin (2013). This will enable the manager to transition the new knowledge more easily into his or her everyday practice.

Pilot Program

A large health care organization implemented a leadership development program for their nurse managers. The training program was effective and may be replicated in other health care organizations. An educational needs assessment for the nurse managers indicated that they were interested in a leadership development program, and the CNE identified leadership development as a topic for an educational program. The program had three elements and encompassed a time span of about four months. The first element was the assignment of the Essentials of Nurse Manager (ENMO) course (American Association of Critical Care Nurses, 2016); this is made up of eight modules in three categories: The Science of the Business of Nursing, The Art of Leading People, and the Leader Within. These

modules were assigned to be completed prior to Weekly Lunch and Learn sessions. The second element was Weekly Lunch and Learn sessions that occurred over a 12-week period. During these sessions, the nurse managers were able to collaborate and discuss real-life situations with each other and with the educators that had previous nursing administrative experience. This enabled them to brainstorm and become confident in their decisions. The third session was a two-day live leadership development program, one week apart from the leadership development program that discussed additional topics identified by the CNE that were important for their role in the organization. Some of these topics included managing the multi-generational workforce, career planning, leadership styles, effective communication, time management, change management, and team building. The activities for these topics were interactive and tools for self-assessment were administered, completed, and discussed.

Results

The evaluation of the program by the nurse managers was very positive. Three months after the program, the nurse managers were able to cite examples of how they used the content from the program in their daily practice as nurse leaders. This demonstrates long-term effects of the educational program. The nurse managers also requested training in additional topics, which were given later that year; this is important for the ongoing leadership development of the nurse managers. Additionally, an annual needs assessment should be administered to determine additional leadership development topics.

Future topics for ongoing leadership development could include preparation to obtain certification as a nurse executive and to obtain an advanced degree in nursing administration. Because nurse managers are the role models for the staff, obtaining specialty certification can enable a culture of certification to be created on the units. Pursuing an advanced degree could also be positively viewed by the staff and may encourage the staff to continue their education as well. Nurses with specialty certification and advanced education contribute positively to the future of nursing.

Implications for Future Practice

Implications from this program are that it can be replicated in other organizations. The ENMO course is readily available and the modules can be used with case studies and situations that nurse managers may contend with in

Continued

CLINICAL CORNER—cont'd

their practice. This will foster the development of tools and skills to solve issues that may occur on the units. The content for the live course could be determined in collaboration with Nursing Administration and Nursing Education.

It would be beneficial to measure the effect of the leadership development program over the long term, such as six months and annually. Demographic data about the participants and their level of experience in the nurse manager role should be obtained. Additional measurements could be to determine the effect of leadership development on staff satisfaction, retention rates, patient satisfaction and quality outcomes for the organization, and the leadership ability as perceived by the directors of nursing and CNE.

Conclusion

The nurse manager has a critical role in health care organizations. There are many responsibilities that are key to quality functioning and performance. The nurse manager ensures that patients are provided with care that is compassionate, safe, and fiscally responsible. The nurse manager is also directly linked to patient and staff satisfaction, and a healthy work environment. Because the role of nurse manager is such an important one, preparation for this role is imperative. This pilot leadership development program adds value to support the necessity of leadership development. Appropriate leadership development and education for the nurse managers is essential to ensure that quality outcomes are attained for the health care organizations and to ensure the future success of the nursing profession.

Anne Marie Flatekval
Leadership Development for Nurse Managers
Ramapo College of New Jersey, Mahwah, NJ

EVIDENCE-BASED PRACTICE

Dyess, S., Sherman, R., Pratt, B., & Chiang-Hanisko, L. (2016). Growing nurse leaders: their perspectives on nursing leadership and today's practice environment. *Online Journal of Issues in Nursing, 21*(1), 7.

Growing Nurse Leaders: Their Perspectives on Nursing Leadership and Today's Practice Environment

With the growing complexity of health care practice environments and pending nurse leader retirements, the development of future nurse leaders is increasingly important. This article reports on focus group research conducted with Generation Y nurses prior to their initiating coursework in a master's degree program designed to support the development of future nurse leaders. Forty-four emerging nurse leaders across three program cohorts participated in this qualitative study conducted to capture perspectives about nursing leaders and leadership.

Three major categories were identified:
- Idealistic expectations of leaders
- Leading in a challenging practice environment
- Cautious but optimistic outlook about their own leadership and future and study limitations

The conclusion offers implications for future nurse leader development. The findings provide important insight into the viewpoints of nurses today about leaders and leadership.

The absence of an adequate leadership pipeline has been cited as a key challenge in nursing today.

Turnover in the first year of employment among new nurses is a persistent problem in many organizations. These nurses are less accepting and more critical about workplace practices than the generations who have preceded them.

They also report more interest in pursuing higher education in nursing. Generation Y nurses are just beginning to move into leadership roles. Retiring nurses should take responsibility for leadership succession.

Research Methodology

The qualitative findings presented in this article were part of a larger action research design promoted by that guided a three-year funded project. A focus group was conducted with cohort members prior to the beginning of their coursework in a master's degree program for nursing administration and financial leadership. Each group was asked the same seven questions related to their perceptions about nursing leadership, the practice environment, health care challenges, and the future of health care (see Table 1).

The focus groups were audiotaped and transcribed verbatim.

Continued

EVIDENCE-BASED PRACTICE—cont'd

TABLE 1   Focus Group Questions

Seven Lead Questions

1. Can you tell me about your understanding of leadership?
2. What do you hope to gain from leadership education?
3. What concerns do you have that might prevent you from entering a formal leadership position?
4. How do you think leadership influences practice, practice environments, and patient outcomes?
5. What is the practice environment like for you and your coworkers?
6. Can you describe your leadership vision for health care in 2020?
7. Is there anything else that you would like to share?

The Sample

The sample included 44 students who were enrolled in an emerging nurse leader master's degree program. Prior to the beginning of their academic coursework, students were invited to participate in a focus group with other members of their program cohort. The majority (54%) were in nursing practice for three years or less; whereas 86% were in practice for six years or less. The cohorts were predominantly female (96%). More than half (55%) of the students identified themselves as a member of an ethnic minority. The age range was 23 to 53 with a majority of the sample in the Generation Y cohort born between 1980 and 2000. The mean age for all participants was 31 years; however, this number was skewed by several older participants who entered nursing as a second career. A majority (84%) worked in the hospital environment. Of the 13 different hospital institutions represented, none had achieved Magnet designation. Some of the participants had been in a charge or relief charge position prior to entering the program. Very few (8%) held formal leadership roles, and those who did were in the equivalent of an assistant nurse manager role.

Study Findings

Three major thematic categories were identified from analysis of the data. These categories included: idealistic expectations of leaders, leading in a challenging practice environment, and cautious but optimistic outlook about their own leadership and future.

They expect their leaders to be available and present on the unit to assist with patient care when needed.

Their comments indicated a limited understanding of the range of responsibilities and time commitment associated with the role of nurse leader.

Despite challenges noted, they are willing to take leadership roles because they see the potential to change their environments.

They expressed enthusiasm about their own abilities to lead in a different way.

Discussion

In the midst of their expression of idealism and challenges, the participants recognize that they are the future of nursing leadership. A key concern for nurse leaders today is who will replace them when they retire.

Conclusion: Implications for Nurse Leaders

The most significant contribution today's leaders can make for the future is to develop their successors so they will adapt, prosper, and grow. With the expected large-scale retirements of many Baby Boomer nurses, the future of nursing leadership will be in the hands of Generation Y nurses early in the next decade.

Acknowledgment

The project described in this article is funded, in part, with the Health Resources and Services Administration (HRSA) Advanced Nursing Education Grant D09HP22615-01-00. The authors have no financial claims or conflicts of interest associated with this manuscript.

References

American Hospital Association. (2014). *Managing an intergenerational workforce: strategies for health care transformation.* <https://www.aha.org/about/cpi/managing-intergenerational-workforce.shtml>

American Psychological Association. (2012). *Stress by generation.* https://www.apa.org/news/press/releases/stress/2012/generation.pdf>

American Organization of Nurse Executives. (2014). *AONL position statement on the educational preparation for nurse leaders.* <https://www.aone.org/resources/leadership%20tools/PDFs/EducationPreparationofNurseLeaders%5FFINAL.pdf>

NCLEX® EXAMINATION QUESTIONS

Chapter 1 Leadership and Management

1. A nurse enters the room and finds a patient on the floor. What should the nurse do first?
   A. Assess the patient for injuries
   B. Call for help
   C. Call the physician
   D. Tell the patient to call when getting out of bed

2. What task can the RN assign to an LPN?
   A. Administer blood to a patient
   B. Do intake on a new admission
   C. Develop a care plan
   D. Observe the patient hourly if he is a fall risk

3. Which of the following is described as the use of individual traits and personal power to influence and guide strategy development and be future oriented and visionary?
   A. Leadership
   B. Management
   C. Team leader
   D. Nurse manager

4. Which of the following describes the act of planning, organizing, staffing, and directing?
   A. Management
   B. Leadership
   C. Mentoring
   D. Supervising

5. Leadership traits include drive, persistence, creative problem solving, initiative, self-confidence, ability to influence others, and intelligence. The thought is that these traits when put into practice will result in positive outcomes. What theory considers that leaders are presumed to possess certain traits that are leadership specific?
   A. Trait theory
   B. Behavioral theory
   C. Contingency theory
   D. Contemporary

6. Which of the following lists balancing efficiency and patient safety, promoting trust, creating and managing change; implementing shared decision making around work design and flow; and establishing a learning environment?
   A. Institute of Medicine
   B. Board of Nursing
   C. Institutional Review Board
   D. American Nurses Credentialing Center

7. Identify the problem, gather relevant information, identify the alternatives, weigh the evidence, choose among alternatives, take action, and review your decision and evaluate the consequence are the steps in:
   A. Decision making
   B. Nursing process
   C. Plan of care
   D. Autonomy

8. The nurse manager, or head nurse, that is responsible for supervising the work of nonmanagerial personnel and the day-to-day activities of a specific work unit or units is the:
   A. Middle-level manager
   B. First-level manager
   C. Middle-level manager
   D. Upper-level manager

9. A program that will support a nurse during a move into a management role is:
   A. Mentorship
   B. Transition to practice
   C. Orientation
   D. Proctoring

10. Which of the following is a structure and process for partnership, equity, accountability, and ownership?
    A. Transformational leadership
    B. Inspirational motivation
    C. Shared governance
    D. Nursing theory

Answers: 1. A   2. D   3. A   4. A   5. A   6. A   7. A
8. B   9. B   10. C

REFERENCES

American Association of Critical Care Nurses. Essentials of Nurse Manager Orientation. 2016. www.aacn.org/education/online-courses/essentials-of-nurse-manager-orientation.

American Nurses Association (2016). Scope and standards of practice—Nurse administration. Silver Spring, MD: American Nurses Association.

American Nurses Credentialing Center (2019). Magnet application manual. Silver Spring, MD: ANCC.

American Organization of Nurse Leaders (2019). Nurse Leader Competencies. American Organization of Nurse Leaders. Accessed September 24, 2019.

Bass, B.M., & Riggio, R.E. (2005). Transformational leadership (2nd ed.). Mahwah, NJ: Lawrence Erlbaum Associates, Inc.

Batson, V (2004). Shared governance in an integrated health care network. AORN, 80(3), 498, 501–504, 506, 509–512.

Carroll, P. (2006). Nursing leadership and management: A practical guide. Clifton Park, NY: Thomson Delmar Learning.

Chism, L. A. (2013). *The Doctor of Nursing Practice* (2nd ed.). Burlington, MA: Jones and Bartlett Learning.

Cipriani, P. (2011). Move up to the role of nurse manager. American Nurse Today, 6(3), 61–61.

Fennimore, L., & Wolf, G. (2011). Nurse manager leadership development. *The Journal of Nursing Administration, 41,* 204–210. https://doi.org/10.1097-nna.0b013e3182171aff.

Guanci, G (2018). The nurse manager's role in shared governance culture. Nursing Management, 49(6), 46–50.

Institute of Medicine (2004). Keeping patients safe. Washington, DC: National Academies Press.

Kerr, J (2015). Leader or manager? These 10 important distinctions can help you out. Kerr, J. Accessed September 24, 2019.

Kouzes, J.M, & Posner, B.Z (2017). The leadership challenge (6th ed.). John Wily and Sons.

Mackoff, B. L., Glassman, K., & Budin, W. (2013). Developing a leadership laboratory for nurse managers based on lived experiences: A participatory action research model for leadership development. *JONA: The Journal of Nursing Administration, 43,* 447–454. https://doi.org/10.1097/NNA.0b013e3182a23bc1.

Marquis, B., & Huston, C. (2017). Leadership roles and management functions in nursing. Philadelphia, PA: Wolters Kluwer.

Martin, J. S., McCormack, B., Fitzsimons, D., & Spirig, R. (2012). Evaluation of a clinical leadership programme for nurse managers. *Journal of Nursing Management, 20,* 72–80. https://doi.org/10.1111/j.1365-2834.2011.01271.x.

McNamara, M. S., Fealy, G. M., Casey, M., O'Connor, T., Patton, D., Doyle, L., & Quinlan, C. (2014). Mentoring, coaching, and action learning: Interventions in a national clinical leadership development program. *Journal of Clinical Nursing, 23,* 2533–2541. https://doi.org/10.1111/jocn.12461.

Moore, L. W., Sublett, C., & Leahy, C. (2016). Nurse managers' insights regarding their role highlight the need for practice changes. *Applied Nursing Research, 30,* 98–103. https://doi.org/10.1016/j.apnr.2015.11.006.

Northouse, P. (2007). Leadership theory and practice. Thousand Oaks, CA: Sage Publications.

Parry, J., Calarco, M. M., Hensinger, B., Kearly, G., & Shakarjian, L. (2012). An online portal to support the role of the nurse manager. *Nursing Economic$, 30,* 230–232.

Porter-O'Grady, T. (2001). Is shared governance still relevant? Journal of Nursing Administration, 31(10), 468–473.

Porter-O'Grady, T (2003). A different age for leadership 105-110. Journal of Nursing Administration, 33, 105–110.

Porter-O'Grady, T., & Mallach, K. (2015). Quantum leadership. Building better partnerships for sustainable health (4th ed.). Burlington, MA: Jones & Bar.

Quinn-O'Neil, B., Kilgallen, M., & Terlizzi, J. (2011). Creating a unit-based resource nurse program. American Journal of Nursing, 111(9), 46–51.

Rees, S., Glynn, M., Moore, R., Rankin, R., & Stevens, L. (2014, June). Supporting nurse manager certification. *JONA: The Journal of Nursing Administration, 44,* 368–371. https://doi.org/10.1097/NNA.0000000000000083.

Scully. N. J. (2014). Leadership in nursing: The importance of recognizing inherent values and attributes to secure a positive future for the profession. *Australian Journal of Nursing Practice, Scholarship and Research, 22,* 439–444.

Sherrod, D., & Harper- Harrison, A. (2010). Get equipped to navigate the waters of healthcare change. *Nursing Management, 41,* 51–53. https://doi.org/10.1097/01.NUMA.0000368569.12845.22.

St. Luke's Medical Center (2015). Resource nurse job description. St. Luke's Medical Center. http://jobs.stlukesmedcenter.com/registered-nurse-clinical-resource-nurse/job/3303764.

Stringer, E.T. (2007). Action Research Sage Thousand Oaks. Thousand Oaks, CA: Sage.

Sullivan, E., E., & Decker, P. (2001). Effective leadership and management in nursing (5th ed.). Upper Saddle River, NJ: Prentice Hall.

Wilson, V., Paterson, S., & Kornman, K. (2013, December 10). Leadership development: An essential ingredient in supporting nursing unit managers. *Journal of Healthcare Leadership, 5,* 53–62. https://doi.org/10.2147/JHL.S52719.

Zwink, J., Dzialo, M., Fink, R., Oman, K., Shiskowsky, K., Waite, K., … Le-Lezar, J. (2013). Nurse manager perceptions of role satisfaction and retention at an academic medical center. *JONA: The Journal of Nursing Administra-*

tion, 43(3), 135–141. https://doi.org/10.1097/NNA.0b013 e318283dc56.

BIBLIOGRAPHY

American Nurses Credentialing Center [ANCC]. (2019, 2013). *Magnet application manual.* Silver Spring, MD: Author.

American Nurses Association. (2016). *Scope and standards of practice—Nurse administration.* Silver Spring, MD: Author.

American Organization of Nurse Leaders. (2019). American Organization of Nurse Leaders. *Nurse Leader Competencies.* Retrieved September 24, 2019 from https://www.aonl.org/resources/nurse-leader-competencies.

Bass, B. M., & Riggio, R. E. (2005). *Transformational leadership* (2nd ed). Mahwah, NJ: Lawrence Erlbaum Associates, Inc.

Batson, V. (2004). Shared governance in an integrated health care network. Denver, CO: American Association of PeriOperative Nurses. 498, 501-504, 506, 509-512 AORN 80 (3) 493–496. 498, 501-504, 506, 509-512.

Carroll, P. (2006). *Nursing leadership and management: A practical guide.* Clifton Park, NY: Thomson Delmar Learning.

Cipriani, P. (2011). Move up to the role of nurse manager. *American Nurse Today*, March 2011. 6(3), 61–62.

Institute of Medicine. (2004). *Keeping patients safe.* Washington, DC: National Academies Press.

Kerr, J (2015). *Leader or manager? These 10 important distinctions can help you out.* Denver, CO. Retrieved September 24, 2019 from http://www.inc.com/james-kerr/leading-v-managing-ten-important-distinctions-that-can-help-you-to become-better.html

Kotter, J. (1996). *Leading change.* Boston, MA: Harvard Business School.

Marquis, B., & Huston, C. (2017). *Leadership roles and management functions in nursing.* Philadelphia, PA: Wolters Kluwer.

Northouse, P. (2007). *Leadership theory and practice.* Thousand Oaks, CA.: Sage Publications.

Porter-O'Grady, T., & Mallach, K. (2015). *Quantum leadership. Building better partnerships for sustainable health* (4th ed.). Burlington, MA: Jones & Bartlett.

Porter-O'Grady. T. (2001). Is shared governance still relevant? *Journal of Nursing Administration, 31*(10), 468–473.

Quinn-O'Neil, B., Kilgallen, M., & Terlizzi, J. (2011). Creating a unit-based resource nurse program. *American Journal of Nursing, 111*(9), 46–51.

St. Luke's Medical Center. (2015). *Resource nurse job description.* http://jobs.stlukesmedcenter.com/registered-nurse-clinical-resource-nurse/job/3303764.

Sullivan, E., & Decker, P. (2001). *Effective leadership and management in nursing* (5th ed.). Upper Saddle River, NJ: Prentice Hall.

Zenger, J., & Folkman, J. (2009). *Ten fatal flaws that derail leaders. Harvard Business Review, 87*(6), 18. Retrieved September 24, 2019 from https://hbr.org/2009/06/ten-fatal-flaws-that-derail-leaders/sb1.

Organizational Structure of Health Care

OBJECTIVES

- Differentiate between a care delivery model and a professional practice model.
- Describe the various organizational structures in health care.
- Identify the management structures of patient care.
- Describe the various modes of patient care delivery systems.

- Discuss the pros and cons of each of the delivery systems.
- Determine the responsibility of the nurse in the various care delivery systems.
- Relate a clinical scenario to each of the delivery models.

KEY TERMS

care coordination function that helps ensure that the patient's needs and preferences for health services and information sharing across people, functions, and sites are met over time (National Quality Forum, 2012; as quoted in (American Nurses Credentialling Center, 2019) [ANCC])

care delivery system a system for the delivery of care that delineates the nurse's authority and accountability for clinical decision making and outcomes. The care delivery system is integrated with the professional practice model and promotes continuous, consistent, efficient, and accountable delivery of nursing care. The care delivery

system is adapted to meet evidence-based practice standards, national patient safety goals, affordable and value-based outcomes, and regulatory requirements. It describes the manner in which care is delivered, the skill set required, the context of care, and the expected outcomes of care (ANCC, 2019)

case/care management model of care in which the nurse integrates delivery of clinical services across the various transitions of care

functional nursing model of care in which nursing work is allocated according to specific tasks and skills primary nursing model of care in which one nurse assumes accountability for care delivered by other personnel in a 24-hour period

professional practice model the driving force of nursing care. It is a schematic description of a theory, phenomenon, or system that depicts how nurses practice, collaborate, communicate, and develop professionally to provide the highest level of care for those served by the organization

(e.g., patients, families, communities). Professional practice models illustrate the alignment and integration of nursing practice with the mission, vision, and values that nursing has adopted (ANCC, 2019)

team nursing model of care in which a group of staff members led by a nurse provides care

total patient care model of care in which the nurse assumes full accountability for care of a group of patients

LEADERSHIP STRUCTURE IN HEALTH CARE

The health care industry is a complex web of patient care facilities and workers with the chief goal of caring for patients in a safe, cost-effective manner. Improving the U.S. health care system requires the pursuit of three aims: improving the experience of care, improving the health of the population, and reducing per capita costs (Berwick, Nolan, & Whittington, 2008). To this end, the organizational structures of most health care organizations tend to focus on oversight, efficiency, and stakeholder satisfaction.

Health care institutions are usually organized according to lines of authority, power, and communication. Structures are defined as centralized or decentralized depending on the degree to which the organization has spread its lines of authority.

Integrative Structures in Health Care

With the dramatic changes that have occurred in health care since 2010, health care systems are now being reorganized to provide for care throughout the various transitions of care. Single acute care institutions have partnered or merged with health care agencies and facilities providing broader care, for example, the relationship between an acute care hospital with a long-term care facility, a rehabilitation agency, and a home health care organization. These reorganizations also provide increased efficiency and financial stability of services. Large health care systems have been formed with statewide mega mergers of multiple acute care institutions, medical offices, long-term care facilities, and home care and community-based health services. Organizations may be vertically integrated or horizontally integrated. Vertical integration (affiliation of a particular health

care facility with the health maintenance organization) provides for different but complementary services among the organizations involved. Horizontal integration (shared services or reciprocal services across two or more institutions) allows for shared provision to be made, for instance, the provision of maternal/child services by one affiliate and orthopedic surgery services by another.

Organizational Structures

An organizational chart is a visual means of determining the level of centralization or decentralization. A centralized organization is a typical hierarchy that follows a chain of command and is characterized by top-down decision making. The more decision making is "pushed down" through the organizational levels, the more decentralized the organization becomes. A flat organizational structure signifies the removal of hierarchical layers, demonstrating that the authority for action occurs at the point of service (Fig. 2.1). In a more decentralized organization, lower-level managers and staff have an increased opportunity for shared governance and often report greater job satisfaction (Rundio & Wilson, 2010).

Functional Structures

Functional structures arrange services and departments according to what they do (Fig. 2.2). Departments providing similar functions would all report to a common manager or vice president. In such a structure, nursing units would report to the larger nursing services. Other services in support of patient care, such as respiratory and dietary, might report to a nonnursing manager or vice president. This type of structure supports professional expertise but can result in the "silo" effect, in which departments become separate entities with little interaction.

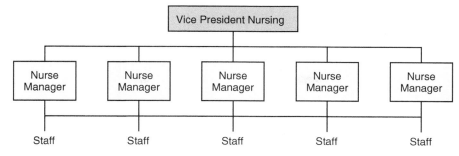

Fig. 2.1 Organizational structure. (From Yoder-Wise, P. S. [2007]. *Leading and managing in nursing* [4th ed.]. St. Louis: Mosby.)

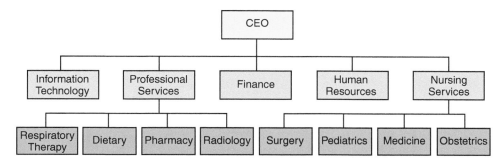

Fig. 2.2 Functional structure. (From Yoder-Wise, P. S. [2007]. *Leading and managing in nursing* [4th ed.]. St. Louis: Mosby.) *CEO*, Chief executive officer.

Product Line Structures

In product line structures, the functions necessary to produce a specific service are brought together into an integrated unit under the control of a single manager (Fig. 2.3). For example, the orthopedic service line at a hospital would include all personnel providing services to the orthopedic service population. This might include the orthopedic ambulatory care service, the orthopedic operating rooms, the orthopedic trauma center of the emergency department, and the orthopedic rehabilitation center. Benefits of this model include coordination of all services within the specialty and a similarity of focus. A limitation would be increased expense caused by duplication of services.

Matrix Structures

Matrix structures combine both function and service line in an integrated service structure (Fig. 2.4). In a matrix organization, the manager of a unit responsible

for a service reports both to a functional manager (vice president for nursing) and a service manager (directors of the services: cardiovascular services, trauma services, surgical services, or women's and children's services). Such a structure requires a collaborative relationship between the service line and functional manager. The nurse is responsible to the nurse manager and vice president of nursing for nursing care and to the program director when working within the matrix.

Integrated Structures

In an integrated health care system (e.g., networks), providers agree to accept the risk of caring for a particular patient segment or population for a pre-established fee. They provide care across the continuum. Preventative care is inherent in this structure, with primary care providers, not the hospital, at the center of the structure. Keeping people healthy is the goal of this type of structure, thereby decreasing the need for hospitalization.

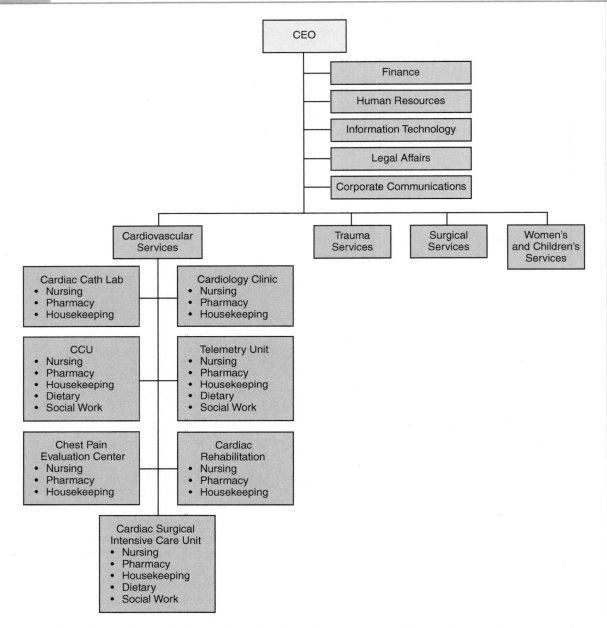

Fig. 2.3 Product line structure. (From Yoder-Wise, P. S. [2007]. *Leading and managing in nursing* [4th ed.]. St. Louis: Mosby.) *CCU,* Cardiac care unit; *CEO,* Chief executive officer.

In vertically and horizontally integrated structures (health care systems), hospitals, delivery systems, medical groups, and health care workers are brought together under one umbrella with shared purpose and unity of control. Potential challenges include relatively high overheads and internal power struggles (Rundio & Wilson, 2010).

In the organizational structure, the nursing department is usually listed on the senior leadership level. The chief nursing officer (chief nursing executive, senior

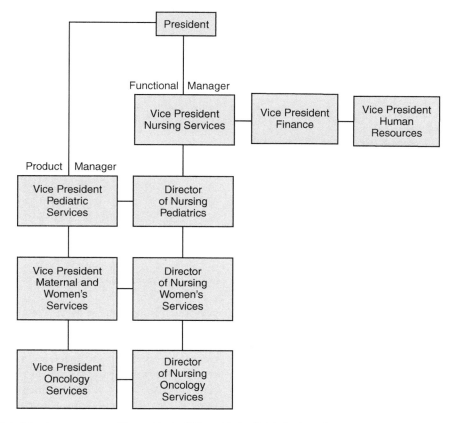

Fig. 2.4 Matrix structure. (From Yoder-Wise, P. S. [2007]. *Leading and managing in nursing* [4th ed.]. St. Louis: Mosby.)

vice president of patient care, vice president of nursing, chief nursing officer, etc.) is the highest-level reporting nursing officer in an organization. As a new staff nurse, you will report to a unit-based manager. Although you will be ultimately responsible to the chief nursing officer, on a day-to-day basis you might report to a shift charge nurse. This charge nurse (patient care manager) will have the overall responsibility for the patient care delivered during the work shift. There are many delivery systems, and the titles and responsibilities of the nurse and nurse manager vary according to the system used.

MAJOR TYPES OF CARE DELIVERY SYSTEMS

A patient care delivery model is the method used to deliver care to patients. There are multiple care delivery models, and the choice of a model within an organization is dependent on many factors: financial, staffing capability, patient population, organizational mission, and philosophy. The **care delivery system** delineates the nurses' authority and accountability for clinical decision making and outcomes (ANCC, 2019). It is adapted to regulatory requirements and describes the context of care, the manner in which care is delivered, and the skill set required. The fundamental element of any patient care delivery system (Manthey, 1990) is a combination of the following:

- Clinical decision making
- Work allocation
- Communication
- Management
- Coordination
- Accountability

The following are the models associated with nursing practice:

- Total patient care
- Functional nursing
- Team nursing
- Modular nursing
- Primary nursing
- **Case/care management**

With the changes in health care brought about in the COVID-19 pandemic, there have been calls for changes to the present structures of patient care (Berhaus, 2021).

Total Patient Care

Total patient care is the oldest method of providing care to a patient. It is sometimes called case method (not to be confused with case management). It was the primary care delivery model until the 1930s, and it had a resurgence in the 1990s. In this model one nurse assumes accountability for the complete care of a group of patients. It has been described as a type of primary nursing (Reverby, 1987), but in total patient care the accountability for coordination of care does not extend beyond the assigned shift. This is the type of care seen in private duty nursing and some intensive care units, and it was the model of care used by Florence Nightingale.

Advantages of total patient care:

- Quality of care; all care is delivered by a registered nurse
- Continuity of care for a given shift
- High patient satisfaction
- Decreases communication time required between staff
- Reduces the need for supervision
- Allows one person to perform more than one task
  Disadvantages of total patient care:
- May not be cost-effective because of the number of registered nurses needed to provide care
- Some nurses dislike this model because they believe that some of the patient care activities could be done safely and effectively by others with less skill

An example of a patient care assignment using the total patient care model is shown in Table 2.1.

Functional Nursing

Functional nursing is a model in which work is allocated according to specific tasks and technical skills. This model was popular from the late 1800s to the end of World War II. In this model the "charge nurse" identifies the tasks/work that need to be completed during the shift. These tasks/work are then divided and assigned to

TABLE 2.1   Patient Care Assignment Using the Total Care Model

Hester B., RN, MSN	Patient Care Manager 4 West
Joseph Z., RN, BSN	Full patient care, documentation, orders, admissions, discharges: rooms 410–414
Maria C., RN	Full patient care, documentation, orders, admissions, discharges: rooms 415–417
Joy T., RN, BSN	Full patient care, documentation, orders, admissions, discharges: rooms 418–420
Michael Y., RN	Full patient care, documentation, orders, admissions, discharges: rooms 421 and 422
Clarisa T., RN	Full patient care, documentation, orders, admissions, discharges: rooms 423–425

personnel. In this model there would be a "medication nurse," a "dressing nurse," etc. This model of care delivery is oriented to the accomplishment of tasks. It is efficient in times of staff shortages, and you will see patient care units reverting to this delivery mode in times of staff shortage, such as "snow emergencies" when the number of staff is limited. Some institutions with a large variation in the classification of staff (registered nurses, licensed practical nurses, nurse aides, and technicians) to care for patients may also use functional nursing.

Advantages of functional nursing:

- A large number of tasks can be completed in a shift
- The ability to mix staff classifications
- Efficient financially
- Staff members can be trained to master one task
  Disadvantages of functional nursing:
- Charge nurse may be the only one with a total view of patient
- Decreased patient satisfaction
- Decreased nurse satisfaction
- Fragmented communication
- Unit coordination becomes the responsibility of the charge nurse
- Fragmented accountability

An example of a patient care assignment using the functional nursing method is shown in Table 2.2. In this assignment, everyone is accountable for a portion of care. The challenge is that all aspects of patient care need to be communicated to the next shift, and the charge

TABLE 2.2 Patient Care Assignment Using the Functional Nursing Model	
Unit 4 West Telemetry: 30 Patients	
Mary L., RN, BSN, charge nurse	All orders, rounds, report
Bob W., telemetry technician	All monitors, rhythm strips q4h, and chart
Lisa N., RN	Medications: rooms 401–415, oversee nurse aide Tom R: rooms 401–415, charting for rooms 401–415, admissions/discharges: rooms 401–415
Tom R., nurse aide	Hygienic care: rooms 401–415, feeding, line cart restock

TABLE 2.3 Patient Care Assignment Using the Team Nursing Model	
Mary B., RN, BSN	Charge nurse Oversight of patients Rooms 410–422
Team A	
Betty K., RN	Team leader, Team A Rooms 410–416 Documentation, orders admissions/discharges, charting for PCA; restocks cardiac arrest cart
Maria B., RN	Rooms 410–412 patient care Medications Team A
Sara N., LPN	Rooms 413–416 Blood sugars: rooms 414, 416
Edith W., PCA	Hygienic care: rooms 410, 412, 414, 415 Assists patients: rooms 411, 413, 416 Vital signs 8 a.m. and 12 noon
Team B	
Tom A., RN	Team leader, Team B Rooms 417–422 Documentation, orders admissions/discharges, charting for PCA
Marci S., RN	Rooms 418, 420 patient care
Michael T., PCA	Hygienic care: rooms 417, 422 Vital signs 8 a.m. and 12 noon Blood sugars: rooms 417, 422

nurse must make sure that all pertinent information is known by them and that they are then able to communicate it to the next shift. This can lead to fragmented patient knowledge and a lack of holistic care.

Team Nursing

Team nursing is a delivery approach that uses a group of staff members led by a nurse to provide care. The team is composed of health care workers with a diversity of skills, education, licensure, and ability who work collaboratively to provide care to a group of patients. The registered nurse is the team leader, and she supervises and evaluates the team members delivering care. The team leader can provide care to a patient with complex care needs but usually does not provide hands-on care. Strong communication skills are essential. This model supports group work and productivity.

Advantages of team nursing:
- Facilitation and overseeing of novice nurses
- Smaller group of patients allows for a higher quality of care than with functional nursing
- Team leader has knowledge of patient needs and can provide coordination of care
- Fixed teams relate to higher quality patient care
Disadvantages of team nursing:
- Increased time needed to communicate within the team
- Expensive because of the increased number of staff needed
- Increased time required to supervise, coordinate, and delegate
- Can lead to omissions in care
- Most educated staff relegated to role of supervision, not direct delivery of care

An example of a patient care assignment using the team nursing model is shown in Table 2.3. In this assignment, care is delivered by a group of staff, all of whom report back to the team leader. It is the team leader who has the decision-making responsibility for the care delivered to the group of patients.

Modular Nursing

A variation of team nursing is modular nursing (Anderson & Hughes, 1993). Modular nursing is based on the physical layout of the unit. Some hospital units were designed to house a number of smaller patient "pods" and as such are structurally divided into smaller patient care areas or substations. Nurses are stationed near the patients. The essential components of modular nursing:
- A module consists of a group of staff members and a group of patients

- Patients are grouped by spatial or floor plan clustering
- Nurse/patient assignment is standardized by cluster

Advantages of this model center on the physical layout of the assignment and the ease of working in such an environment. Disadvantages center on the need to have consistent numbers of staff members in such a physical environment.

Primary Nursing

Primary nursing is a one-to-one approach to patient care. Each patient is assigned a specific nurse, who assumes 24-hour responsibility for the delivery, implementation, evaluation, and coordination of care. The primary nurse works in conjunction with nurses (associate nurses) on the other shifts to coordinate all care for the patient and family. The primary nurse is responsible for the development and evaluation of the plan of care for the patient. Decision making is decentralized and takes place at the patient's bedside. This is a flexible model and can include a variety of skill mixes. It does not mean that only registered nurses care for patients. The primary nurse plans, coordinates, and evaluates the plan of care, but the care can be delegated to appropriate staff members depending on the patient acuity.

Advantages of primary nursing:
- Improved quality and continuity of care
- Simplified communication
- Increased nurse satisfaction in nurses prepared for the role
- Patients perceive care to be more personalized
Disadvantages of primary nursing:
- Increased number of hours of care per day requires a greater number of registered nurses
- Overall patient satisfaction results are inconclusive
- Can be difficult to implement if patient has multiple unit transfers

An example of a patient care assignment using the primary nursing model is shown in Table 2.4.

Case Management

Case management is a model that mixes both process and care delivery. In hospital nursing it focuses on the achievement of patient outcomes within an effective and appropriate time frame. It is focused on the entire illness episode and can cross all units in which the patient receives care. It is associated with the use of care pathways/order sets/care maps/protocols/clinical practice guidelines, which are written plans that

TABLE 2.4 Patient Care Assignment Using the Primary Nursing Model	
Hester A., RN, MSN	Patient Care Manager 4 West
Joseph T., RN, BSN (primary nurse) 7 a.m. to 3 p.m. Jody N. (associate nurse) 3 p.m. to 11 p.m. Evelyn B. (associate nurse) 11 p.m. to 7 a.m.	Full patient care, documentation, orders, admissions, discharges: rooms 410–414
Maria C., RN 7 a.m. to 3 p.m. Cathy C., RN, BSN (primary nurse) 3 p.m. to 11 p.m. Evelyn L. (associate nurse) 11 p.m. to 7 a.m.	Full patient care, documentation, orders, admissions, discharges: rooms 415–417
Joy T., RN, BSN (primary nurse) 7 a.m. to 3 p.m. Peter U., RN (associate nurse) 3 p.m. to 11 p.m. Barbara S., RN (associate nurse) 11 p.m. to 7 a.m.	Full patient care, documentation, orders, admissions, discharges: rooms 418–420
Michael T., RN, BSN (primary nurse) 7 a.m. to 3 p.m. Peter B., RN (associate nurse) 3 p.m. to 11 p.m. Barbara S., RN (associate nurse) 11 p.m. to 7 a.m.	Full patient care, documentation, orders, admissions, discharges: rooms 421 and 422
Clarisa I., RN 7 a.m. to 3 p.m. Diane O. (associate nurse) 3 p.m. to 11 p.m. Erline P., RN, BSN (primary nurse) 11 p.m. to 7 a.m.	Full patient care, documentation, orders, admissions, discharges: rooms 423–425

identify critical and predictable events that must occur throughout a hospitalization and after the hospitalization. The assigned case manager works with the assigned nursing staff to coordinate patient progress through the transition of care pathway. The Case Management Society of America defines case management as "a collaborative process of assessment, planning, facilitation and advocacy for options and services to meet an individual's health needs through communication and available resources to promote cost-effective outcomes" (Case Management Society of America CSMA, 2010). The case management model also extends beyond the hospital setting, with case managers working with patients and families in all transitions of care. Some institutions use case managers in partnership with chronically ill patients at high risk for continued hospital readmissions. The case managers work with the patients to coordinate the entire spectrum of care in all settings (acute care, long-term care, subacute, ambulatory, insurance companies, community). Case management has been associated with decreased readmissions for chronically ill patients.

Case managers are often population based, so that one case manager may work with all surgical patients within a hospital, although some institutions do use unit-based case managers. The case manager is assigned to the patient on admission and follows the patient for the entire hospital stay and performs all posthospital care coordination. Not all case managers are nurses.

The Standards of Practice for Case Managers (Case Management Society, 2010) include:

1. Addressing the total individual concerns, including medical, psychosocial, behavioral, and spiritual needs
2. Collaborating to focus on moving the individual to self-care whenever possible
3. Increasing the involvement of individual and caregivers in the decision-making process
4. Minimizing the fragmentation of care within the health care system
5. Using evidence-based guidelines, as available, in the daily practice of case management
6. Focusing on transitions of care, which includes a complete transfer to the next care setting or provider that is effective, safe, timely, and complete
7. Improving outcomes by using adherence guidelines, standardized tools, and prevention processes to measure a client's understanding and acceptance of proposed plans, his or her willingness to change, and his or her support to maintain health behaviors
8. Expanding the interdisciplinary team to increase clients and/or their identified support system
9. Moving clients to optimal levels of health and well-being
10. Improving medication reconciliation for a client through collaborative efforts with medical staff
11. Improving adherence to the plan of care for the client, including medical differences
    Advantages of case management:
- Provides a professional practice model for nurses
- Is cost-effective
  Disadvantages of case management:
- May lead to fragmented communication

- Needs to be integrated into the care delivery model
- May lead to nurses caring for patients to become more skills focused if the case manager makes all the decisions

Table 2.5 provides an overview of the major types of nursing care delivery models.

The care delivery system delineates the nurses' authority and accountability for practice and outcomes. The care delivery system is integrated with the professional practice model. According to the ANCC (2019, p. 158), the professional practice model is the "driving force of nursing care." It is a schematic description that depicts how nurses practice, collaborate, communicate, and develop professionally to provide high-quality care for those served by the organization. It is integrated with the care delivery model and promotes continuous, consistent, efficient, and accountable nursing care.

There is confusion about the differences between care delivery and professional practice models. Care delivery models are the operational mechanisms and processes used to actually provide care to the patient and family. Professional practice models depict how nurses collaborate, communicate, and develop within the organization (Murphy, Hinch, Llewellyn, Dillon, & Carlson, 2011). One important predictor of registered nurse job satisfaction is the presence of a professional practice model (Hayes, O'Brien-Pallas, Duffield, Shamian, & Hughes, 2012).

Some of the professional practice models that have been embraced by nursing over the past few years include:

Relationship-based care (RBC): Relationships are built with the patient and family. The goal of this model is to work collaboratively with the patient and family to effect positive outcomes.

Transforming care at the bedside: The goal of this model is to empower nurses to improve care processes, delivery, and outcomes at the bedside by identifying initiatives for quality improvement.

Family-centered care: The goal of this model is to care not only for the patient but also for the family by including the family in all aspects of care and decision making as allowed by the patient.

Synergy model of patient care: This model was developed by the American Association of Critical-Care Nurses (AACN). It places the needs of the patient at the core of the model, with a matching of the needs of the patient to the competencies of the nurses. The ideal outcome of this model is the patient moving safely and effectively through the health care delivery system.

TABLE 2.5 Overview of Major Types of Nursing Care Delivery Models

Model	Focus	Clinical Decision Making	Work Allocation	Time Span
Total patient care	Total patient care	Nurse at bedside, charge nurse makes some decisions	Assigning patients	One shift
Functional	Tasks	Charge nurses make most decisions	Assigning tasks	One shift
Team	Group task	Team leader makes most decisions	Assigning tasks	One shift
Primary	Total patient care	Nurse at bedside	Assigning patients	24 hours/7 days a week

(From Tiedman, M., & Lookinland, S. (2004). Traditional models of care delivery: What have we learned? *Journal of Nursing Administration, 34*(6), 291–297.)

TABLE 2.6

Model	Communication	Documentation	Outcomes	Quality
Total patient care	Hierarchical: charge nurse gives and receives report	Unknown	May lack continuity of care between caregivers	High: all care delivered by RN
Functional	Hierarchical: charge nurse gives and receives report	Tasks	Fragmented care	Omissions and errors can occur
Team	Hierarchical: charge nurse to charge nurse, or charge nurse to team leaders, or team leaders to team members	Tasks and care plan	Fragmented care	Omissions and errors can occur
Primary	Lateral: caregiver to caregiver	Individualized plan	Continuity of care	Process oriented

SUMMARY

The manner in which patient care is delivered to patients and families is reflective of the nursing philosophy of the organization. Each model of patient care delivery has advantages and disadvantages for both the patient and the nurse. The role of the nurse in each type of model differs according to the delivery system. It is important to acknowledge your role and responsibilities in the model used in your institution.

New models of patient care delivery and professional practice are being developed and used across the United States. Some of the newer models combine aspects of the models already in existence. As research and evidence concerning the successes and challenges of the new models evolve, care delivery will change.

EVIDENCE-BASED PRACTICE

(Agency for Healthcare Research and Quality. *Making Care Transitions Safer: The Pivotal Role of Nurses*. (2016). <https://www.ahrq.gov/news/blog/ahrqviews/pivotal-role-nurses.html> Accessed September 2016.)

Making Care Transitions Safer: The Pivotal Role of Nurses

By Jeffrey Brady, MD, MPH; Richard Ricciardi, PhD, NP, AHRQ

As frontline practitioners, nurses are highly attuned to the fact that patients' needs can be very different depending on their setting of care. This insight gives nurses a unique role in making care transitions safer, a long-standing goal of the Agency for Healthcare Research and Quality (AHRQ), along with our local and federal patient safety counterparts, and one in which nurses play a pivotal role.

Care transitions occur when a patient is transferred to a different setting or level of care. They can occur when the patient moves to a different unit within the hospital, when a patient moves to a rehabilitation or skilled nursing facility, or when a patient is discharged back home. Among older patients or those with complex

EVIDENCE-BASED PRACTICE—cont'd

conditions, our research shows that care transitions can be associated with adverse events, poorer outcomes, and higher overall costs, if not managed well. They can also lead to an increase in potentially preventable hospital readmissions.

Nurses are typically the first to ask about or notice changes in a patient's health condition, such as mental status, medication routine, or vital signs, when a patient is transferred to a different hospital unit or care setting. The American Nurses Association (ANA), has identified transitions of care as a key component of its 2016 Culture of Safety campaign. At AHRQ, we support this priority and nurses' efforts to make transitions safer, both at the local level and through federal efforts.

The Partnership for Patients' (PfP) Community-based Care Transitions Program was launched in 2012. The goal was to improve care when Medicare patients move from hospitals to home or to other settings. Of the sites that participated in the project, those that successfully lowered hospital readmissions implemented nurses or coaches and offered at least two support services for older patients.

Hospitals participating in PfP efforts have used AHRQ's Re-Engineered Discharge Toolkit (RED) to successfully reduce readmissions and improve care transitions. The RED Toolkit describes a process in which nurses or health coaches lead efforts to oversee the discharge process.

Care transitions between units within a facility can also be problematic, especially when teamwork breaks down. AHRQ's TeamSTEPPS® is a curriculum that promotes a culture of safety by improving communications and teamwork skills among nurses and others on health care teams.

Promoting safe and effective care across the many settings where patients receive care is a complex challenge; it is one that can be addressed only with the input and leadership of nurses. Working together with nurses and other frontline clinicians, AHRQ will continue to develop tools and resources to ensure that all patients receive the safest care possible, no matter where it is delivered.

NCLEX® EXAMINATION QUESTIONS

1. Which type of structure is a hierarchy that follows a chain of command concept and is characterized by top-down decision making?
   A. Decentralized
   B. Organizational
   C. Functional
   D. Matrix
2. You are the charge nurse on the night shift. One of your tasks is to assign both direct patient care activities and indirect patient care activities to staff members. You are aware that one of the direct patient care activities is:
   A. Restocking supplies
   B. Transporting patients
   C. Clerical activities
   D. Electrocardiogram tracing
3. You are the nurse supervisor listening to report and observe a nurse delegating a task to a nursing assistant that should be done by a nurse. What should you do?
   A. Discuss with charge nurse
   B. Discuss at the next staff meeting
   C. Openly discuss that she is wrong
   D. Discuss why the task is not appropriate for the nursing assistant
4. Which of the following is a list of delegation factors?
   A. Your state's nurse practice act, hospital policies and procedures, job descriptions, patient needs, staff competencies, clinical situation, professional standards
   B. Your state's nurse practice act, hospital policies and procedures, job descriptions, patient needs, staff competencies, clinical situation
   C. Your state's nurse practice act, hospital policies and procedures, job descriptions, patient needs, staff competencies, professional standards
   D. Your state's nurse practice act, hospital policies and procedures, patient needs, staff competencies, clinical situation, professional standards
5. A model of care in which the nurse assumes full accountability for care of a group of patients is:
   A. Case management
   B. Total patient care
   C. Primary care
   D. Functional nursing

6. The type of patient care in which the nurse caring for the patient makes most decisions is:
   A. Functional
   B. Team
   C. Case management
   D. Total patient care

7. What type of structure combines both function and service line in an integrated service structure?
   A. Matrix structure
   B. Integrated structure
   C. Product line structure
   D. Point of care structure

8. Which of the following is a disadvantage of team nursing?
   A. Facilitation and oversight of novice nurses
   B. Increase time to communicate within the team
   C. Fixed teams relate to higher-quality patient care
   D. Team leader has knowledge of patient needs and can provide coordination of care

9. The fundamental elements of any patient care delivery system decision making are with:
   A. Leadership style
   B. Work allocation
   C. Nursing productivity
   D. Patient acuity

10. The nurse manager is planning a meeting with the staff members on group process. Which of the following functional roles should be discussed?
   A. Each group needs an individual with responsibility to coordinate and maintain records
   B. An effective team needs a spokesperson
   C. The group needs to have equal roles with their leader
   D. The team rallies around group leader

Answers: 1. A   2. D   3. D   4. D   5. B   6. D   7. A
8. B   9. B   10. A

BIBLIOGRAPHY

American Nurses Credentialling Center. (2019). 2019). Magnet Application Manual. Spring, MD: ANCC: Silver.

Anderson, C., & Hughes, E. (1993). Implementing modular nursing in a long term facility. Journal of Nursing Administration, 23(6), 23–35.

Berhaus, P. (2021). Current nursing shortages could have long lasting consequences: Time to change our present course. Nursing Economics, 39(5), 247–250.

Berwick, D. M., Nolan, T., & Whittington, J. (2008). The triple Aim: Care, Health, and Cost. Health Affairs, 27(3), 759–69.

Case Management Society of America (CSMA). (2010). Standards of Practice for Case Management (3rd edition). AR: Little RockCSMA.

Hayes, L, O'Brien-Pallas, L., Duffield, C., Shamian, J., & Hughes, F. (2012). Nurse turnover; a literature review – An Update. International Journal of Nursing Studies, 49, 887–905.

Manthey, M (1990) Definitions and basic elements of a patient care delivery system with an emphasis on primary nursing.

In G. Meyer, M. Madden, & E. Lawrence (Eds). *Patient care delivery models* (pp 201-211). Rockville, MD:Aspen)

Murphy, M., Hinch, B., Llewellyn, J., Dillon, P. & Carlson, E. (2011). Promoting Professional Nursing Practice: Linking a Professional Practice Model to Performance Expectations. *Nursing Clinics of North America*. 46(2011) 67-79.

O'Conno, B., Bennett, M., Crawford, S., & Korfiatis, V. (2006). The Trials and Tribulations of Team Nursing. Collegian, 13(3), 11–7.

Reverby, S (1987). *Ordered to Care: the Dilemna of American nursing 1850-1945*. Cambridge, MA: Cambridge University Press.

Rundio, A., & Wilson, V. (2010). Nurse Executive Review and Resource Manual. Spring, MD: ANCC, Silver.

Rundio, Wilson, V., & Meloy, F. (2016). Nurse Executive Review and Resource Manual. Spring, MD: ANCC, Silver.

Tiedman, M. & Lookinland, S. (2004). Traditional models of care delivery: what have we learned? *Journal of Nursing Adminsitration*. 34(6), 291–7

Yoder-Wise, P. (2007). Leading and Managing in Nursing. St Louis, MO: Elsevier Mosby.

Strategic Management and Planning

OUTLINE

OBJECTIVES

- Define strategic management and strategic planning.
- Discuss the importance of the strategic planning process.
- Identify the components of the strategic plan.
- Compare and contrast the various types of strategic planning processes.
- Distinguish between short- and long-term plans and objectives.
- Identify the role of the nurse manager in the strategic planning process.

KEY TERMS

environmental scan analysis of the political, demographic, social, regulatory, and technologic environments of the organization

goals statements of direction of the organization

mission statement statement defining the purpose of the organization

objectives measurable statements related to the goals of the organization

performance measures quantitative tools that allow for measurement of the achievement of goals

stakeholders all groups that may be affected by an organization's services, actions, and outcomes

strategic context competitive environment of the organization

values philosophy or behaviors determined to be vital to the organization

vision future-oriented statement of where the organization sees itself

WHAT IS STRATEGIC PLANNING?

Simply put, strategic planning is the process by which an organization/nursing department or unit decides where it is going over the next year or longer and how it is going to get there. Typically, the process is organization wide and the outcome of the process, on an organizational level, cascades down to the patient care department and the individual units and employees. The strategic plan is the "map" of where the organization, department, or unit is going over the next year or longer.

Strategic management is the process of setting goals and objectives for the organization/department/unit, determining the resources that are necessary to meet the goals, creating an action plan, and evaluating progress toward meeting the goals. It involves defining the long-term objectives of the organization and setting priorities. The timeline is future oriented and predicts organizational activities over several years (Rundio & Wilson, 2013, p. 37).

Strategic planning used to be the domain of the financial managers of many institutions. This philosophy has changed, and strategic planning now includes all stakeholders of the organization. Nurse managers have an important role in the strategic plan of the organization and in the implementation of action plans at the unit level that assist the organization in meeting its goals.

Leaders of an organization need to focus on a series of key questions as they begin the strategic planning process (Finkler, Kovner, & Jones, 2007, p. 216):

- Why does the organization exist?
- What is the organization currently?
- What would it like to be?
- How can we make the transformation to what we want to be?
- How will we know when the transformation is done?

In answering these questions, the leaders will find that the answers lead to other questions, such as: What are the strengths and challenges faced by the organization? What is its competitive status? Who are the primary stakeholders for the organization? How does the organization measure its performance? How does it learn from its performance? Do we make a difference? What is the value to our stakeholders?

The strategic planning process is similar to the nursing process. The components of the process are as follows:

- Creation of a shared mission and vision
- Assessment of current state and environment
- Setting of objectives
- Development of short- and long-term objectives and strategies
- Statement of needed resources
- Plan for implementation
- Plan for evaluation

ELEMENTS OF A STRATEGIC PLAN

Mission and Vision Statements

The first step in strategic management is the development of a mission statement for the organization. The mission statement focuses on the definition of what the organization does and aspires to do. The mission statement for some organizations is further divided into a vision, which tells the reader where the organization wants to be in the future. Many organizations also create a values statement, which includes the behaviors of importance within the organization. Some organizations include the mission, vision, and values statement in one document. An example is the Mission, Vision, and Values of the Henry Ford Health System (HFHS) (2011):

Mission: To improve human life through excellence in the science and art of health care and healing.

Vision: Transforming lives and communities through health and wellness; one person at a time.

Values: We serve our patients and our community through our actions that always demonstrate each patient first, respect for people, high performance, learning and continuous improvement, and a social conscience.

This mission, vision, and values set the direction for HFHS and serve as the basis for their strategic planning and management of operations.

The mission and vision of an organization are consistent with the organizational structure. For example, the mission statement for a small critical access hospital with no primary care services will reflect that reality. Large academic medical centers will have statements that focus on their teaching and research role.

Statement of Competitive Environment and Strategy

As part of the strategic planning process, it is vital for an organization to be aware of its competitive environment. This is accomplished through strategic analysis.

Sometimes this is called an environmental scan. This activity can include conducting a review of the organization's environment (e.g., a review of the political, social, economic, and technical environment). Planners carefully consider various driving forces in the environment, such as increasing competition, changing demographics, and so forth. Planners also look at the various strengths, weaknesses, opportunities, and threats (SWOT) regarding the organization; such information forms the strategic context of the organization. As nurse managers, you will participate in the patient satisfaction initiatives of your institution. Most nurses are aware of the performance of the other units in the hospital in relation to patient satisfaction, and some are aware of the performance of the similar units in the area. An example of changing demographics and their effect on hospital planning would be a population shift to large numbers of families moving into the local area served by the institution. This information from the environmental scan might result in a facility increasing the number of services for a pediatric population. An example of technical and regulatory changes occurring is the introduction of electronic medical records and their meaningful use.

Other information collected for the strategic planning process comes from past performance and information collected from all stakeholders through a variety of means. These involve satisfaction surveys (patient, employees, physicians, community), focus groups with members of the community to determine issues of importance, and other means of listening to the expressed desires of the local community.

The organization then determines its strategic challenges and strategic opportunities. Examples of such challenges and opportunities from the HFHS (2011) are as follows:

Strategic Challenges and Advantages
Challenges

SC1: Accelerating pressures requiring cost control, revenue growth, and diversification

SC2: Growing transparency of results and aligning physicians to drive accountability for improvement

SC3: Potential increasing competition caused by possible mergers and acquisitions.

SC4: Increase of publicly available information and the effect on consumer decision making

SC5: Redesigning care to maximize health and effective outcomes while reducing costs

SC6: Addressing health care needs of our diverse population including the uninsured and underinsured

SC7: Retaining, training, and engaging an effective, collaborative workforce and developing leaders

Advantages

SA1: "Can Do" spirit: A focus on workforce engagement, talent development, and recognition creates unique energy and a "can do" culture to continuously improve the quality and safety of our services.

SA2: Strategic geographic positioning: The HFHS provider and insurance representation in all Southeast Michigan (SEM) regions, growing into other Michigan markets, is fundamental to the integration model and growth.

SA3: Long-term presence in and support of our communities: HFHS has been an active community member in Detroit since 1915 while also creating relationships and facilities in each of our suburbs.

SA4: Commitment to diversity and equity: HFHS is located in a highly diverse community, and this commitment creates a desirable environment in which to work and receive care.

SA5: System integration: A vast continuum of services, unique in health care, provides a means of achieving success across all seven performance pillars.

SA6: Academic mission: Our extensive clinical training and research programs attract physicians and allied professionals to HFHS from around the globe.

Many organizations use pillars to organize and measure performance. HFHS uses seven pillars that represent the areas most important to our success: people, service, quality and safety, growth, research and education, community, and finance. The framework aligns system strategic objectives, strategic initiatives, and related performance measures and targets for the system and within business units from the top of the organization to the individual employee. Most organizations use six pillars, people, service, quality, community, finance, and growth (Studer, 2003), but with the academic teaching role of this medical center, a seventh pillar was added reflecting that activity.

The competitive strategy is the organization's plan for achieving its goals. It states what services will be provided to whom. It is decided on as a direct result of the information provided by the strategic analysis and environmental scan. The organization evaluates its mission, vision, and goals in light of the information provided by the environmental scan, the identified strengths and challenges, and the demand for service. Based on this competitive strategy, the organization makes a plan that allows it to take advantage of the identified strengths and needs of the various stakeholders. The product of this process is conclusions about what the organization must do as a result of the major issues and opportunities facing the organization. These conclusions include the overall accomplishments (or strategic goals) the organization should achieve.

Statement of Short-Term and Long-Term Goals

According to Carter McNamara (2006), the long- and short-term goals are the overall methods (or strategies) to achieve the strategic goals of the organization. An example of a short-term goal of an organization might be to improve performance on the core measures for cardiac failure, increasing from 80% to 85% compliance by the end of the year. A long-term goal might be to consistently perform at 98% to 100% at the end of 3 years. Goals should be designed and worded as much as possible to be Specific, Measurable, Acceptable to those working to achieve the goals, Realistic, Timely, Extending the capabilities of those working to achieve the goals, and Rewarding to them (SMARTER).

Action Planning

Action planning is the process by which the specific goals are matched with each strategic goal. The overall organization-wide strategic goals cascade down to all departments and units and, in some cases, the individual employees. Action planning requires specifying expected outcomes with each strategic goal. These outcomes then form the basis of the performance scorecards used in most organizations. The anticipated outcomes are usually based on the competitive strategy of the organization and are often benchmarked against "best in class performers" or to where the organization wants to be in terms of performance.

Often, each objective is associated with a tactic, which is one of the methods needed to achieve an objective. Therefore, implementing a strategy typically involves implementing a set of tactics along the way; in that sense, a tactic is still a strategy but on a smaller scale.

Action planning also includes specifying responsibilities and timelines with each objective, or who needs to do what and by when. It should also include methods to monitor and evaluate the plan, which includes knowing how the organization will know who has done what and by when.

It is common to develop an annual plan (sometimes called the operational plan or management plan), which includes the strategic goals, strategies, objectives, responsibilities, and timelines that should be implemented in the coming year. These are the short-term goals of the organization. The difference between short- and long-term plans and objectives relates to the time expected to accomplish them. These times vary from institution to institution, but short-term plans usually extend up to 1 year. Long-term plans vary from 3 to 5 years.

Usually, budgets are included in the strategic and annual plan and with individual departmental and unit plans. Budgets specify the funds needed for the resources that are necessary to implement the annual plan. Budgets also show how the funds will be spent. (See Chapter 4 for information on budgets.)

The strategic planning process of HFHS is diagrammed in Fig. 3.1 and an example of their broad strategic plan is shown in Fig. 3.2. Note that the goals are organized by the seven pillars identified by HFHS. The goals relate to the strategic challenges and opportunities developed by the organization. The performance indicators list the measures that will be used to measure progress toward achievement of the goals. The benchmarks relate the performance of the competitors or "best in class," and the targets are the short- and long-term goals.

As this organizational plan cascades down to the departments and units, it becomes more specific with action plans and timelines for measures of achievement. The action plan in Fig. 3.3 is a departmental action plan for another organization. Note that it is also organized according to the pillars, but it is much more department specific than a broader organization-wide strategic plan. Also note the action steps and the outcome results.

UNIT-BASED PLANNING PROCESS

Planning typically includes several major activities or steps in the process. Different organizations often have different names for these major activities and often conduct them in different orders. Strategic planning is very individualized according to the organization. The organizational strategic plan cascades down to the departmental plans, which cascade to the unit plans and end with the individual employee performance plan.

Strategic Challenge/Advant.*	Strategic Objectives by Pillar (Key Stakeholders*)	System Strategic Initiatives (Core Competencies*)	Key Short-Term (ST) and Long-Term (LT) Plans (Bold = most important)	Key Performance Measures (Results Figures) (Bold = most important)	Performance Targets 2011	Stretch 2013	Best Comp 2013
SC7	People: National leader in healthcare employee retention and engagement (KS1,2)	Develop a competent, agile workforce and build a culture of development (C1, C2, C3)	Develop & implement a flexible staffing model; internal staffing pool (ST); Enhance 1st yr. retention programs (LT)	Overall Employee Turnover (Fig. 7.3-3)			7.3%
SA1, 4, 6		Develop a high-performance work environment with a highly engaged workforce (C1, C3)	Focus on increasing engagement scores for bottom quartile leaders (ST); Conduct semi-annual pulse surveys for employees, including toolkits and support for all managers (LT)	Overall & Nursing Engagement Index, 1-5 scale (Fig. 7.3-15)			4.35
SC3,4	Service: Best-in-class service to our customers among U.S. healthcare organizations (KS1,2,3)	Create consistency of The Henry Ford Experience at all HFHS facilities (C1, C2, C3)	Share lessons and customer feedback to spread best practices (ST); Roll-out Culture of Service plan (LT)	HCAHPS results at/above national benchmarks (Fig.7.2-5)			100%
SA1, 4, 5				% Top Box, "Likelihood to Recommend" (Fig. 7.2-3,8,10)			90%ile
SC2, 5	Quality & Safety: National leader in delivering safe, reliable, high-quality, & highly coordinated care to each individual patient (KS1,2,3)	Fully implement the HFHS No Harm Campaign via System and local collaborative teams (C1,C2,C3)	Implement best practices for reducing harm in each of the 6 harm categories (LT)	Harm events per 1000 acute care patient days (Fig.7.1-1)			n/a
SA1, 4, 5		Reduce readmissions via discharge and post-acute coordination (C2)	Implement readmissions avoidance tactics at all sites (ST); System-wide case management system (LT)	Readmissions within 30 Days (Fig. 7.1-13)			8.0%
SC1, 2 3, 6	Growth: Dominant health system in Michigan (KS1,2,3)	Execute growth plans for hospitals to capture market share (C2, C3)	Implement strategies to attract new business to HFWBH and HFH (LT) and HFMH-WC (ST)	Tri-County IP Market Share (Fig. 7.5-11)			20.2%
SA1 - 5		Execute physician integration and access improvements (C1, C2, C3)	Expand HFMG ambulatory centers in high growth markets; recruit needed physicians (LT)	IP Admissions (Fig. 7.5-9)			116,686
				OP Visit Volume (Fig. 7.5-14)			n/a
		Alter insurance product mix to offset shrinking HMO market (C1, C2, C3)	Launch new HAP products in preparation for 2012-2013 enrollment periods (LT)	Total HAP membership (Fig. 7.5-15)			n/a
SC 2, 5, 7	Research & Education: Leading independent academic medical center and nationally preferred clinical research partner (KS1,2,3)	Strengthen research and education programs through new medical school affiliation(s) and fully integrated allopathic and osteopathic GME programs (C1, C3)	Expand research capabilities and clinical trials to attract new NIH and other external funding (LT)	NIH research grants and contracts (7.1b(1)✱)			$33M
SA1, 2, 4, 5, 6			Integrate Medical Education System-wide (LT)	Trainee Satisfaction (Fig. 7.3-14)			n/a
				Ready for independent practice (Fig. 7.3-14)			n/a
SC5, 6	Community: National leader in community health advocacy and involvement (KS1,2,3)	Improve access to care/services for the Underinsured/Uninsured (C2, C3)	Increase support and utilization of community clinics	Visits to Community Clinics (Fig. 7.4-8)			n/a
SA1, 3, 4		Leverage the refreshed CHNA report at all BUs and address identified community needs. (C2,C3)	Implement Community Benefit management and reporting structures for all BUs (ST); link to CHNA (LT)	Community Benefit (Fig. 7.4-11)			n/a
SC1, 2, 3, 5, 6	Finance: Financial strength to fund clinical services, health management, people, research, and education strategies (KS1,2,3)	Achieve operating profit and philanthropic donations sufficient to fund 3-year capital plans (C3)	Continue revenue and cost management programs at all sites (LT)	System Operating Net Income (Fig. 7.5-1)			n/a
SA1 - 5			Continue philanthropic campaigns targeting external donors and employee contributors (ST)	Cost per Unit of Service (Fig. 7.5-2)			n/a
				% Philanthropic Donor Renewal (Fig. 7.4-7)			n/a
				Philanthropy Cash Collected (Fig. 7.5-8)			n/a

*Strategic Challenges: SC1=Cost Control/Revenue Growth, SC2= Phys. Align/Accountable, SC3=Increased Competition, SC4=Increased Consumerism SC5= Care Redesign SC6= Care Needs Diverse Population SC7= Workforce Support Strategic Advantages: SA1="Can Do" Spirit, SA2=Strategic Geographic Positioning SA3=Community Support SA4=Commitment to Diversity/Equity SA5=System Integration SA6=Academic Mission Key Stakeholders: KS1=Patients (IP, OP, ED, CCS) KS2=Community (Detroit, Regional service areas), KS3=Purchasers (Employers, Health Plan Members) Core Competencies: C1=Innovation, C2=Care Coordination, C3=Collaboration/Partnering

Fig. 3.1 The strategic planning process of Henry Ford Health System (2011). (https://nist.gov/system/files/documents/2017/10/10/2011_Henry_Ford_Health_System_Award_Application_Summary.pdf. Fig. 2.1-1, p. 8.)

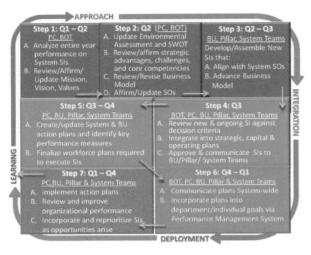

Fig. 3.2 An example of the HFHS broad strategic plan. (https://www.nist.gov/system/files/documents/2017/10/11/2011_Henry_Ford_Health_System_Award_Application_Summary.pdf. Fig. 2.1-2.2, p. 8).

On a unit-based level, the nurse manager will oversee the unit-based planning process. Things to accomplish include the following:

1. Identify your purpose (mission statement): The mission statement for your unit should carefully mirror that of the overall organization. Remember, it is important that all levels of the organization are "on the same page." If the unit goals are different than those of the organization, there is a potential conflict.
2. Select the goals your organization must reach if it is to accomplish your mission: The unit and personal goals of each employee must relate to accomplishment of the mission of the unit and organization.
3. Identify specific approaches or strategies that must be implemented to reach each goal: Identify realistic activities that you and your staff will do to accomplish the goals.
4. Identify specific action plans to implement each strategy: Identify the things necessary for you and your staff to achieve the goals. This is related to the development of the budget to assist you in the identification of resources necessary to achieve the goals.

Sample 90-Day Action Plan • Women's and Children's Service Line (1/06-3/06)			
CSF	**Goal**	**Action steps**	**90-Day result report**
People	Maintain FT turnover rate	• Leader rounding x2 areas each day • Review rounding information at weekly manager meetings. • Implement 90-day AP with direct reports.	• Turnover rate at >1.6% • One 90-day AP per unit
Service	Acheive 90th percentile on inpatient satisfaction	• Nurse rounding • Bi-weekly meeting with Women/Children's patient satisfaction team	• 90th percentile or higher in patient satisfaction
Quality	Reduce practice variation in DRG 372, 373	• Physician champion identified • OM to perform CPA DRG 372-373 • PA to perform documentation analysis	• Decrease DRG 372 LOS • Assure appropriate DRG assignment
	Pediatric asthma	• Physician champion identified • Perform CPA on asthma DRG	• Decrease readmissions for pediatric asthma patients
Financial	Maintain expenses within budget	• Review OB/GYN financials with OBs • Nurse managers analyze and report OT needs to SLL	• BAR at or above 80 • Overtime below 3.0% • Expenses below budget
Growth	Develop a vision for pediatric services	• Set up meeting with LeBonheur Children's Hospital to discuss increase in pediatric subspecialties • Develop cost-benefit analysis with marketing for branding of pediatric services	• Presented draft of vision to March SLOG • Pediatric branding identified and cost-benefit reported to SLOG w/in 30 days
	Implement Women/Children's Community Advisory Board	• Recruit Advisory Board members • Develop agenda for first meeting	• First Advisory Board meeting March, 2006

Fig. 3.3 Action plan (North Mississippi Medical Center, 2006). Application for the Malcolm Baldrige Performance Excellence Award. (http://baldrige.nist.gov/PDF_files/NMMC_Application_Summary.pdf.)

5. Monitor and update the plan: As you see in the department plan, there is a 90-day monitoring of results. The careful monitoring of performance allows you and your unit to determine whether your action plans are working or if they need reworking. Most strategic plans are fluid documents allowing for changes to be made as necessary.

As a nurse, you will also deal with action plans that address the Joint Commission Core Measures (see Chapter 5), the National Patient Safety Goals (see Chapter 10), the Centers for Medicare & Medicaid Services (CMS) Hospital Consumer Assessment of Healthcare Providers and Systems (HCAHPS) measures, the National Database of Nursing Quality Indicators (NDNQI) nursing outcome measures, Magnet requirements, infection control measures, patient satisfaction, and particular issues of concern within your institution. Action plans for specific clinical concerns are usually managed by the performance improvement department of the clinical department, but the nurse manager and staff should be aware of these action plans and their role in the achievement of the overall organizational goal. An example of an action plan for a clinical goal is shown in Fig. 3.4.

Purposes of Planning

- Increases the chances of success by focusing on results and not on activities
- Forces analytical thinking, knowledge of current evidence, and evaluation of alternatives
- Establishes a framework for decision making that is consistent with organizational strategic objectives
- Orients people to action rather than reaction
- Includes day-to-day and future-focused managing
- Helps to avoid crisis management and provides decision-making flexibility

Sample APs for Clinical Goal (Others AOS) Goal

Overall: Improve clinical processes and outcomes
Specific: Improve tracheostomy management and outcomes

▼

Action Plans

Overall: Analyze and manage tracheostomy (perform CPA)
Specific:
- Implement structured monitoring of processes
- Analyze and improve processes with physicians and team
- Automate process improvements through order sets and protocols
- Educate staff on changes

▼

Performance Indicators

In-Process: patients receive:
- DVT and stress ulcer prophylaxis
- Ventilator weaning protocol
- Nutrition protocol
- Multidisciplinary team rounds
Outcomes: Inpatient mortality (decreased), CCU and overall LOS (decreased), cost of care (decreased)

Fig. 3.4 An example of an action plan for a clinical goal (North Mississippi Medical Center, 2006). Application for the Malcolm Baldrige Performance Excellence Award. http://baldrige.nist.gov/PDF_files/NMMC_Application_Summary.pdf.

- Provides a basis for managing organizational and individual performance
- Is cost-effective
  (Adapted from Rousel, 2013)

▮ SUMMARY

Strategic planning is a continually evolving process in most organizations, with constant monitoring of performance of goals, achievement of strategic objectives, and updating of the plan as changes occur within the environment. As a nurse manager, it is your responsibility to always be aware of the plan and your role in the plan and, as a staff nurse, to be aware of your role in assisting the organization and your unit in the achievement of the strategic goals.

CLINICAL CORNER

Strategy is a concept not always well understood by nurses. However, the nursing department, typically the largest component of the workforce in hospitals, has a pivotal role in achieving strategic objectives. Strategic initiatives take on many forms. Theoretically, care planning outlines a strategy for providing care to a particular patient. Strategies are used to implement evidence-based practice, professional practice models, nursing councils, or to achieve Magnet status. Although strategies may be reflective of departmental-level initiatives, they usually have some connection to strategies for the organization developed in the C-suite. Understanding different types of strategies will allow the nursing department(s) to develop goals (strategies) that are consistent with the organization's plan.

Types of Strategies

There is a decision logic of strategy development that includes five categories of strategy: directional, adaptive, market entry, competitive, and implementations. Directional strategies are the broadest and set the mission for the organization and determine the values and strategies goals of the organization. Adaptive strategies provide the organization with the mechanisms by which to achieve the broad directional strategies. Market entry strategies provide the process for achieving the adaptive strategies. Competitive strategies determine which approach the organization will take to remain competitive within the industry. Lastly, implementation strategies, which are the most precise, are specific to value-added services. This sequence of strategy decision represents a specific sensibleness in strategy development. In review of each stage of decision making, it makes perfect sense to approach this process in such a systematic, rationale matter. Each phase represents a step for which the end result is a comprehensive strategy for the organization. Without this approach, executives risk crucial gaps in their planning.

Retrenchment Strategy and Penetrations Strategy

A retrenchment strategy may be employed when there is declining profitability of an organization. This is usually precipitated by increasing costs; the most common is increased costs of manufacturing or overstaffing. However, organizations may take a different path in light of these factors. The leadership may look at market penetration strategies instead.

Penetration strategies address better ways to serve the existing markets with existing products or services. This may include such steps as an aggressive advertising campaign, more competitive pricing, or increased publicity for the organization. Rather than addressing the internal mechanism of reducing staff or reducing manufacturing expense, the focus is on external organizational issues. Both strategies are aimed at increasing profitability; one has an internal focus and the other has an external focus. If an organization attempts the market penetration strategy without success, a retrenchment strategy may be the next step.

Other logical combinations of strategies might be related and unrelated diversification. The former looks at adding new related products requiring the establishment of a new division, and the latter adds unrelated products, which also require the establishment of a new division. The market strategies of penetration and retrenchment as explained earlier can be used together as well. Liquidation and harvesting can be a duel strategy in which liquidation refers to selling off part of an organization's assets. Harvesting refers to a late stage of a product cycle in which profitability is determined to decline in the future but will continue to generate profits for a period of time. In addition, product development (improving current products or services) can be used in combination with market development (introducing these products into new geographic areas). There are a number of strategies that can be used in combination depending on the current state of the organization's market share, profitability, or other factors that determine the success of the industry.

A combination of strategies related to achieving the vision of an organization are the directional strategies and the adaptive strategies. defined directional strategies as those which set the fundamental direction of the organization and the vision for the future. Adaptive strategies are more specific and speak to the primary mechanisms for achieving that vision. In addition, there are multiple types of adaptive strategies that can be used in combination to accomplish the vision: related diversification and unrelated diversification, backward and forward vertical integration, market and product development, penetration and enhancement, and in some cases maintaining the status quo. Depending on the organization, the current position in the market and their vision, there can be several combinations of adaptive strategies the organization may employ. If the organization is particularly successful, the leadership may decide to focus on the status quo, that is, maintaining their current position the market. There are many factors that influence strategy development.

Continued

CLINICAL CORNER—cont'd

Mission, Vision, and Values

The mission, vision, and values are part of situational analysis and strategy formation. They describe the current state of the organization and organize the beliefs and philosophy of the organization. These documents also set boundaries and set the broadest direction for the organization. Therefore, they are the foundation on which directional strategies are developed and adaptive strategies, to meet those directional strategies, are established.

Competitor information categories are very useful in conducting a competitive analysis. This information for competitive analysis is categorized into specific types of data that assist strategic planners and organizational leadership to make decisions about the health care services they offer or will offer in the future. First and foremost is the general category, which defines the characteristics of the area: population, nearest alternative health care services, threat of new entrants to the market, and transportation availability. All of these components of this category are important to accurately assess the market and the potential for viability of the current organization's services or new services.

Second is the economic landscape of the area. Median incomes of the population served and employment of the population are indicators of the number of insured patients and other information: other issues such as types of businesses and growth rate are also included. The level of poverty is an indicator in the service area that can give information about potential services to the community. For example, a cosmetic surgery program in an area with a large number of individuals at or below the poverty level is not likely to do well because it is predominantly a self-pay operation. However, clinic services may better serve this population and meet their health care needs.

Demographics of the area is an indicator of potential services. Demographics include issues such as the number of individuals in the targeted service area, age of the population, level of education, and ethnicity. An area with a high population growth is likely to benefit from obstetrics and pediatric services. An area with a predominant aging population may benefit from geriatric specialties. The components of the demographics of specific areas is an essential clue to what services will be successful and what services may not. Strategic planners would be foolish to ignore such important information as the demographics of the area.

Psychographic information is another concept of interest to strategic planners. This category includes the presence of big business within the community, the frequency of summer activities, orientation toward youthfulness, lifestyles, attitudes, and social class. For example, plastic surgery programs may be appealing to a younger, upwardly mobile group. Likewise, a plastic surgery program may also appeal to a community with large sectors of big business where appearance is highly valued. Psychographic information provides details to strategic planners about the buyer's habits, values, or hobbies. This type of information provides the basis for determining what programs or services would appeal to the community.

Lastly, the health status of the targeted service area is also needed and is probably one of the most important. The health of the population discloses the incidence of disease within the community. This category includes such issues as mortality, deaths, motor vehicle accidents, work-related injuries, and infant deaths, among others. For example, the incidence of cancer and the types of cancer may give rise to specific cancer treatment centers. The incidence of heart disease may initiate the development of a comprehensive cardiac program. As also pointed out, the number of birth defects may precipitate a program for orofacial reconstructive surgery. The health status of the currently served community or the targeted market is a vital component to effective strategic planning.

Each of these categories are very important for health care organizations. The categories provide focus for the organization in terms of where to commit resources in the future. Without an accurate assessment of the economic, demographic, psychographic, health status, incidence and types of disease, and the risk indicators of a targeted market for services, it is unlikely that health care organizations can achieve their desired goals. To disregard one or more of these information categories may create larger scale problems for the health care organizations and invite competitors into the service areas to meet those overlooked needs. In summary, poor strategic planning will lead to greater, more intense competition.

Service Area

defined the service area as "the geographic area surrounding the health care provider from which it pulls the majority of its customers/patients." The service area requires a clear definition because it is reflective of the consumer's health care preferences and needs. By determining this service area, the health care facility can tailor services to meet these preferences and community needs. Furthermore, this market determines

CLINICAL CORNER—cont'd

what services will be offered. Caution should be taken, however, as this information can be very subjective and may be determined by patient histories, available technology, organization reputation, and physician affiliation.

Managed care can affect the service area definition just by the structure of the provider's payment contracts. Managed care includes some elements such as explicit standards for selecting providers, health maintenance organizations (HMOs); financial incentives for consumers to use specific providers and procedures that are associated with the plan, preferred provider organizations (PPOs); and point of service plans (POSs) that combine the features of HMOs and PPOs. All of these elements can lead to a redefinition of service areas or a need to contract with specific managed care organizations. For example, if a specific managed care organization provides insurance to a large number of employees in the area, but the local hospital does not have a contract with that organization, consumers are likely to seek services elsewhere to avoid potentially large out-of-pocket financial responsibilities.

Contracting with specific managed care organizations is likely to require changes to the revenue projections of the organization as well, affecting the budget. If revenue projections were based on traditional per diem rates, the influence of a managed care organization entry into the market can be enormous. This is another reason it is so important for strategic planners to conduct accurate assessments of the service area. It is only through a rigorous competitive analysis that a health care organization can develop a strategy that will lead the organization on a successful trajectory.

NCLEX® EXAMINATION QUESTIONS

1. The mission of an organization:
   A. Sets the competitive tone
   B. States what is done by the organization
   C. Measures the performance of a unit
   D. Defines the philosophy of an institution

2. The vision of an organization is:
   A. A statement defining the purpose of the organization
   B. A future-oriented statement of where the organization sees itself
   C. Philosophy or behaviors determined to be vital to the organization
   D. Analysis of the policies, demography, and social environment of the organization

3. Action plans for specific clinical concerns are usually managed by the performance improvement department, but it is also important that the following individuals are aware of these action plans and their role in the achievement of the overall organizational goal:
   A. Nurse managers, clinical department, and staff nurses
   B. Risk managers, purchasing department, and nursing assistants
   C. Nurse manager, risk manager, and president
   D. Nurse manager, nursing assistants, and risk manager

4. A specific action plan should be used for each:
   A. Goal
   B. Strategy
   C. Outcome
   D. Performance improvement

5. On a unit-based level, the nurse manager will oversee the unit-based planning process. Which of the following is seen as an item to be accomplished?
   A. Identify unit-specific policies, procedures, and protocols
   B. Identify your mission statement and specific action plan to implement each strategy
   C. Evaluate staffing needs and change as needed
   D. Evaluate your vision and identify policies

6. The purpose of an environmental scan is to assist the organization in:
   A. Setting of strategic goals
   B. Measuring competitive performance
   C. Developing an awareness of the social and regulatory arena
   D. Determining short- and long-term business objectives

7. Analysis of the political, demographic, social, regulatory, and technologic environments of the organization is:
   A. Performance measures
   B. Environmental scan

C. Strategic context

D. Competitive performance

8. Which of the following is the process by which the specific goals are matched with each strategic goal?

A. Action planning

B. Work strategies

C. Expected outcomes

D. Performance indicators

9. Accelerating pressures requiring cost control, revenue growth, and diversification is referred to as:

A. Strategic challenge

B. Strategic advantage

C. Strategic disadvantage

D. Corporate goal

10. A focus on workforce engagement, talent development, and recognition creates unique energy and a culture to continuously improve the quality and safety of services is considered:

A. Corporate goal

B. Strategic advantage

C. "Can Do" culture

D. Process improvement

Answers: 1. A   2. A   3. A   4. B   5. B   6. C   7. B   8. A
9. A   10. B

REFERENCES

Center for Disease Control (2013). Stats in the state of New Jersey. Retrieved (date need), from http://www.cdc.gov/nchs/pressroom/states/NJ_2014.pdf

BIBLIOGRAPHY

Finkler, S., Kovner, C., & Jones, C. (2007). *Financial management for nurse managers* (3rd ed.). Philadelphia, PA: W. B. Saunders.

Henry Ford Health System. (2011). Application for the Malcolm Baldrige Performance Excellence Award. https://www.nist.gov/system/files/documents/2017/10/11/2011_Henry_Ford_Health_System_Award_Application_Summary.pdf.

McNamara, C. (Authenticity Consulting, LLC). Copyright © 1997-2006. Adapted from the *Field Guide to Nonprofit Strategic Planning and Facilitation*. www.managementhelp.org/plan_dec/str_plan/models.htm.

North Mississippi Medical Center. (2006). Application for the Malcolm Baldrige Performance Excellence Award. http://baldrige.nist.gov/PDF_files/NMMC_Application_Summary.pdf.

Rousel. L. (2013). *Management and leadership for nurse administrators*. Sudbury, MA: Jones & Bartlett.

Rundio, V., & Wilson, A. (2013). *Nurse executive review and resource manual* (3rd ed.). Silver Spring, MD.

Studer. Q. (2003). *Hardwiring excellence: Purpose, worthwhile work, making a difference*. Gulf Breeze, FL: Fire Starter Publishing.

Financial Management in Health Care

OBJECTIVES

- Define health care.
- Identify factors influencing today's health care system.
- Discuss the economic realities of U.S. health care.
- Identify the major forms of reimbursement for health care.
- Describe the U.S. health care system.
- Define budgeting.

- Differentiate between types of budgets.
- Discuss the advantages of various budget processes.
- Describe the key elements of budget preparation.
- Identify the responsibilities of the nurse manager in budget preparation.
- Discuss the responsibilities of the nurse manager in budget review.

KEY TERMS

Accountable Care Organization (ACO) one billing occurs across the transition of care; generally the better the quality of care, the better the reimbursement

bottom line income of an organization that is the result of revenue (money earned) minus expenses

budget detailed financial plan for carrying out the activities of an organization or unit

budget variance difference between actual budget and actual spending

capital budget financial plan that deals with purchases of capital assets (equipment, land, etc.)

cash budget financial plan that tracks cash received and spent

cash on hand amount of cash readily available to the organization

Centers for Medicare & Medicaid Services (CMS) formerly known as the Healthcare Financing Administration, the federal agency that administers Medicare, Medicaid, State Children's Health Insurance Program (SCHIP), and several other health-related programs

continuum of care matching an individual's ongoing needs with the appropriate level and type of medical, psychological, health, or social care or service within an organization or across multiple organizations

for-profit organizations organizations with stated financial structures that include profit goals and tax liabilities

health care systems all of the structures, organizations, and services designed to deliver professional health and wellness services to consumers

health maintenance organization (HMO) geographically organized system that provides an agreed-on package of health maintenance and treatment services

indirect costs generalized costs (housekeeping, information technology, etc.) for support of the program and billed to the program; often called support costs

managed care linkage between the financing and delivery of services in such a way as to permit payers to exercise control over the delivery of services

Medicaid joint federal and state assistance program designed to pay for medical long-term care assistance for individuals and families with low income and limited resources

Medicare health insurance program for people age 65 and older or under age 65 with certain disabilities or any age with end-stage renal disease

not-for-profit organizations organizations with financial structures that project financial goals with particular tax and legislative protection or shelters

operating (expense) budget financial plan for the day-to-day activities of the organization

personnel budget part of the operating budget that deals with personnel needed to deliver care; composed of salary and benefit costs

preferred provider organization (PPO) managed care company that contracts with health care providers (both physicians and hospitals) and payers (self-insured employers, insurance companies, or managed care organizations) to provide health care services to a defined population for predetermined fixed fees

revenues income received for goods or services provided

value-based purchasing reimbursement for health care services based on quality of care

variable costs costs that vary in relation to volume and productivity

HEALTH

With the advent of health care delivery services organized under hospitals and care giving facilities in the early 19th century, there has been movement toward standardizing care and financial practices within these institutions. It was not until the early 20th century that hospitals began a pay-for-service financial plan. In this arrangement, the patient pays for services received (fee for service) with no ceiling placed on the total amount that could be charged. Insurance companies paid for the services rendered by most institutions. As the cost of health care in the United States rose exponentially, insurers began exploring more cost-effective ways to pay for health care. This has resulted in the health care plans, insurance plans, and federal plans that exist today.

This change in reimbursement for health care services has dramatically affected all aspects of health care delivery in the United States driven by changes in Medicare reimbursement. Reimbursement is now based on the quality of care (value-based purchasing), whereby hospitals are fined if they do not meet the benchmark level of performance for identified patient outcomes.

This has also affected the way nursing care is provided. For example, today, patients who are hospitalized have a much higher acuity than they did 20 years ago. Today, the norm is for many patients to be treated at home or in ambulatory care settings; only the critically ill remain in the hospital. Nursing has been expected to meet these challenges both in acute care and in home care. Today there are more ambulatory services, shorter inpatient stays, and an increase in care for chronic illnesses. The greatest challenge facing the U.S. health care system is the high cost of care and services. Technology enables the survival of premature infants weighing 2499 g or less. Some of the infants are kept alive with life support, which may include ventilators and/or feeding tubes. These infants may have a lifetime connection with pediatricians, nurses, specialists, and therapists. Many of them are placed in early intervention programs, whereby the nurses and therapists visit the child and family in the home setting. Once these "preemies" are 3 years-old, they are placed in preschool programs for children with special needs. There are also transitions in the continuum of care in which patients with chronic illnesses, such as congestive heart failure, receive care of various levels of acuity during the transitions of the chronic condition. The more recent role of the nurse navigator working with these single populations of patients (such as congestive heart failure) has an expected outcome of increasing the quality of care for that population and decreasing the readmission rates. These are two examples of the trend of health care in the United States: health care is paramount but at what expense, and health care at an insurmountable expense. So not only are older adults living longer, the chronically ill are living longer, and the preemies are kept alive on life support. Individuals in severe motor vehicle accidents are air lifted to trauma centers and kept alive. What is the cost to the families and to the nation? The costs affect employers, health care providers, the government, and the public sector.

In 2012, the Institute for Healthcare Improvement (IHI) described an approach to optimizing health system performance. It is the IHI's belief that new designs must be developed to simultaneously pursue three dimensions called the "Triple Aim":
- Improving the patient experience of care (including quality and satisfaction)
- Improving the health of populations
- Reducing the per capita cost of health care

Health care systems in attempting to meet the Triple Aim must focus on the individuals and families that use their services, design and integrate services to meet patient and family needs across the continuum of care, and do all in a cost-effective manner while delivering high-quality care as evidenced by patient and organizational outcomes. Many of the megamergers that have been seen in the last 5 years are a result of the required delivery of care across all transitions.

FACTORS THAT INFLUENCE THE FINANCIAL BURDEN OF HEALTH CARE IN THE UNITED STATES

There are numerous factors that influence the continuing financial burden of health care within the United States.

Demographic Influences

The United States is culturally diverse. There is a continuous influx of people from all countries of the world. It is crucial for the U.S. health care system to deliver culturally competent care. The United States spends more on health care per capita than any other industrialized Western nation, yet the United States has disproportionately more people without access to appropriate health care (Yoder-Wise, 2011). The numbers of individuals without health care insurance has dropped since the implementation of the Affordable Care Act in 2013, and the health care system is changing to meet the current demands of the health care environment.

Steep population growth and an aging population will increase the need for health care services in the future. The U.S. population age 65 years and over is predicted to reach 82 million in 2050, a 137% increase over 1999. Between 2011 and 2030, the number of older adults could rise from 40.4 million (13% of the population) to 70.3 million (20% of the population) as Baby Boomers begin turning 65 (U.S. Census Bureau, 2010).

The U.S. health care system is the most costly in the world, accounting for 17% of the gross domestic product with estimates that this percentage will grow to nearly 20% by 2020 (National Healthcare Expenditure Projections, 2010–2020). Prescription drug costs are also expected to jump by double digits (Baugh, 2015).

Health care costs are a function of the prices of materials, personnel, and services and the use of health care services. Economic interests shape the evolution of technology and health care. The types of health care services delivered continue to be limited by multiple factors, most notably cost constraints and reimbursement (Wywialowski, 2004, p. 33). Financial resources have become the focus of much of the clinical decision making within health care, and the success or failure of a health care organization depends on the extent that its structures have changed to the extent necessary to deliver high-quality care.

Uninsured Individuals

The number of uninsured nonelderly Americans decreased from over 44 million in 2013 (the year before the Affordable Care Act [ACA] provisions) to just below 27 million in 2016. However, in 2017, the number of uninsured people increased by nearly 700,000 people; the first increase since implementation of the ACA. Ongoing efforts to alter the ACA or to make receipt of Medicaid contingent on work may further erode coverage gains seen under the ACA (Tolbert, 2020).

One reason for lack of insurance is that their place of employment does not provide health care coverage; another reason is that they cannot afford the high cost of health care. The uninsured and underinsured populations affect hospitals and the communities in which health care is sought.

This places an added burden on the facilities to provide "charity care." When a patient who is uninsured receives care, the cost of the care trickles down to other payers, to the government, or to private insurance companies. This added cost is then passed down to the customers and to taxpayers. In the end, the uninsured population affects everyone not just the uninsured. Bankruptcy in the United States has had a direct correlation to medical expenses and depleted savings.

Medical Technology

The expansion of medical technology and specialty medicine also affects the economics of health care. For example, diagnostic and therapeutic techniques such as magnetic resonance imaging, organ transplantation, and electronic medical records enhance the capabilities of health care while increasing costs.

Health Care Payment Sources

There are rising expectations about the value of health care services in the United States. It is the cultural norm in America that we will all expect to receive the highest quality of health care at all times. To this end, the United States spends a great deal of money on health care services. The people of the United States are covered by Medicare, Medicaid, insurance companies, and managed care companies although 16.1% of the U.S. population was not insured as of January 2014, which is down from 17.3% before the American Affordable Care Act's requirement for Americans to have health insurance took effect on January 1, 2014. The numbers of uninsured have been increasing since the assaults on the ACA (Tolbert, 2020).

The United States continues to rely on a free-market approach to health care, with the private sector providing insurance coverage (through employers) and the federal sector providing for some individuals who are unable to pay.

Medical insurance began in 1847 with payments made to offset income loss that resulted after an accident. Blue Cross Blue Shield originated the reimbursement of general health costs in the 1930s. The private health care industry has changed dramatically with the advent of managed care. In the private sector, the following five types of organizations fund health care costs:

- Traditional insurance companies, which includes Blue Cross Blue Shield for-profit commercial insurance companies
- Preferred provider organizations (PPOs), which act as brokers between insurers and health care providers
- Health maintenance organizations (HMOs), which are independent prepayment plans
- Point of service (POS) plans, which combined features of classic HMOs with client choice characteristics of PPOs
- Self-funded plans in which the employer takes on the role of insurer

PRIVATE INSURANCE

The majority of insured Americans received health care insurance through their place of employment. The focus of such coverage has moved from the straight fee-for-services rendered model to managed health care. Managed health care organizations provide for both the delivery and the financing of health care for their members. The principal force behind the movement away from fee-for-service was the belief that health care costs can be controlled by "managing" the way in which health care is delivered and used.

The foundation of the managed care organization is the primary care provider (PCP). The PCP can be a physician or a nurse practitioner. This provider serves as the gatekeeper to coordinate and manage the patient's use of resources and referrals and protects the patient from unnecessary overtreatment.

HMOs deliver comprehensive health maintenance and treatment services for a group of enrolled individuals. Several models of the HMO structure have evolved. The group model is one in which practitioners employed by the insurer spend all their time caring for patients of that particular HMO. An example of this model is the Kaiser-Permanente health care system. Another model is Independent Practice Associations (IPAs) in which independent practitioners (not employed by the HMO) provide care for HMO members and are reimbursed for that care. Practitioners in an IPA contract may be restricted to caring only for members enrolled in that IPA, but some contracts allow practitioners to provide for nonmembers as well. Many IPAs have ceased existence because they were unable to remain financially viable. In a network model, HMOs contract with individual practitioners and practitioner groups for both primary and specialty services. In a capitation system, each organization is paid a fixed negotiated rate per member per month for each patient regardless of how often services are used. Box 4.1 provides various types of HMOs.

BOX 4.1 **Types of Health Maintenance Organizations**	
Staff model	Self-contained organization Majority of physicians are on staff and paid by HMOs
Group model	Single, large multispecialty group that is the sole or major source of care for enrollees
Network model	Two or more group practices contract to care for the majority of patients enrolled in HMO plan
Independent practice association	Contractual agreements with a wide variety of care providers Members have greater choice

HMO, Health maintenance organization.

SOCIAL HEALTH MAINTENANCE ORGANIZATION

A social health maintenance organization (SHMO) is a demonstration model conducted under Medicare to determine the value and feasibility of combining health and medical services in one payment. Services provided include those of traditional Medicare and Medicaid and adult day care, homemaker services, respite care, hospice care, transportation, and chronic care in a nursing facility without prior hospitalization (Rundio & Wilson, 2013).

POINT OF SERVICE PLANS

POS plans evolved in response to patient concerns about their lack of choice in choosing providers in the previously mentioned plans. These plans allow members to pay additional fees to use providers outside of the individual network.

PPOs agree to deliver services to members for a fee-for-service negotiated price. Members must receive care exclusively from within the PPO or incur additional costs. To control costs, the health care agency must receive preauthorization from the PPO for a member to be hospitalized and second opinions are required before all major procedures.

Bundled Payments

Bundled payments provide for all payers along the care continuum to share the payment for the total care provided regardless of the location of care and the number of providers. As an example, a 90-year-old individual presents at an emergency department (ED) with a fall and a urinary tract infection. After 3 days on an inpatient unit with intravenous (IV) antibiotic infusions, the patient is transferred to a skilled rehabilitation facility for continued treatment before returning home with home care follow-up. In a bundled care reimbursement system, reimbursement with be shared by all providers. Such payments will become the norm, as opposed to the current delivery model in which each location and provider receives reimbursement (Cleverley & Cleverley, 2018). This is a major reason for the mergers of facilities providing full transition of care services.

U.S. GOVERNMENT

The federal government oversees plans that assist older adults, the disabled, and some uninsured individuals.

Medicaid

Medicaid is a joint federal and state assistance program designed to pay for medical long-term care assistance for individuals and families with low income and limited resources. Medicaid is available only to certain low-income individuals and families who fit into an eligibility group that is recognized by federal and state laws. It sends payments directly to health care providers. Over time amendments to the Social Security Act, popularly known as the Medicare Bill (1965), have been made to include people with developmental disabilities and other low-income groups including the elderly, children, and pregnant women. Medicaid went into effect in 1966 and is known as Title XIX of the Social Security Act. Each state sets its own guidelines regarding eligibility and services. These may include age, disabilities, income, financial resources (e.g., bank accounts, real property, or other items that can be sold for cash), and citizenship status (whether the individual is a U.S. citizen or a lawfully admitted immigrant). There are special rules for those who live in nursing homes and for children with disabilities living at home. Children may be eligible for coverage if they are U.S. citizens or lawfully admitted immigrants. Eligibility for children is based on the child's status not that of the parents.

State Children's Health Insurance Program

Of all developed countries, the United States continues to have a high proportion of uninsured individuals. The lack of health insurance is greatest for blacks and Hispanics, younger Americans age 18 to 34, and men more than women. Most of the uninsured have at least one family member who is working full time, but they do not obtain coverage because the cost of premiums is high. The State Children's Health Insurance Program (SCHIP) is a plan that targets uninsured children who are not eligible for Medicaid. These programs were implemented at the state level to provide insurance for all children.

Medicare

Medicare is the government's largest health care financing program. Medicare is the name given to a health insurance program administered by the U.S. government, covering people who are either age 65 and over or who meet other special criteria. Medicare currently provides coverage for services for more than 49 million beneficiaries. Approximately 81% of the enrollees are elderly, 19% are disabled, and less that 1% have end-stage renal disease (Kaiser Family Foundation, 2016). There have been numerous changes to the Medicare system since its introduction. It was expanded in 1972 to include people of any age with end-stage renal disease. Many of these changes have been attempts to deal with the high cost of Medicare expenditures.

Administration of Federal Insurers

The Centers for Medicare & Medicaid Services (CMS), a component of the Department of Health and Human Services (HHS), administers Medicare, Medicaid, and SCHIP. The Social Security Administration is responsible for determining Medicare eligibility and processing premium payments for the Medicare program.

Benefits

The "Original Medicare" program has two parts: Part A (Hospital Insurance) and Part B (Medical Insurance). Only a few special cases exist where prescription drugs are covered by Original Medicare, but as of January 2006, Medicare Part D provides more comprehensive drug coverage. Medicare Advantage (MA) plans are another way for beneficiaries to receive their Part A, B, and D benefits.

Part A: Hospital Insurance

Part A covers hospital stays. It will also pay for stays in a skilled nursing facility if certain criteria are met.
1. The hospital admission must be at least 3 days, 3 midnights, not counting the discharge date.
2. The nursing home admission must be for a condition diagnosed during the hospital stay or for the main cause of hospital stay. For instance, a hospital stay for a broken hip and then nursing home stay for physical therapy would be covered.
3. If the patient is not receiving rehabilitation, but has some other ailment that requires skilled nursing supervision then the nursing home condition would be covered.
4. The care being rendered by the nursing home must be skilled. Medicare Part A does not pay for custodial, nonskilled, or long-term care activities including activities of daily living (ADLs) such as personal hygiene, cooking, cleaning, etc.

The maximum length of stay (LOS) that Medicare Part A will cover in a skilled nursing facility per diagnosis is 100 days. The first 20 days would be paid for in full by Medicare with the remaining 80 days requiring a copayment. Many insurance companies have a provision for skilled nursing care in the policies they sell.

If a beneficiary uses some portion of their Part A benefit and then goes at least 60 days without receiving skilled services, the 100-day clock is reset and they qualify for a new 100-day benefit period.

Part A is financed by taxes paid by employers and working individuals. Medicare Part A (Hospital Insurance) helps cover inpatient care in hospitals, including critical access hospitals and skilled nursing facilities (not custodial or long-term care). It also helps cover hospice care and some home health care. Beneficiaries must meet certain conditions to get these benefits.

Part B: Medical Insurance

Part B medical insurance helps pay for some services and products not covered by Part A, generally on an outpatient basis. Part B is optional and may be deferred if the beneficiary or their spouse is still actively working. There is a lifetime penalty (10% per year) imposed for not taking Part B if not actively working.

Part B coverage includes physician and nursing services; radiographs; laboratory and diagnostic tests; influenza and pneumonia vaccinations; blood transfusions; renal dialysis; outpatient hospital procedures; limited ambulance transportation; immunosuppressive drugs for organ transplant recipients; chemotherapy; hormonal treatments, such as Lupron; and other outpatient medical treatments administered in a physician's office. Medication administration is covered under Part B only if it is administered by the physician during an office visit.

Part B also helps with durable medical equipment (DME), including canes, walkers, wheelchairs, and mobility scooters for those with mobility impairments. Prosthetic devices, such as artificial limbs and breast prostheses after mastectomy, one pair of eyeglasses after cataract surgery, and oxygen for home use are also covered. As with all Medicare benefits, Part B coverage is subject to medical necessity. Complex rules are used to manage the benefit, and advisories are periodically issued that describe coverage criteria. On the national level, these advisories are issued by CMS and are known as national coverage determinations (NCDs). Local coverage determinations (LCDs) only apply within the multistate area managed by a specific regional Medicare Part B contractor. Local medical review policies (LMRPs) were superseded by LCDs in 2003.

Part B medical insurance is a supplementary voluntary medical insurance financed by general tax revenues and by required premium contributions. Medicare Part B (Medical Insurance) helps cover physicians' services and outpatient care. These may include the following:

- Outpatient surgery
- Diagnostic tests
- Radiology and pathology services
- Emergency services
- Outpatient rehabilitation services
- Renal dialysis
- Medical equipment and supplies
- Preventive services (mammography)

Part C: Medicare Advantage Plans

With the passage of the Balanced Budget Act of 1997, Medicare beneficiaries were given the option to receive their Medicare benefits through private health insurance plans instead of through the Original Medicare plan (Parts A and B). These programs were known as "Medicare+Choice" or "Part C" plans. Pursuant to the Medicare Prescription Drug, Improvement, and Modernization Act of 2003, the compensation and business practices changed for insurers that offer these plans, and Medicare+Choice plans became known as MA plans. In addition to offering comparable coverage to Part A and Part B, MA plans may also offer Part D coverage.

Part D: Prescription Drug Plans

Medicare Part D went into effect on January 1, 2006. Anyone with Part A or B is eligible for Part D. It was made possible by the passage of the Medicare Prescription Drug, Improvement, and Modernization Act in 2003. To receive this benefit, a person with Medicare must enroll in a stand-alone prescription drug plan (PDP) or MA plan with prescription drug coverage (MA-PD). These plans are approved and regulated by the Medicare program, but they are actually designed and administered by private health insurance companies. Unlike Original Medicare (Parts A and B), Part D coverage is not standardized. Plans choose which drugs (or even classes of drugs) they wish to cover and at what level (or tier) they wish to cover. Likewise, they are free to choose which drugs and what level (tier) not to cover, and to choose not to cover some drugs at all. The exception to this is drugs that Medicare specifically excludes from coverage, including, but not limited to benzodiazepines, cough suppressants, and barbiturates. Plans that cover excluded drugs are not allowed to pass those costs on to Medicare, and plans are required to repay CMS if they are found to have billed Medicare in these cases.

Prescription Drug Coverage

Most people pay a monthly premium for this coverage. Since 2006, Medicare prescription drug coverage has been available to everyone with Medicare. Medicare prescription drug coverage is insurance.

Private companies provide the coverage. Beneficiaries choose the drug plan and pay a monthly premium. Like other insurance, if a beneficiary decides not to enroll in a drug plan when they are first eligible, they may pay a penalty if they choose to join later.

Hospice

In 1983, Medicare added hospice benefits for the last 6 months of life to cover services for the patient who is terminally ill. An organized program consists of services provided and coordinated by an interdisciplinary team at a frequency appropriate to meet the needs of individuals who are diagnosed with terminal illnesses and have a limited life span. Hospice workers view death as a normal part of the life cycle. Hospice emphasizes living the remaining months of life as fully and as comfortably as possible.

Hospice care specializes in management of pain and other physical symptoms of a dying patient, and meeting the psychosocial and spiritual needs of the individual and of the individual's family or other primary care person(s). The program also includes a continuum of interdisciplinary team services across all settings in which hospice care is provided, availability of 24-hour access to care, utilization of volunteers, and bereavement care to the survivors, as needed, for an appropriate period of time.

Ambulatory Payment Classifications

The Hospital Outpatient Prospective Payment System (HOPPS) "applies to designated hospital outpatient services furnished in all classes of hospitals..." The unit of payment is based on the assignment on the similar clinical characteristics and costs within the Healthcare Common Procedure Coding System (HCPCS). There is present pressure on hospital outpatient services, especially ambulatory surgery, in the area of costs. Costs for hospital-connected outpatient surgery is higher than costs incurred through more independent ambulatory surgery centers.

CHARITY CARE ASSISTANCE

As an example, the New Jersey Hospital Care Payment Assistance Program (Charity Care Assistance) provides free or reduced-charge care to patients who receive inpatient and outpatient services or care in an acute care hospital throughout New Jersey. Hospital assistance and reduced-charge care are available only for necessary hospital care.

Hospital care payment assistance is available to New Jersey residents who

- Have no health coverage or have coverage that pays for only part of the bill,
- Are ineligible for any private or government-sponsored coverage, and
- Meet both the listed income and assets eligibility criteria.

The reimbursement for charity care varies from state to state, so be aware of the charity care regulations at your workplace. A sample of income criteria that is related to the percentage of hospital charge to be paid by patients is listed in Box 4.2.

The federal government also operates health care networks, such as the Veterans Health Administration (VHA) and the Indian Health Service (IHS).

BOX 4.2 Income Criteria for Health and Human Services Poverty Income Guidelines	
Income as a Percentage of HHS Poverty Income Guidelines	Percentage of Charge Paid by Patient
≤200%	0
>200% but ≤225%	20
>225% but ≤250%	40
>250% but ≤275%	60
>275% but ≤300%	80
>300%	100

(From *New Jersey State Department of Health. New Jersey Hospital care payment assistance fact sheet.* (August 2016). <www.state.nj.us/health/charitycare/documents/charitycare_factsheet_en.pdf>.
HHS, Department of Health and Human Services.

VETERANS HEALTH ADMINISTRATION

The goal of the VHA is to provide excellence in patient care, veterans' benefits, and customer satisfaction. The VHA strives for high-quality, prompt, and seamless service to U.S. veterans. Of the 25 million veterans currently alive, nearly three of every four served during a war or an official period of hostility. About a quarter of the nation's population (approximately 70 million people) are potentially eligible for VA benefits and services because they are veterans or family members or survivors of veterans.

INDIAN HEALTH SERVICE

IHS, an agency within the HHS, is responsible for providing federal health services to American Indians and Alaska Natives. The IHS is the principal federal health care provider and health advocate for Indian people, and its goal is to raise their health status to the highest possible level. The IHS provides a comprehensive health service delivery system for American Indians and Alaska Natives who are members of 566 federally recognized tribes across the United States.

TYPES OF HEALTH CARE SERVICES

With the continuing focus on the cost-effectiveness of delivery of care, health care has moved from the acute care hospital to a full continuum of services within the community and the hospital. Twenty years ago, it was not uncommon for a community hospital to attempt to provide all services for a majority of patients, and LOSs were long and expensive. As the cost improvement model advanced, health care services have been divided into primary, secondary, and tertiary centers of care.

Health promotion and disease prevention are a focus of many HMOs. Practitioners' offices provide many health maintenance activities, as do community centers for education and health assessment.

There are three types of health care services: primary, secondary, and tertiary care (Box 4.3). Primary care is health maintenance that decreases the risk for disease. Secondary care encourages disease prevention through early intervention. Tertiary care is long-term care.

BOX 4.3	Types of Health Care Services	
Type of Care	**Description**	**Examples**
Primary	Decreases risk for disease	Immunizations
	Health maintenance	Nutrition counseling
Secondary	Disease prevention through early intervention	Surgery
Tertiary	Long-term care	Durable medical equipment
		Education

Many diagnostic services, such as colonoscopies, are now being provided in ambulatory care settings and physicians' offices. Many surgical procedures are also now being provided in ambulatory care settings. Secondary and tertiary care is provided in a number of settings across the health care continuum. Health care is provided by the types of agencies and facilities listed in Box 4.4.

It is important for you as a nurse to realize that different levels of care are paid for at differing rates by both private and federal insurers. This differentiation in financial reimbursement for these services results in "type-specific" staffing, standards of care, and services rendered. Each type of service also has to meet differing accreditation requirements (see Chapter 5).

FOR-PROFIT AND NOT-FOR-PROFIT HEALTH CARE AGENCIES

Although the majority of the health care facilities in the United States function as not-for-profit organizations, there is a movement toward hospitals becoming for-profit organizations. An example of a for-profit entity would be a physician group opening their own same-day surgery center. There are examples of hospitals that have become for-profit institutions where the profit is funneled back to either the hospital or an overseeing corporation.

With health care costs continuing to escalate, it will be important for you as a nurse to be aware of the economic forces that affect your day-to-day nursing care.

BOX 4.4 Agencies and Facilities That Provide Health Care

Health Care Facility	Examples	Health Care Facility	Examples
Acute care	Hospitalization for episode of illness *Example: patient suffering an acute myocardial infarction*	Rehabilitation	Post-injury focus on restoration of function *Example: patient with spinal cord injury relearning activities of daily living*
Subacute care	Continued hospitalization after initial acute stage has passed *Example: patient requiring long-term ventilatory assistance*	Home health care	Post-hospitalization support within the home *Example: post-congestive heart failure patient requiring medication and dietary follow-up*
Long-term care	Continued hospitalization after stabilization of chronic long-term condition *Example: patient in end-stage Alzheimer disease*	Hospice services • Inpatient	Care of the dying patient and family *Example: in-home care for dying patient*
Residential care	Living facilities for patients in need of basic support *Example: group home for individual with mental retardation*	• Outpatient	*Example: in-home care for dying patient*
Assisted living	Living facilities with an option of basic support *Example: 85-year-old independent patient with occasional falls*	Health care centers Local health departments	Full range of preventative health care services *Example: federally qualified health care center* Preventative health services in support of *Healthy People 2020* *Examples: blood pressure screenings, immunizations*
Ambulatory care	Diagnostic testing screenings Low-acuity surgery *Example: same-day operations*	Urgent care centers	Treatment of nonurgent injuries *Examples: physical examinations and first aid*

BUDGETING PROCESS

Budget review and management represent one of the most important responsibilities of the nurse manager in this era of escalating health care costs and decreasing reimbursements. The economic stability of an organization depends on the management of the resources that are required to deliver care in a cost-effective and safe manner. The earlier content of this chapter provided a review of the essentials of health care reimbursement.

Health care institutions are businesses, and one of the largest costs is the actual delivery of patient care. The resources required to deliver that patient care are costly and most often managed at the point of service (the unit). Nurses need to understand how to manage the cost of patient care as it relates to their clinical practice and to the workings of their particular unit. Also, accrediting agencies require collaborative input from staff in the development of annual budgets (The Joint Commission, 2019).

In most institutions, there is a well-defined process for the development, implementation, and evaluation of the budget. The budgeting process is a part of the overall strategic planning process (see Chapter 3). The organizational budget cascades down to individual departments and units. Budgets are usually developed annually for a 12-month period. The budget cycle is based on the organization's definition of the fiscal year (calendar [January 1 to December 31] or fiscal [July 1 to June 30]).

There are two major types of budgeting processes: zero-based and incremental. Zero-based budgeting requires the entire budget to be recreated annually starting from zero. This type of budgeting allows for the consideration of alternatives in the delivery of the service. All portions of the zero-based budget need to be justified annually. This type of budgeting also demands the proactive evaluation of the need for the services. Incremental budgeting is the more traditional approach, building on the previous year's budget. If a 10% increase in funds is available, the budget may be increased by 10%. This is an easier process, but at times it allows budgets to become bloated with minimal justification of the service or at times it does not reflect the actual changes that may be anticipated for the unit.

The budgeting process can be divided into phases (Finkler, Kovner, & Jones, 2007):

- Information gathering and planning
- Development of organizational and unit budgets
- Development of cash budgets, negotiation, and revision
- Evaluation

Information Gathering and Planning

In the information gathering and planning phase, the nurse manager is provided with data necessary to the development of the budget. An environmental assessment is done, which provides the organization and the nurse manager with information about the changing needs of the community, changing professional requirements, economic changes that will affect the unit's function, community demographics, stakeholder needs and requirements, regulatory changes, and other items. This assessment provides the context of the needs that the unit budgets for during the next fiscal year. This environmental assessment provides the materials for the reassessment of the organization's mission, goals, and priorities. As organizational priorities are set, financial objectives are created, allocating resources to all units.

Development of Organizational and Unit Budgets

Organizational and unit budgets are then created to match the financial objectives of the organization. It is important that both the financial and overall objectives of the particular unit are in concert with the organization-wide objectives and goals. The basic assumptions of the organization need to be part of the development of both organizational and unit objectives. Such assumptions may be the negotiated union contract raise for all employees, the cost of a new electronic record system, or similar items. Such assumptions are an important part of the development of the unit budget.

Development of Cash Budgets, Negotiation, and Revision

The cash budget is developed after the operating and capital budgets of the unit or department are developed. It is at this stage that the unit manager's negotiating and revising skills come into play. This cash budget is usually prepared by the chief financial officer, and is the plan for the actual anticipated cash receipts and disbursements of the organization (the cash flow). An organization must have sufficient cash to meet its monthly obligations. This reflects the cash on hand. Ideally, the nurse manager needs to be able to predict when budgeted items will be needed. Unexpected expenditures do occur and may put a strain on a cash-poor system.

Evaluation

Evaluation of the budget occurs at both the organizational and unit levels. Many organizations have created dashboards that allow for the monitoring of progress in meeting department goals. These dashboards provide a quick visual display of the unit's performance. An example of an organization-wide financial dashboard is shown in Fig. 4.1. Evaluation of the budget performance is usually obtained through a process known as variance analysis. A variance is the difference between planned and actual costs. A positive variance (favorable) may be seen when the budgeted amount was greater than that which was actually spent. A negative variance may be seen if the budgeted amount was less than the actual spending. Variance analysis is a complex process in which the unit environment is fully investigated. Variances may be characterized in five ways. A volume variance in a hospital setting may occur in response to fluctuating *in-patient days*. An efficiency variance may be expressed in changes from the anticipated hours per patient day (HPPD). A rate variance reflects the difference between the budgeted hourly rate of pay and the actual rate paid. A nonsalary expenditure variance may be caused by changes in patient mix, supply quantities and costs, and price paid. A negative variance may be seen in the number of staff required during a 2-week period. However, on further investigation, it may be determined that the patient acuity was higher than anticipated, and expenses were increased in response to this increased acuity. It is the role of the nurse manager to be aware of the variances related to the unit and the reasons for the alteration in expected performance. These variance data are often used in the

HELPING HANDS HOSPITAL DASHBOARD RESULTS

	Q1	Q2	Q3	Annual Goal	Top 10%
QUALITY					
1. Overall patient satisfaction	88%	90%	93%	92%	95%
CORE MEASURES					
2. Acute Myocardial Infarction					
A. AMI Beta Blocker on discharge	90%	95%	98%	100%	100%
B. Smoking Cessation Advice/Counseling	98%	98%	100%	100%	100%
C. Heart Attack patients given aspirin on arrival	99%	98%	97%	100%	100%
D. Heart Attack patients given aspirin on discharge	100%	100%	100%	100%	100%
E. Heart Attack patients given thrombolytic medication within 30 min of arrival	100%	99%	100%	99%	100%
3. Surgical Care Improvement Project (SCIP)					
A. Surgery patients who received preventative antibiotic 1 hour before incision	94%	92%	91%	96%	98%
B. Surgery patients whose preventative antibiotic are appropriately selected	98%	92%	94%	96%	96%
FINANCIAL					
Days Cash on Hand	150	175	170	180	184
Inpatient net receivables (000s)	69,500	65,000	68,000	69,000 (per Qtr)	73,000 (per Qtr)
Average L.O.S.	4.1	3.9	4.3	3.9	3.85
Inpatient gross charges (000s)	70,000	68,000	69,500	70,050 (per Qtr)	75,000 (per Qtr)
Market Share	42%	48%	47%	49%	56%
PEOPLE					
Nursing Full-Time Equivalents	400	385	396	400	400
Employee satisfaction (overall)	79%	82%	81%	88%	91%
Injury/Illness Last Time per 100 employees	5%	6%	4%	4%	2%

Interpretation   Red – below goal   Orange – within 2% of goal   Green – at goal   Blue – top 10% at goal

Fig. 4.1 An example of an organization-wide financial dashboard. (From Indiana Rural Health Association. (2008). *Inpatient scorecards.* <www.indianaruralhealth.org/Sample%20Dashboard%20_(3_).pdf>.

preparation of the next year's budget. Examples of such variable costs seen in unit budgets are as follows:

- Increased overtime related to greater-than-anticipated use of sick time
- Increased use of part-time personnel related to an unanticipated increase in patient acuity
- Increased expense for minor equipment because of an electrical malfunction that destroyed equipment
- Increased expenses caused by resignation of staff and orientation of replacement staff

Many health care organizations have flexible budgets that automatically adjust to environmental changes. A goal of most organizations is to proactively anticipate challenges through the collection of the information in an environmental assessment. An example of a proactive budget process would be the budgeting of increased staff during the influenza season.

Most organizations provide the nurse manager with fiscal reports on a routine basis (weekly, monthly, or quarterly depending on the organization). This allows each cost center manager to carefully monitor the financial activity of the unit. The budget process is continually evolving work, requiring evaluation and continual improvement.

TYPES OF BUDGETS

The overall budget is composed of a number of smaller budgets that represent specific areas of concern in the financial objective setting of an organization. The operating (expense) budget includes: (1) the personnel budget, (2) costs other than for personnel, and (3) the revenue budget. Not all units prepare a revenue budget, and it may be done by the finance department.

The personnel budget requires that the nurse manager forecast the anticipated workload for the year. This is done based on information gathered from the environmental assessment, review of the previous workload, and identification of the services to be provided. The calculation of staff needs is a complex procedure. First, the average daily census and occupancy rate are calculated. The total required patient-care hours are calculated (Fig. 4.2). Then, the number of full-time equivalents (FTEs) required to provide care is calculated based on the expected number of hours. A FTE is calculated as 2080 hours of work per year. Then, the number of full-time employees, part-time employees, and shifts needs to be calculated. Adjustments need to be made for employee benefits and nonproductive time (vacation, orientation, education, sick time, etc. Fig. 4.3).

The next step is to prepare a daily staffing plan. This plan includes the staff mix of individuals required to provide the patient care (registered nurses, licensed practical nurses, unit clerks, patient care associates, etc.). Remember that the skill mix of staff and the staffing requirements are regulated. It is important that the nurse manager maintain compliance with all regulatory boards while determining the budget. Once the nurse manager has decided on the positions required to deliver care, the other labor costs can be included in the personnel budget. These other labor costs include benefits, shift differential, overtime, raises, premium pay, and so forth. Benefits are often calculated at close to an additional 40% to 50% of an individual's pay.

For costs other than personnel costs, the nurse manager will have to calculate supply and expense costs, such as supplies, education, travel to conferences, telephone, electricity, and minor equipment. Some health care institutions also require support services (indirect costs) to be included in the budget, for example, information technology services provided by an in-house department to a unit. These are all examples of indirect costs.

The nurse manager is dealing with only minor equipment purchases in this budget. For major items there is a capital expenditure budget. A capital expenditure must have a life span of at least 1 year, and there is usually a dollar limit for determining whether an equipment request is capital or minor. A capital expenditure usually costs more than $500 or $1000 (depending on the institution) and includes equipment and renovation expenses needed to meet long-term goals. Organizations often perform long-term planning with capital expenditures. In this manner, the organization determines priorities for such expenditures.

Each nursing unit is usually called a cost center. The cost center is the organizational unit for which costs

WORKLOAD CALCULATION (TOTAL REQUIRED PATIENT-CARE HOURS)						
Patient Acuity Level*	Hours of Care Per Patient Day (HPPD)†	×	Patient Days‡	=	Workload§
1	3.0		900		2,700
2	5.2		3,100		16,120
3	8.8		4,000		35,200
4	13.0		1,600		20,800
5	19.0		400		7,600
Total			10,000		82,420

*1, Low; 5, high.
†HPPD is the number of hours of care on average for a given acuity level.
‡1 patient per 1 day = 1 patient day.
§Total number of hours of care needed based on acuity levels and numbers of patient days.

Fig. 4.2 Calculation of patient-care hours.

Productive Hours Calculation

Method 1: Add all nonproductive hours/FTE and subtract from paid hours/FTE
Example: Vacation 15 days
Holiday 7 days
Average sick time 4 days
TOTAL 26 days

26 × 8* hours = 208 nonproductive hours/FTE
2080 − 208 = 1872 productive hours/FTE

Method 2: Multiply paid hours/FTE by percentage of productive hours/FTE
Example: Productive hours = 90%/FTE
(1872 productive hours of total 2080 = 90%)
2080 × 0.90 = 1872 productive hours/FTE

Total FTE Calculation

Required Patient-Care Hours ÷ Productive Hours Per FTE = Total FTEs Needed

82,420 ÷ 1872 = 44 FTEs

*Based on an 8-hour shift pattern.

Fig. 4.3 Productivity calculation. *FTE, Full-time Equivalent.*

can be identified and managed. Although in most large health care organizations the revenue budget is prepared by the chief financial officer, the nurse manager must be aware of the revenue anticipated by the unit. Nurses working in smaller outpatient centers may be responsible for the development of the revenue budget. The calculation of the revenue budget requires knowledge of the anticipated reimbursement expected for patient care and the time of the expected reimbursement.

The majority of health care institutions orient the nurse manager to the financial aspects of the position. This also includes an orientation to the budget process of the institution and the role of the nurse manager in this process. Some health care agencies have changed the organizational structure of the unit management to include a clinical nurse manager and a business manager. The business manager may not be a nurse, but they work with the unit director to maintain financial efficiency in operations.

STAFF NURSE ROLE IN BUDGET PROCESS

Although the nurse manager or director oversees the budget, the staff nurse also has a role in the financial management of the unit. The clinical nurse, through the organization's shared governance process, participates in the budget process. In Magnet institutions, the

TABLE 4.1 Strategies for Cost-Conscious Nursing Practice

1. Understanding what is required to remain financially sound
2. Knowing costs and reimbursement practices
3. Capturing all possible charges in a timely manner
4. Using time efficiently and effectively
5. Discussing the costs of care with the patient
6. Meeting patient rather than provider needs
7. Evaluating cost-effectiveness of new technologies and equipment
8. Predicting and using nursing resources efficiently
9. Using research to evaluate standard nursing practice
10. Consistently evaluating practice based on evidence

(Adapted from Yoder-Wise, P. S. (2011). *Lending and managing in nursing.* (4th ed., p. 239). Mosby: St. Louis).

clinical nurse is expected to advocate for resources that result in actual allocation of such resources to support a nursing unit goal (American Nurses Credentialing Center, 2018). The staff nurse needs to be aware of the financial costs and reimbursement of the care delivered on the unit. Table 4.1 delineates strategies for cost-conscious nursing practice.

SUMMARY

Health care has undergone many changes in the last 10 years. The rapid pace of change shows no signs of abating, and it is important for nurses to be aware of the rules and regulations of payment, reimbursement, and the various types of health care systems and care available to patients and their families. The nurse usually is the advocate for the care that the patient receives and works with the case manager to determine the level of services necessary for the patient. Sadly, the reimbursement method often dictates much of the care available to the patient. It is imperative for nurses to be aware of all of the ramifications of the payers, so that appropriate care can be planned and implemented for the duration of the patient's need.

The financial management of a clinical unit, and the entire health care institution, is the responsibility of the nurse leaders and clinical nurses. The careful balance of delivery of quality health care and financial stewardship is a delicate balance that nurse leaders juggle daily. This is a goal of the Triple Aim. It is a learning system that all nurses work with on a daily basis.

CLINICAL CORNER

Changing Reimbursements for Accountable Care Organization—Nursing Perspective

The structure of the Accountable Care Act (ACA) is changing reimbursements for **Accountable Care Organizations** (ACOs) through a system of quality and financial incentives to encourage improvement of care while lowering cost to consumers and payers. These reimbursement modifications significantly increase demands on the role of nursing as we are in the forefront to improve overall care for health care consumers in the hospital and the community. Nursing's potential to improve and eliminate complications along with lowering LOS directly influences the ACO's ability to receive enhanced reimbursement. By demonstrating our value to improve patient outcomes, nursing is in an excellent position to become leaders in the ACO's ability to provide services to patients and enable it to remain a viable organization while thriving in today's ever-changing health care environment.

The most significant changes that effect reductions in reimbursement are based on preventing hospital-acquired infections, other quality outcomes, and **Hospital Consumer Assessment of Healthcare Providers and Systems [HCAHPS])**. Preventing hospital-acquired infections gives the role of the nurse greater importance. Hospital quality performance is coupled to its financial reimbursement; therefore nursing's role must be to improve the overall care that we give to our patients by using best practices and research to demonstrate our ability to make comprehensive contributions to the financial **bottom line** of the ACO.

Advanced nursing research has brought more scientific models of nursing care to our arsenal of health care delivery and practice. With each intellectual investigation, evaluation, and improvement, we expand our body of knowledge while building new foundations of our professional nursing practice. In these pursuits, not only are we improving the vocation of nursing, but we are fulfilling nursing's responsibility to humanity within the art and science of nursing: caring, compassion, and knowledge.

Infections acquired by patients while in the hospital, such as catheter-associated urinary tract infections (CAUTIs) and central line–associated bloodstream infections (CLABSIs), take a significant toll on the health of a patient who is already dealing with a comprising illness. These infections place the ACO at substantial risk of lost revenue in the form of extra costs to care for the patient, for which hospitals do not receive reimbursement. A report from the Centers for Disease Control and Prevention stated that an estimated cost for each CLABSI is around $17,000 per case (Centers for Disease Control and Prevention (CDC), 2011).

Reducing clinical variation by all clinicians through the use of established interventions and best practices enhances the overall quality outcome for the patient and brings other cost savings. Nurses can help lead their reluctant colleagues into improvement in practices by means of protocols, pathways, and care plans, which nursing has used for many years now. Standardization in practices to eliminate variability of the care that each patient receives will represent a cost saving for the patient and the ACO.

Along with educating nursing staff and caregivers in best practices to improve the nursing process and skill level, we have an obligation to improve accurate documentation for the electronic health record (EHR).

Continued

The EHR has become an even more important tool for the documentation of care provided to the patient. Health care medical records continue to evolve; nevertheless the massive amount of money to build EHR systems and the inconsistency of different IT systems throughout the country demonstrate the vulnerability of documentation. There is no prefect EHR technology system, at least not yet.

Certainly, one can argue the EHR gives the interdisciplinary team, the nurse, and other care partners the ability to communicate better and have more timely information that can lead to more appropriate changes in the care for each patient. But at what cost? Many clinicians feel they cannot spend as much time interacting with their patient because of the need to spend so much time at the computer. Point of care documentation is here to stay; therefore, there needs to be more standardization of EHRs to optimize the documentation process.

It is no longer acceptable to not perform a thorough head-to-toe assessment of the patient at admission to look for and document any existing conditions, such as decubitus ulcers and urinary tract infections and to evaluate the patient's fall rate score. Any preventable condition discovered after entry into the hospital that was not documented at the time of admission will lead the organization to be charged with a hospital-acquired adverse event. The inevitable outcome of the failure to complete documentation is loss of reimbursement.

The same EHR documentation requirement applies to the education of the patient and their family and/ or partner, which should start at time of admission. Discharge instructions, which have been viewed in the past by nurses as an onerous chore to be rushed through as quickly as possible to get the patient out the door, become an even more important method to prevent readmission. We cannot think only of what happens inside the walls of our organization, we must now think "outside the walls." (This is a term I created several years ago. My intent was to demonstrate to clinicians the necessity of realizing patient outcomes and readmissions have a severe reimbursement impact on the ACO. Clinicians must partner with all levels of care providers for continuity of care.)

ACOs are penalized with lost reimbursement for readmissions within 30 days after hospital discharge. If nurses are thinking outside the walls of the hospital, then patients and their caregivers should receive comprehensive aftercare education to prevent hospital readmission and to assist the patient to return to optimal health. Several methods can be used to follow up with the patient after discharge, for instance, by the use of discharge phone calls, home visits from a nurse, and online communication (chat) with a nurse. Furthermore, effective communication after discharge should include the next level of care where the patient will be living; this must include nursing homes and assisted-living situations. All strata of patient care have a responsibility for linkage of care.

Link together all the documentation nurses need to do along with all the quality nursing indicators now required, and it is a wonder nurses have any time to provide actual nursing care for a patient. Currently, with the loss of reimbursement, ACOs are in the unenviable positions of having to reduce their most valuable assets, employees. Nurses are not immune to having their positions eliminated, and they are currently being required to work harder with reduced amounts of resources. With all the requirements for added value, HCAHPS, patient safety, quality, and prevention measures, one can safely justify that more and better educated nurses are needed at the bedside, not fewer. ACOs should invest in continuous education for nurses and other hands-on caregivers.

Nursing leaders have an obligation to team up with their colleagues, nurse managers, and nursing staff to combine our talents and other resources to articulate the importance of additional nurses at the bedside, which adds value to the ACO. If the ACO will fully acknowledge that nurses have the ability to contribute by developing and implementing plans, and reinventing how care is delivered to the patient on multiple levels, then nurses will significantly demonstrate that increasing nursing staff will help the ACO reach expected quality and financial performance goals.

Shirley Bennett Thompson, RN, BSN, BSBA, MSHA, FACHE

(Bennett Thompson LLC, February 1, 2015)

Reference

Centers for Disease Control and Prevention (CDC). (2011). Morbidity and Mortality Weekly Report (MMWR), Vital Signs: Central Line-Associated Blood Stream Infections–United States, 2001, 2008, and 2009. March 2011. <www.cdc.gov/mmwr/pdf/wk/mm60e0301.pdf>.

EVIDENCE-BASED PRACTICE

EBP Budgeting for a Video Monitoring System to Reduce Patient Falls and Sitter

Costs: A Quality Improvement Project

(Kowalski, S. L., Burson, R., Webber, E., & Freundl, M. (2018). Budgeting for a video monitoring system to reduce patient falls and sitter costs: A quality improvement project. *Nursing Economics*, *36*(6), 291.)

A Midwest medical center has had an interprofessional fall prevention taskforce in place for several years. The group formulated a fall prevention protocol based on findings from the Morse scale assessment scores. Additionally, bedside sitters were used to monitor patients identified as having the highest risk of falling. The taskforce accomplished early gains in fall prevention, but over time fall rates began to level out with minor variations over several years, based on data from this facility's incident report tool. It was determined that use of bedside sitters did not lead to an appreciable decrease in patient falls. Inpatient sitter costs have been rising and may be as high as $3 million per year (Rochefort et al., 2011)

Bedside sitters were typically used after the patient's first fall if fall prevention measures were considered likely to be ineffective because of patient characteristics, such as impulsivity or dementia. Incident reports indicated patients continued to fall even with 1:1 bedside sitters in attendance. The medical center did not have a pool of available bedside sitters, therefore, it used existing staff to function as sitters. The personnel used were nurse technicians, licensed vocational nurses, or registered nurses. When a staff member was used as a sitter, either the employee worked overtime or was removed from the unit's staffing model. The use of staff as direct observation sitters was ineffective and expensive, contributing to staff fatigue and dissatisfaction. The use of video monitoring to replace direct observation bedside sitters to reduce patient falls was identified as a possible solution.

Available Knowledge

A literature review was conducted searching for fall-reduction technologies, including video monitors. Only a few peer-reviewed, evidence-based articles were available to support the use of video monitors to improve patient safety and reduce fall rates. The next step was developing a plan to demonstrate the potential benefits within the local health care facility. Facility adoption of a video monitoring system (VMS) was viewed as necessary to provide regionally equitable levels of monitoring for at-risk patients. Because of this hospital system's budget planning constraints, it was anticipated that if the budget proposal was accepted, the time frame until implementation could be greater than a year. This article is designed to create a blueprint for assembling clinically based data and working with an interprofessional team including medical center leadership, nurse managers, fall-prevention committee, biomedical engineering, and quality and safety managers to create a budget proposal for this health care innovation aimed at reducing patient falls. The clinical questions proposed were if the typical sitter model of staffing were to be replaced with the video monitor model of staffing at this medical center then

1. What could be the sitter and fall-related cost savings to the facility?
2. How could fall rates and fall injury rates be affected?
3. How much staff could be returned to the unit?

Financial Narrative

A financial narrative was completed and presented to facility stakeholders to gain support for the project. The cost of the VMS was estimated to produce an overall savings to the facility within less than a year after implementation. Therefore, a reduction of bedside sitter use of 75% was anticipated. After budget approval, system installation, staff training, and preimplementation data collection the VMS would be implemented with an initial capacity of eight patients. Based on reports from other facilities, it would be beneficial to use staff with experience in bedside care, such as nurse aids or caregivers on physical work restrictions, to monitor video systems because staff with bedside experience can better anticipate patient activity and are already skilled in direct communication with patients. The budget proposal was presented and accepted by the facility management team. Subsequently a facility walkthrough was conducted with the vendor and biomedical engineer to obtain a formal quote to move forward with procurement and implementation of the VMS. The video monitoring company included staff training and technology support as part of the installation package.

Continued

EVIDENCE-BASED PRACTICE—cont'd

Budget Item	Year 1 VM	Year 1 Sitters	Year 2 VM	Year 2 Sitters	Year 3 VM	Year 3 Sitters
Eight monitors at $10,000 each	$80,000	0	0	0	0	0
Central monitoring station	$30,000	0	0	0	0	0
4.2 FTE VMT staffing (pulled from existing model)	(0)	(0)	(0)	(0)	(0)	(0)
8 hours of training for five CNAs as VMTs	$764.00	0	0	0	0	0
8 hours of training for two CNAs as VMTs	$0	0	$305.60	0	$305.60	0
Licensing/system support contracts	$20,000	0	$20,000	0	$20,000	0
Managers, technical, biomedical support	(0)	(0)	(0)	(0)	(0)	(0)
Use of direct observation sitters (Average daily sitter cost × 365)	—	$422,086	—	$422,086	—	$422,086
Use of VM observation	$105,521.50		$105,521.50		$105,521.50	
Fall-related injury costs	$201,864 (50% reduction)	$403,728	$201,864	$403,728	$201,864	$403,728
Total estimated costs	$438,149.50	$825,814	$327,691.10	$825,814	$327,691.10	$825,814

Note: As evidenced by the cost analysis, the video monitoring can be a cost-effective means of reducing patient falls and returning staff to the unit.
CNA, Certified nursing assistant; FTE, full-time equivalent; VM, video monitoring; VMT, video monitor technician.

▮ NCLEX® EXAMINATION QUESTIONS

1. Which of the following promotes cost-effective resource management?
   A. Using all levels of personnel to their fullest when making assignments
   B. Providing necessary equipment and properly charging patients
   C. Returning uncontaminated, unused equipment to the appropriate department for credit
   D. All of the above are correct

2. _____ includes budgeting and resource allocation. Human, financial, and material resources must be considered:
   A. Resource management
   B. Cost-effective care
   C. Cost containment
   D. Process improvement

3. The majority of health care institutions:
   A. Orient the nurse manager to the financial aspects of the position

   B. Do not orient the nurse manager to the financial aspects of the position
   C. Orient the staff nurse to the budget process of the institution
   D. Do not orient the night supervisor to the financial aspects of the position

4. In preparation for creation of a unit budget, the nurse manager will:
   A. Work with staff to set priorities
   B. Develop a cash budget for the unit
   C. Orient all staff to cost-conscious practices
   D. Create a spreadsheet to track spending

5. As a manager, you are attempting to evaluate the present status of the capital expense budget. You would look at:
   A. The cost of benefits for your staff compared with the budget
   B. The amount of money spent to date on equipment
   C. The variance reports sent to the unit on a weekly basis
   D. Productivity scorecard results for staffing

6. When developing an incremental-type budget, the nurse manager understands:
    A. Yearly budgets are dependent on the previous year's budget
    B. Anticipated changes are allowed
    C. Changes must be justified
    D. The yearly budget for the upcoming year will be less than for the present year

7. As the nurse manager you are aware that which of the following is revenue gained?
    A. From patient
    B. Third-party payers
    C. Overtime
    D. Working with less licensed personnel

8. Which of the following is not one of the types of organizations that fund health care costs?
    A. Traditional insurance companies
    B. PPOs
    C. HMOs
    D. Charity care

9. Payments that provide for all payers along the care continuum to share the payment for the total care provided regardless of the location of care and the number of providers is referred to as:
    A. Bundled
    B. PPO
    C. HMO
    D. Medicare/Medicaid

10. Which of the following is a plan that targets uninsured children who are not eligible for Medicaid? The program was implemented at the state level to provide insurance for all children.
    A. Medicaid
    B. Medicaid SSI
    C. The State Children's Health Insurance Program
    D. Centers for Medicaid and Medicare

Answers: 1. D   2. A   3. A   4. A   5. B   6. A   7. B   8. D   9. A   10. C

BIBLIOGRAPHY

American Nurses Credentialing Center. (2018). *2019, Magnet application manual.* Silver Spring, MD: Author.

Baugh, M. (2015) *The 411 on health care benefits: 4 Benefits you can expect for 2016.* Retrieved July 2, 2019, from <http://www.learnvest.com/2015/10/2016-heqlth-care-benefit-changes/>

Cleverly, W., & Cleverly, J. (2018). *Essentials of health care finance* (8th ed.). Burlington, MA: Jones and Bartlett.

Finkler, S., Kovner, C., & Jones, C. (2007). *Financial Management for nurse managers and executives.* St. Louis, MO: Saunders.

Grohar-Murray, M. E., & DiCroce, H. R. (2011). *Leadership and management in nursing* (3rd ed). Upper Saddle River, NJ: Prentice Hall.

Institute for Healthcare Improvement. (2014). Triple aim initiatives, <www.ihi.org/engage/initiatives/TripleAim/Pages/default.aspx>.

Kaiser Family Foundation. (2016). Distribution of Medicare beneficiaries by eligibility category. Retrieved August 4, 2019 from <http://kff.org/medicare/state-indicator/distribution-of-medicare-beneficiaries-by-eligibility-category-2/>

Kelly-Heidenthal. P. (2003). *Nursing leadership and management.* Clifton Park, NY: Delmar Thompson Learning.

National Healthcare Expenditure Projections. (2010–2020). Centers for Medicare & Medicaid Services, Office of the Actuary.

New Jersey Hospital Care Payment Assistance Program (Charity Care Assistance). (2013). www.nj.gov/health/cc/documents/ccfactsh.pdf.

Rundio, A., & Wilson, V. (2013). *Nurse executive: Review and resource manual.* Silver Spring, MD: ANCC.

The Joint Commission. (2019). *Comprehensive accreditation manual—Hospitals.* Oak Book, IL: Author.

Tolbert J, Orgera K. (2020) *Key facts about the uninsured. population.* https://www.kff.org/uninsured/fact-sheet/key-facts-about-the-uninsured-population/.

U.S. Census Bureau. (2010). *U.S. Census Data.* www.census.gov.

Wywialowski, E. F. (2004). *Managing client care* (3rd ed.). St. Louis: Mosby.

Yoder-Wise, P. S. (2011). *Leading and managing in nursing* (4th ed.). St. Louis: Mosby.

5

Health Care Regulatory and Certifying Agencies

OBJECTIVES

- Identify health care regulatory and certifying agencies.
- Explain the nurse's role in relation to hospital surveys.
- Differentiate among The Joint Commission, Det Norske Veritas, and Healthcare Facilities Accreditation.
- Define accreditation.
- Discuss strategies for implementation of proper procedures for an upcoming hospital survey.

- Discuss strategies for implementation of proper procedures using appropriate regulatory and certifying agency guidelines.
- Differentiate between accreditation and awards for performance.
- Discuss the nurse's role in accreditation and awards for excellence.

KEY TERMS

accreditation a self-assessment and external peer assessment process used by health care organizations to accurately assess their level of performance in relation to established standards and to implement ways to continually improve

Accreditation Association for Accreditation of Ambulatory Surgery Facilities (AAAASF) accredits ambulatory surgery centers, outpatient physical therapy, rural health clinics

Accreditation Association for Ambulatory Health Care (AAAHC) accredits ambulatory surgery centers

American Osteopathic Association (AOA) Healthcare Facilities Accreditation Program osteopathic accreditation program that ensures health care facilities meet standards of care while also meeting the Medicare conditions of participation for ambulatory surgery centers, critical access hospitals, and hospitals

Centers for Disease Control and Prevention (CDC) agency charged with the promotion of health and quality of life by preventing and controlling disease, injury, and disability; has created multiple infection control standards that are now part of standards for The Joint Commission accreditation

Community Health Accreditation Partner (CHAP) accredits home health agencies, hospice care

compliance to act in accordance with stated requirements, such as standards; levels of compliance include noncompliance, partial compliance, and substantial compliance

Det Norske Veritas (DNV) a health care accreditation agency that integrates the International Organization for Standardization's 9001 quality management system with the Medicare conditions of participation

National Institute for Occupational Safety and Health (NIOSH) federal agency responsible for conducting research and making recommendations for the prevention of work-related injury and illness.

NIOSH is part of the CDC within the U.S. Department of Health and Human Services

Occupational Safety and Health Administration (OSHA) U.S. Department of Labor agency that ensures the safety and health of America's workers by setting and enforcing standards; providing training, outreach, and education; establishing partnerships; and encouraging continual improvement in workplace safety and health

state departments of health departments that foster accessible and high-quality health and senior services to help all people to achieve optimal health, dignity, and independence in an attempt to prevent disease, promote and protect well-being at all life stages, and encourage informed choices that enrich the quality of life for individuals and communities

The Joint Commission (TJC) accreditation organization that strives to continuously improve the safety and quality of care provided to the public through the provision of health care accreditation and related services that support performance improvement in health care organizations

U.S. Department of Health and Human Services (USDHHS) U.S. government's principal agency for protecting the health of all Americans and providing essential human services, especially for those who are least able to help themselves

REGULATORY AGENCIES

Health care organizations work with myriad accrediting and regulatory agencies so that optimum standards of care and delivery of care can be met. Regulatory agencies are charged by federal and state governments to

- set standards for the operation of health care organizations,
- ensure compliance with federal and state regulations developed by government administrative agencies, and
- investigate and make judgments regarding complaints brought by consumers of the services and the public.

Licensing of health care agencies to maintain practice occurs through state departments of health. State

departments of health usually oversee outcomes of care within health care facilities, investigate consumer complaints, and deal with issues of importance to the public health. These agencies monitor basic compliance with the specific health care regulations of that state. Compliance with regulatory standards on both national and state levels is mandatory, and fines can be leveled against organizations for noncompliance.

Accreditation agencies evaluate health care organizations against a set of standards that have been validated against best practice. Accreditation is voluntary but mandatory for continued Centers for Medicare & Medicaid Services (CMS) reimbursement. The Medicare conditions of participation require that hospitals be accredited by an organization with "deeming authority." Deeming authority is authority granted by CMS to accrediting organizations to determine, on the behalf of CMS, whether an organization evaluated by the accreditor is in compliance with corresponding Medicare regulations.

ACCREDITATION

Accreditation agencies were initially founded to set a minimum of standard of care. As they have matured, their mission has expanded to "continuously improve health care for the public, in collaboration with other stakeholders, by evaluating health care organizations and inspiring them to excel in providing safe and effective care of the highest quality and value" (The Joint Commission, 2019a, b). They have moved from compliance agencies to agencies that hope to drive improvement and quality of care.

Accrediting agencies move beyond basic compliance and look to the continual improvement of operational systems critical to patient care and safety. Although accreditation is listed as a voluntary process, federal reimbursement of health care is dependent on accreditation. The three major health care organization accrediting agencies are The Joint Commission (TJC), Det Norske Veritas (DNV), and the American Osteopathic Association (AOA) Healthcare Facilities Accreditation Program.

THE JOINT COMMISSION

The mission of TJC (previously known as the Joint Commission on Accreditation of Healthcare Organizations) is to continuously improve the safety and quality of care provided to the public through the provision of health care accreditation and related services that support performance improvement in health care organizations. TJC evaluates and accredits more than 25,000 health care organizations and programs in the United States. An independent, not-for-profit organization, TJC is the country's predominant standards-setting and accrediting body in health care. Since 1951, it has maintained state-of-the-art standards that focus on improving the quality and safety of care provided by health care organizations. TJC's comprehensive accreditation process evaluates an organization's compliance with these standards and other accreditation requirements.

Its evaluation and accreditation services are provided for the following types of organizations:
- General, psychiatric, children's, and rehabilitation hospitals
- Critical access hospitals
- Health care networks, including managed care plans, preferred provider organizations, integrated delivery networks, and managed behavioral health care organizations
- Home care organizations, including those that provide home health services, personal care and support services, home infusion and other pharmacy services, durable medical equipment services, and hospice services
- Nursing homes and other long-term care facilities, including subacute care programs, dementia special care programs, and long-term care pharmacies
- Assisted living facilities that provide or coordinate personal services, 24-hour supervision and assistance (scheduled and unscheduled), activities, and health-related services
- Behavioral health care organizations, including those that provide mental health and addiction services, and services to persons with developmental disabilities of various ages in various organized service settings
- Ambulatory care providers, such as outpatient surgery facilities, rehabilitation centers, infusion centers, group practices, and office-based surgery
- Clinical laboratories, including independent or freestanding laboratories, blood transfusion and donor centers, and public health laboratories
- Palliative care programs
- Comprehensive cardiac care programs
- Health care staffing services
- Office-based surgery centers

Accreditation by TJC is recognized nationwide as a symbol of quality that reflects an organization's commitment to meeting certain performance standards. To earn and maintain TJC's Gold Seal of Approval, an organization must undergo an on-site survey conducted by TJC at least every 3 years. Laboratories must be surveyed every 2 years.

Benefits of Accreditation

There are many benefits to accreditation, but those specific to health care accreditation
- lead to improved patient care;
- demonstrate the organization's commitment to safety and quality;

- offer an educational on-site survey experience;
- support and enhance safety and quality improvement efforts;
- strengthen and support recruitment and retention efforts;
- may substitute for federal certification surveys for Medicare and Medicaid;
- help secure managed care contracts;
- facilitate the organization's business strategies;
- provide a competitive advantage;
- enhance the organization's image to the public, purchasers, and payors;
- fulfill licensure requirements in many states;
- are recognized by insurers and other third parties; and
- strengthen community confidence.

Standards and Performance Measurement

TJC standards address an organization's level of performance in key functional areas, such as patient rights, patient treatment, and infection control. The standards focus not simply on an organization's ability to provide safe, high-quality care, but also on its actual performance. Standards set forth performance expectations for activities that affect the safety and quality of patient care. If an organization does the right things and does them well, there is a strong likelihood that its patients will experience good outcomes. TJC develops its standards in consultation with health care experts, providers, measurement experts, purchasers, and consumers.

There are also disease-specific certifications, such as TJC's certificate of distinction for primary stroke centers. This certification program was developed in collaboration with the American Stroke Association. The disease-specific certifications evaluate programs that provide clinical care directly to participants. Examples include, but are not limited to, services provided in hospitals, long-term care health care settings, home care organizations, health plans, integrated delivery systems, rehabilitation centers, physician groups, and disease management service companies. They also evaluate programs that provide comprehensive clinical support and that interact directly with participants on-site, by telephone, or through online services or other electronic resources. Examples include, but are not limited to, disease management

companies and health care plans with disease management services. There are 143 disease-specific certifications available from TJC.

Disease-specific care certifications focus on
- creating an organized comprehensive approach to disease-specific performance improvement,
- using comparative data to evaluate disease-specific program processes and patient outcomes,
- evaluating the patients' perception of care quality, and
- maintaining data quality and integrity.

The Joint Commission (or any accrediting agency) survey is considered a "rite of passage" for any new nurse manager. Before 2008, the survey would occur every 3 years and was announced. In 2008, TJC started making unannounced visits. This change requires that all health care institutions be in a state of "constant readiness." As a consequence, nurses are required to be aware of accreditation standards, best practice, and current evidence and to deliver nursing care that meets and exceeds standards at all times.

The importance of the nurse's role in ensuring patient safety and delivering quality care is emphasized through key nursing activities such as:
- Influencing improved design of care processes
- Creating a nonpunitive environment to enhance error reporting
- Participating in error reporting and analysis
- Maintaining knowledge of current levels of performance and relationship to goals and benchmarks
- Practicing based on most current evidence

The importance of the nurse's position is further elaborated by his or her leadership role in complying with the necessary standards for medication management, infection control, pain management, and the environment of care. Daily adherence to current standards is of the utmost importance. During a site visit from the accrediting agencies, nurses will be asked to participate in interviews or team meetings with representatives from the accrediting bodies. These site evaluators will also talk with patients to evaluate the patient-centeredness of the care delivered.

One of the most common standards of TJC that affects nursing care deals with the management of pain. The standard includes the following:
- Documentation of assessment of pain
- Documentation of the relief of pain

- Use of therapeutics to manage pain
- Assessment of the use of therapeutics

Documentation of this standard will be reviewed for compliance with the standard. Under this standard, organizations will be required to (TJC, February 2001; (Hospital Consumer Assessment of Healthcare Providers and Systems, 2019):

- Recognize patients' rights to the assessment and management of pain
- Assess the nature and intensity of pain in all patients
- Establish safe medication prescription and ordering procedures
- Ensure staff competency and orient new staff in pain assessment and management
- Monitor patients postprocedurally and reassess patient problems appropriately
- Educate patients on the role of pain management in treatment
- Address patients' needs for symptom management in the discharge planning process
- Collect data to monitor performance

This information is used to inform the HCHAPS assessment used as part of value-based reimbursement.

Accreditation surveyors measure an institution's compliance through the following:

- Interviews with patients, families, and clinical staff
- Review of policies, procedures, protocols, and practices for effective pain management
- Review of clinical records
- Educational materials for patients, family, and staff
- Statement of patient rights or other statements reflecting the organization's commitment to effective pain management

As a nurse, it is important for you to remember that you may be interviewed and your patient charts may be reviewed and evaluated by the team.

DET NORSKE VERITAS

Hospitals across the United States are choosing DNV Healthcare for a new approach to accreditation, one that focuses on quality, innovation, and continual improvement. Although the standards are similar to those of TJC, there is an integration of ISO 9001 standards moving the institution toward continual improvement. There are also disease-specific certifications, such as primary stroke center, comprehensive stroke center, and management of infection risk. There are 364 health care institutions that participate in DNV accreditations.

DNV accreditation requires an annual survey, with a focus on the improvements made since the last survey and the organization's continual compliance with the DNV accreditation process.

THE AMERICAN OSTEOPATHIC ASSOCIATION

The AOA Healthcare Facilities Accreditation is a recognized alternative to accreditation by TJC or DNV. This accrediting agency deals primarily with osteopathic hospitals with approximately 174 accredited institutions across the United States participating. It also certifies institutions as "stroke ready" and as primary stroke centers and comprehensive stroke centers.

OTHER ACCREDITING AGENCIES

There are also the following specialty certifications for specialty care units, and nurses will be asked to participate in these evaluations.

- American College of Surgeons Commission on Cancer: Accrediting agency that evaluates cancer treatment in hospitals and outpatient and freestanding facilities. In addition to participating in a TJC and state licensing survey, nurses may also be asked to participate in a specialty survey such as this depending on their area of practice or expertise.
- Commission on Accreditation of Rehabilitation Facilities (CARF): Accrediting agency that evaluates hospital-based or freestanding medical rehabilitation, employment, and community services.
- Community Health Accreditation Partner (CHAP): Evaluates home care and community health organizations.
- Accreditation Association for Ambulatory Health Care (AAAHC): Evaluates ambulatory surgery centers, medical and dental group practices, diagnostic imaging centers, and student health centers.
- American Association for Accreditation of Ambulatory Surgery Facilities (AAAASF): Accreditation of ambulatory surgery settings.

- Commission on Accreditation of Ambulance Services (CAAS): Accreditation of medical transportation services.
- National Commission for Correctional Health Care (NCCHC): Accreditation of U.S. prisons, jails, and juvenile detention facilities.
- National Committee for Quality Assurance (NCQA): Accreditation and evaluation of quality management systems and managed care organizations.

EDUCATIONAL ACCREDITATION

If your hospital participates in the education of health care personnel, nurses, and physicians, nurses will also be exposed to visits by the accrediting agencies used by the schools working with your hospital. The schools are usually responsible for the compliance with standards in these situations. Your role will be to respond to the role of the students in the provision of care on your unit. Examples of such agencies include the Accreditation Commission of Education in Nursing (ACEN), the Commission on Collegiate Nursing Education (CCNE), the Liaison Committee on Medical Education (LCME; medical schools), the AOA (osteopathic schools), and the Commission on Accreditation in Physical Therapy (CAPTE).

REGULATORY AGENCIES

In addition to these accrediting agencies, there are multiple regulatory and advisory agencies that have an effect on standards of health care. As discussed in Chapter 9, agencies, such as the Occupational Safety and Health Administration (OSHA), regulate the manner in which a hospital implements workplace safety standards. These standards then become part of the accreditor's management of the environment of care standard. The Centers for Disease Control and Prevention (CDC), an agency charged with the promotion of health and quality of life through the prevention and control of disease, injury, and disability has created multiple infection control standards that are now part of standard accreditation and the practice standards of most hospitals. The U.S. Food and Drug Administration (FDA) is a federal agency that regulates drugs, medical devices, and radiation-emitting products. These regulations also form the basis of the medication management standard of the accreditors.

LICENSING BODIES

Health care organizations are licensed to perform services by the state department of health. Most state departments of health undertake the following:

- Regulate a wide range of health care settings for quality of care, such as hospitals, nursing homes, assisted living residences, ambulatory care centers, home health care, medical day care, and others
- Investigate complaints received from patients, other consumers, and other state and federal agencies
- Provide consumer information in the form of report cards and other performance information

Nurses are often called to assist hospital administrators regarding complaints lodged with the state department of health.

GOVERNMENT AGENCIES

There are a number of government agencies that will provide oversight for some of the functions within health care. The following are examples of these agencies.

Occupational Safety and Health Administration

OSHA's mission is to ensure the safety and health of America's workers by setting and enforcing standards; providing training, outreach, and education; establishing partnerships; and encouraging continual improvement in workplace safety and health.

OSHA staff establish protective standards, enforce those standards, and reach out to employers and employees through technical assistance and consultation programs. An example of an OSHA guideline of importance to nursing was the September 12, 2005, guideline for the recommendation to minimize patient lifting to prevent health care musculoskeletal injuries. OSHA recommended that manual lifting of patients be minimized in all cases and eliminated where feasible (Occupational Safety and Health Administration (OSHA) guideline, 2003). This standard has also been implemented in the work safety standards and has resulted in a decline in nursing back injuries.

The U.S. Department of Health and Human Services

The U.S. Department of Health and Human Services (USDHHS) provides 115 programs across 11 divisions covering a wide spectrum of activities including the following (U.S. Department of Health and Human Services (HHS), 2015):

- Health and social science research
- Preventing disease, including immunization services
- Ensuring food and drug safety
- Medicare (health insurance for older adults and disabled Americans) and Medicaid (health insurance for low-income people)
- Health information technology
- Financial assistance and services for low-income families
- Improving maternal and infant health
- Head Start (preschool education and services)
- Faith-based and community initiatives
- Prevention of child abuse and domestic violence
- Substance abuse treatment and prevention
- Services for older Americans, including home-delivered meals
- Comprehensive health services for Native Americans
- Medical preparedness for emergencies, including potential terrorism

CENTERS FOR DISEASE CONTROL AND PREVENTION

The CDC, an agency within the USDHHS, is charged with the promotion of health and quality of life by preventing and controlling disease, injury, and disability. The CDC seeks to accomplish its mission by working with partners throughout the country and the world to

- monitor health,
- detect and investigate health problems,
- conduct research to enhance prevention,
- develop and advocate sound public health policies,
- implement prevention strategies,
- promote healthy behaviors,
- foster safe and healthful environments, and
- provide leadership and training.

Nurses come in contact with the CDC in the development of policies and in the possible investigation of disease outbreaks. One notable example was the 2014/2015 Ebola outbreak in West Africa. Nurses in the United States were called on to treat nurses and health care workers who had contracted the disease. The CDC developed specific policies for the care of such patients.

Other agencies with health care oversight are known by the acronyms shown in Table 5.1.

TABLE 5.1   Glossary of Acronyms

Acronym	Full Name
AAAASF	American Association for Accreditation of Ambulatory Surgery Facilities
AAAHC	Accreditation Association for Ambulatory Health Care
AAHCC	American Accreditation Health Care Commission
ACHC	Accreditation Commission for Health Care
ACR	American College of Radiology
ACS-CoC	American College of Surgeons Commission on Cancer
ALS	American Lithotripsy Society
AOA	The American Osteopathic Association
CAAS	Commission on Accreditation of Ambulance Services
CAP	College of American Pathologists Commission on Inspections and Accreditation
CARF	Commission on Accreditation of Rehabilitation Facilities
CCAC	Continuing Care Accreditation Commission
CDC	Centers for Disease Control and Prevention
CHAP	Community Health Accreditation Program
CMS	Centers for Medicare & Medicaid Services
COA	Council on Accreditation
COLA	Commission on Office Laboratory Accreditation for Blood Banks and Transfusion Services
USDHHS	U.S. Department of Health and Human Services
DNV	Det Norske Veritas
FDA	United States Food and Drug Administration
FEMA	Federal Emergency Management Agency
HAP	Hospital Accreditation Program
NCCHC	National Commission for Correctional Health Care
NIOSH	The National Institute for Occupational Safety and Health
OSHA	Occupational Safety and Health Administration
TJC	The Joint Commission
URAC	Utilization Review Accreditation Commission

(Modified from George Mason University. (2007). *Accreditation agencies in United States.* <http://gunston.gmu.edu/healthscience/547/MajorAccreditationAgencies.asp> [Accessed 18 October 2019.])

OTHER GROUPS RECOGNIZING HEALTH CARE PERFORMANCE AND EXCELLENCE

In this time of heated hospital competition, many institutions are attempting to differentiate their performance from the norm through recognition in other areas of performance. Such levels of recognition demonstrate excellence beyond accreditation, regulatory, and licensing areas.

- The most significant group, in terms of nursing performance, is the American Nurses Credentialing Center (ANCC) that oversees the Magnet Award, which is the highest level of recognition that the ANCC can award to organized nursing services in the national and international arena. Through this award, the ANCC recognizes nursing-sensitive outcomes as a predictor of quality of patient care, and values the retention and recruitment of highly competent nurses (ANCC, 2019).
- The Malcolm Baldrige National Award for Performance Excellence recognizes health care institutions that demonstrate performance excellence across all areas of the organization. The requirements for excellence must exist in seven categories: leadership, strategic planning, customer and market knowledge, information management, workforce focus, process management, and results (Baldrige National Quality Program, 2019).
- *U.S. News and World Report* annually ranks the "best hospitals in the U.S." This ranking rates hospitals across the nation in terms of breadth of expertise and quality. In 2018, almost all community hospitals across the United States were screened and just 165 made it to the rankings (U.S. News and World Reports, 2019). Of the hospitals listed in the "top 10" rankings, all 10 were also Magnet hospitals.
- J. D. Power and Associates recognizes hospitals for service excellence. The firm's Distinguished Hospital Program expands the traditional evaluation of quality by recognizing hospitals that achieve a notable level of satisfaction with services that are provided. This program helps consumers identify hospitals that provide outstanding service excellence and may serve as a competitive advantage when consumers are looking for service excellence (J.D. Power and Associates, 2008, 2019).

TJC accreditation standards, the Malcolm Baldrige National Quality Award, and the ANCC's Magnet Award contain many parallels. All three share the following characteristics:

- Developed using a consensus-building approach
- Built on a core set of values and principles
- Use a framework of important functions (patient care) that cross internal structures (departments) of an organization
- Recognize the "systemness" of organizations
- Focus on continuous improvement and organizational performance
- Are not prescriptive
- Promote the use of organizational self-assessment (TJC, 2013, p. 1)

SUMMARY

It is important to realize that the integration of regulation, accrediting standards, and licensing requirements form a major part of the health care accreditation in the United States. As with all regulatory and accrediting bodies, there are multiple standards for each regulation or level of accreditation. As a nurse, it is your responsibility to understand your role in the accreditation process, your role in the adherence to regulatory standards, and your role in meeting accreditation standards. Although many of the accreditations are "voluntary," hospitals cannot receive reimbursement unless they are accredited. The accreditation process validates the effectiveness and safety of the care rendered. Also, in this era of highly competitive hospitals, the levels and amounts of accreditation may be a way of marketing the excellence of one particular hospital compared with another.

Benefits of DNV GL Healthcare's National Integrated Accreditation for Healthcare Organizations Accreditation

Benefits of DNV GL National Integrated Accreditation for Healthcare Organizations (NIAHO) accreditation can be summarized as follows:

- Integration of the ISO 9001 Quality Management Certification recognizes organizational excellence beyond the minimum requirements of the Centers for Medicare and Medicaid Services' (CMS) Conditions of Participation (CoPs)
- Annual survey drives continuous improvement
- Annual survey encourages a collaborative approach to accreditation
- NIAHO accreditation process fosters a culture that focuses on process improvement and addressing nonconformance rather than criticizing individual performance
- Process improvement encourages the organization to ensure that all employees understand the "why" behind change fostering engagement

Hospitals seek accreditation to demonstrate compliance with the CMS CoPs. Accreditation allows the hospital to receive federal reimbursement for services provided. Most third-party payors require compliance with the CMS CoPs as a prerequisite for reimbursement. Accreditation validates a level of competence appreciated by patients and health care professionals employed by the organization. Nonetheless, compliance with the CMS CoPs is a minimum performance expectation in today's accountable health care environment.

DNV GL-Healthcare (DNV GL) was granted initial deeming authority by CMS in 2008. DNV GL's NIAHO hospital accreditation program is the only accreditation choice that aligns the Quality Management System requirements ISO 9001 with the CMS CoPs.

The ISO 9001 standards, a series of five international criteria, initially published in 1987 and updated in 2105 by the ISO of Geneva, Switzerland, outline the components of a Quality Management System that incorporate W. Edwards Deming's Plan-Do-Study-Act (PDSA) cycle of continuous improvement. ISO 9001 outlines a systematic approach to managing quality (Reid, 2001). NIAHO-accredited hospitals use the ISO 9001 standards to define what requirements an organization needs, in concert with the CoPs, to maintain an efficient quality conformance system. For example, the ISO standards describe the need for an effective quality system, ensure that measuring and testing equipment are calibrated regularly, and maintain an adequate record-keeping system (Schulingkam, 2013).

ISO 9001 requires that all members of the workforce understand the why behind their actions to drive systematic improvement. Nursing, typically the largest segment of the hospital workforce, is central to successful implementation of an integrated Quality Management System. Nurses must participate in the measurement, monitoring, analysis, and improvement of key processes throughout the organization at the bedside, in Quality Management Oversight (an ISO requirement) activities, and as patient (customer) advocates. Nurse leaders are key to encouraging a culture that focuses on process improvement and addressing nonconformance rather than criticizing individual performance.

ISO 9001 registration validates that an organization identifies and complies with its own Quality Management System requirements. Thus, choosing NIAHO accreditation supports a hospital's efforts to create and manage an efficient quality compliance process with a Quality Management System focused on continuous performance improvement and organizational excellence. Adoption of the NIAHO accreditation process can stand alone in a hospital's effort to create and manage an efficient quality conformance system or function as the impetus for developing a holistic system for organizational performance and sustainability, such as that reflected in the Baldrige Criteria for Performance Excellence (Dew, 2014).

The ISO alignment mandates that DNV GL survey (audit) organizations regarding the NIAHO requirements on an annual basis. The annual survey and resulting nonconformance reports enable the actualization of continuous readiness within the organization; there is no "ramp down" because surveyors return to check on progress every year. As a result, there is an urgency for the organization to develop meaningful corrective action plans that drive improvement. Accreditation becomes a management asset for quality and patient safety improvement. Because the focus is on systematic quality management, all employees are empowered to participate in ongoing improvement activities. DNV GL's approach to accreditation has been described as collaborative rather than prescriptive. DNV GL offers training programs related to the NIAHO accreditation process but does not provide consultation services. Customer satisfaction surveys for 2018

Continued

CLINICAL CORNER—Cont'd

indicated that more than 95% of clients responding ranked the NIAHO accreditation program better than their previous accreditation programs (DNV GL Healthcare, 2018).

Compliance with the CMS CoPs is a minimum performance expectation in today's accountable health care environment. Visionary health care leadership knows that a sustainable presence in the hospital management environment relies on an integrated management system that aligns organizational design, strategy, systems, and human capital to create long-term effectiveness in an institutionalized high-performance culture (Dew, 2014).

Five choices are available to hospital organizations seeking to validate compliance with the CMS CoPs. As the health care industry continues to systematically focus on achieving and sustaining quality outcomes, more choices are likely to emerge. For those organizations actively seeking to align accreditation activities with the desire to integrate a sustainable systematic quality management organizational focus with the CoPs, the NIAHO accreditation program is the logical accreditation choice.

References

Dew, L. I., et al. (2014). The changing culture of hospital accreditation and compliance. *ASA Monitor*, *78*(5), 52–54.

Dew, L. I., et al. (2014). The changing culture of hospital accreditation and compliance. *ASA Monitor*, *78*(5), 52–54.

DNV GL Healthcare. (2018). *Customer satisfaction results*. Katy, Texas: DNV GL Healthcare.

Reid, R. D. (2001). *From Deming to ISO 9000:2000. Quality Progress*, *34*/6. <asq.org/quality-progress/2001/06/standards-outlook/from-deming-to-iso-9000-2000.html> Accessed 10.10.19.

Reid, R.D. (2001). From Deming to ISO 9000:2000. Quality Progress, 34/6. Accessed 10.10.19.

Schulingkamp, R. C. (2013). *Study of Malcolm Baldrige Health Care Criteria Effectiveness and Organizational Performance* (pp. 72). New Orleans, Louisiana: Tulane University Theses and Dissertations Archive.

Maureen Washburn, RN, ND, CPHQ, FACHE
Certification and Program Development
DNV GL–Business Assurance,
Healthcare Accreditation Services

EVIDENCE-BASED PRACTICE

A workforce of nurses who develop and use a scholarly nursing practice is critical to the transformation of the health care delivery system. Recommendations from two major reports, the 2015 National Academies of Sciences, Engineering and Medicine's report on the Future of Nursing and the 2016 AACN report Advancing Healthcare Transformation: A New Era for Academic Nursing, included endorsement of increasing the formal education preparation and leadership development for all nurses, the addition of interprofessional learning experiences, a change from the expectation of lifelong learning to a full accountability for continuous learning across the life cycle of a nursing career, and an investment in the preparation of nurse scientists to better integrate research into clinical practice.

For a decade, the program of research concentrated on the examination of what it means to be a nursing scholar in a practice discipline. An analysis of findings about the elements of an optimal clinical practice environment indicated that a workplace that openly values and supports scholarly nursing practice as the expected model of caregiving must provide seamless support and professional development at every level of the organization (Beal, Riley, & Lancaster, 2008). The next step in the program of research was to examine the best organizational practices that support the ongoing development of scholarly nursing practice through full progression of a nurse's career.

A qualitative descriptive design was selected for use with senior nurse leaders of Magnet organizations. Data collection occurred with 32 participants using semistructured audiotaped interviews. Specific questions included the following:

- How does your workplace support the development of clinical nurse scholars?
- What are your expectations for a nurse's engagement in his or her own development?
- What resources do you currently have to support the development of clinical nurse scholars during their career lifetime at your institution?
- What resources do you need to better support the development of clinical nurse scholars during their career lifetime at your institution?
- What do you believe has been the impact of Magnet designation on the development of clinical nurse scholars at your institution?

An analysis of findings revealed an overarching theme: the organization creates and sustains a core culture supportive of scholarly nursing practice. Multidimensional themes also emerged including: expectations for professional development, resources that support scholarly

Continued

EVIDENCE-BASED PRACTICE—Cont'd

nursing practice, and power of the senior nurse leader. The overarching theme is multifaceted and embodies the effect of a Magnet culture and the active relationship between the nursing milieu and the larger institutional environment. Participants indicated that a nursing culture that aligns well with the institutional culture holds out expectations that the nurse workforce will engage in scholarly activity and growth. One senior nurse leader reflected on this perspective "to move an entire organization forward, nurses early on must be fully engaged in the various projects and activities going on in the hospital."

Participants confirmed the key organizational drivers of a clinical practice environment that supports scholarly nursing practice. These included an organizational commitment to professional development that creates a culture and structure of opportunity, a culture of success where employee engagement is high and the core values of the organization drives nurse empowerment, and a vision with dual expectations for equally high standards of patient care and professional development. The power of the senior nurse leader in transforming a culture that supports scholarly clinical nursing practice is strongly supported by the literature. The participants shared that one of their key responsibilities was to serve as role models for others. The nursing literature, Clavelle, Drenkard, Tullai-McGuiness, and Fitzpatrick (2012) reported on the transformational leadership practices of 384 Magnet chief nursing officers (CNOs). Using the five practices of exemplary leadership (Kouzes & Posner, 2012), they found that *enabling others to act* and *modeling the way* were top practices of Magnet CNOs.

It is important to note that the nursing culture in these institutions had a significant and influential effect on the overall organizational culture. Furthermore, it was concluded that the nursing culture that embraced a scholarly practice environment is one that is tightly integrated with organizational culture that supports nursing and its senior leadership.

References

Beal, J., Riley, J., & Lancaster, D. (2008). Essential elements of an optimal clinical practice environment. *Journal of Nursing Administration, 38*(5), 379–387.

Clavelle, J., Drenkard, K., Tullai-McGuiness, S., & Fitzpatrick, J. (2012). Transformational leadership practices of chief nursing officers in Magnet organizations. *Journal of Nursing Administration, 42*(4), 195–201.

Kouzes, J., & Posner, B. (2012). *The leadership challenge: How to make extraordinary things happen in organizations* (5th ed.). San Francisco, CA: Jossey Bass.

▌ NCLEX® EXAMINATION QUESTIONS

1. One of the most common standards of The Joint Commission (TJC) that affects nursing care deals with the management of pain. The standard includes the following:
   A. Documentation of assessment of pain
   B. Documentation of the relief of pain
   C. Use of therapeutics to manage pain and assessment of therapeutics
   D. All of the above

2. Which agency provides national and world leadership to prevent work-related illnesses and injuries and conducts a range of efforts in the areas of research, guidance, information, and service?
   A. Centers for Disease Control and Prevention (CDC)
   B. National Institute for Occupational Safety and Health (NIOSH)
   C. The Joint Commission (TJC)
   D. Centers for Medicare & Medicaid Services (CMS)

3. _____ is a health care accreditation agency that integrates the ISO 9001 quality management system with the Medicare conditions of participation.
   A. DNV
   B. TJC
   C. AOA
   D. NIOSH

4. TJC standards address an organization's level of performance in key functional areas, such as:
   A. Patient rights, patient treatment, high quality care
   B. Patient rights, patient assessment, pain control
   C. Infection control, pain control, falls
   D. Infection control, safe care, injection safety

5. The Occupational Safety and Health Administration (OSHA) has provided guidelines for minimizing patient lifting to prevent health care musculoskeletal injuries. Within these guidelines, OSHA recommends the following:

A. Patients be allowed to decide whether safe lifting equipment should be used when transferring out of bed

B. Manual lifting of residents be minimized and eliminated when feasible

C. Only specific types of lifting equipment be used, such as a ceiling-mounted patient lift with a sling

D. Institutions should be allowed to decide based on patient population whether safe lifting equipment should be used

6. One benefit of accreditation by TJC is that it:

A. Leads to improved patient care and demonstrates the organizations commitment to safety and quality

B. Allows for increased financial gain through Medicare and Medicaid reimbursement and offers employee assistance programs

C. Influences the improved design of care processes, creating a nonpunitive environment to enhance error reporting and allows participation in error reporting and analysis

D. Offers an educational off-site survey experience

7. TJC's evaluation and accreditation services are provided for the following types of organizations:

A. State department of health and town senior housing services

B. Physicians' offices and freestanding laboratory service agencies

C. Home hemodialysis and peritoneal dialysis

D. Critical access hospital, home care organizations, and nursing homes

8. The U.S. Department of Health and Human Services (USDHHS) is the most important federal actor in health care. What are some of the other federal agencies with major health services roles?

A. Department of Veterans Affairs

B. Department of Treasury and Taxation

C. Department of Corrections and Law

D. Department of Agriculture and Taxation

9. An example of what the CDC would evaluate is:

A. A toxic spill on a state highway

B. An outbreak of rubella at a school

C. A flu shot clinic at a pharmaceutical company

D. An outbreak of respiratory syncytial virus in a neonatal intensive care unit

10. NIOSH is:

A. The agency that works closely with TJC and hospital accreditation

B. A local agency that coordinates patient care and patient services

C. A state agency that is part of the CDC in the USDHHS

D. The federal agency responsible for conducting research and making recommendations for the prevention of work-related injury

Answers: 1. D   2. B   3. A   4. C   5. B   6. B   7. D
8. A   9. B   10. D

BIBLIOGRAPHY

American Nurses Credentialing Center [ANCC]. (2019). www.nursecredentialing.org/Magnet/ProgramOverview.aspx. (Accessed 18 October 2019).

Baldrige National Quality Program. (2019-20). *Health care criteria for performance excellence*. Gaithersburg, MD: Baldrige National Quality Program.

Dew, L.I, et al. (2014). The changing culture of hospital accreditation and compliance. ASA Monitor, 78(5), 52–54.

DNV GL Healthcare (2018). Customer satisfaction results. Katy, Texas: DNV GL Healthcare.

Hospital Consumer Assessment of Healthcare Providers and Systems (2019). Hospital consumer assessment of healthcare providers and systems. CMS. https://www.cms.gov/Medicare/Quality-Initiatives-Patient-Assessment-Instruments/HospitalQualityInits/HospitalHCAHPS. (Accessed 24 August 2019).

J.D. Power and Associates. (2008). *Turning information into action*. www.jdpower.com/corporate/healthcare/hospital.aspx. (Accessed 18 October 2019).

Occupational Safety and Health Administration (OSHA) guideline. (2003). www.osha.gov/ergonomics/guidelines/nursinghome/final_nh_guidelines.html. (Accessed 18 October 2019).

Reid, R.D. From Deming to ISO 9000:2000. Qual Prog. June, 2001. http://asq.org/quality-progress/2001/06/standards-outlook/from-deming-to-iso-9000-2000.html. (Accessed 18 October 2019).

Schulingkam, R.C (2013). Study of Malcolm Baldrige Health Care Criteria Effectiveness and Organizational Performance (p. 72). New Orleans, Louisiana: Tulane University Theses and Dissertations Archive.

The Joint Commission. (2019a). Retrieved October 19, 2019 from https://www.jointcommission.org/assets/1/18/2010_DSC_Cert_Guide.pdf. (Accessed 18 October 2019).

The Joint Commission. (2019b). Retrieved. October 19, 2019 from https://www.jointcommission.org/standards_information/tjc_requirements.aspx. (Accessed 18 October 2019).

The Joint Commission. (2001). Pain assessment and management. Oct 2001, 4, 11 Perspectives 8 10. Oct 2001, 4, 11.

The Joint Commission. (2013). *Comparison Between Joint Commission Standards, Malcolm Baldrige National Quality Award Criteria, and Magnet Recognition Program Components.* www.jointcommission.org/assets/1/6/Comparison_Document2013.pdf. (Accessed 18 October 2019).

The Joint Commission. (2014). The Joint Commission mission-related commitments. January 1, 2009

www.jointcommission.org/about_us/about_the_joint_commission_main.aspx. (Accessed 18 October 2019).

U.S. Department of Health and Human Services (HHS). (2015). What we do. www.hhs.gov/about/whatwedo.html/. (Accessed 18 October 2019).

U.S. News and World Reports. (2019). Retrieved October 19, 2019 from hospital consumer assessment of healthcare providers and systems (hcahps) survey. www.asahq.org/resources/publications/newsletter-articles/2014/may-2014/quality-and-regulatory-affairs. (Accessed 18 October 2019).

Case Scenario: An oncology unit's Nursing Team Leader of 25 years is about to retire. The search committee's first candidate reflects on her years of clinical experience, stating that upon graduation she took a job as a medical-surgical nurse on an oncology unit as part of a team providing whole-person care to each patient. The group met each morning and performed interprofessional rounds, bed by bed, including the patient in conversation about the plan of care. After 5 years and a move to another city, she accepted a position doing home care, in which she was the only nurse assigned to several clients that she saw regularly to perform specific tasks such as wound care. Missing the inpatient environment, she returned to bedside nursing in the hospital in a very small community where each registered nurse provided full and total care to four patients.

For their part, the committee explains to the candidate that over the coming year, several of the units need to be physically moved into a new area of the hospital that is currently under construction. They are interested in hearing how the candidate would facilitate the oncology unit's move, once the location is complete.

ITEM TYPE: MATRIX

1. Place an X to indicate which nursing practice model was reflected when this candidate performed duties as a bedside nurse (Chapter 2).

Action	Total Patient Care	Functional Nursing	Primary Nursing
A. Worked as part of a team			
B. Performed interprofessional rounds at the bedside			
C. The only nurse with a total view of the patient			

Action	Total Patient Care	Functional Nursing	Primary Nursing
D. Role was limited to specific wound care			
E. Provided full patient care autonomously			

ITEM TYPE: EXTENDED MULTIPLE RESPONSE

2. Which action will the candidate share with the search committee to competently demonstrate the ability to strategically plan the oncology unit's move? **Check all that apply** (Chapter 3).

A. Gather specific information about features of the oncology unit including amount of equipment and supplies. ☐

B. Assess third-party payers' approval of the new unit. ☐

C. Develop a plan for how each type of supply and capital equipment will be moved. ☐

D. Talk with each type-specific staff member on the unit regarding the person's functional needs in the new environment. ☐

E. Ensure that the move yields revenue for the facility. ☐

F. Allocate staff members from each unit to perform specific moving duties within their ability. ☐

G. Benchmark that future moves will take place on a quarterly basis. ☐

ITEM TYPE: EXTENDED DRAG & DROP

3. The oncology unit will need a nurse leader at the middle management level who can identify how insurers pay based on levels of care that are differentiated into type-specific billable items. What examples of type-specific billable items will the candidate mention to demonstrate knowledge in this area? **Place an X next to each factor that may result in type-specific differentiation for financial reimbursement** (Chapter 4).

Reimbursement Factors	Results in Type-Specific Billing
A. Staffing	
B. Standards of care	
C. Services rendered	
D. Bundled payments	
E. Accreditation requirements	
F. Incremental budgeting	

ANSWERS

1. Total Patient Care: E / Functional Nursing: C, D / Primary Nursing: A, B
2. A, C, D, F
3. A, B, C, E

Structural Empowerment

SECTION OUTLINE

Nurses within Magnet organizations are actively involved in shared governance and decision making to establish standards of care and opportunities for improvement. The flow of information and decision making among professional nurses with Magnet institutions is multidirectional among nurses at the bedside, nursing leadership, interdisciplinary teams, and senior leadership. Nurses throughout such organizations are "empowered" to continually advocate for superior patient and nursing outcomes through structures and processes that are designed to encourage the voice of the nurse in decision making.

This section will deal with shared governance structures, professional decision-making structures, flow of information and policy, and professional development structures that support nursing autonomy.

6

Organizational Decision Making and Shared Governance

OBJECTIVES

- Differentiate among the various structures of shared governance.
- Identify the types of decisions made at the various levels of the organization.
- Recognize the role of senior nursing leadership in the clinical decision making.

- Identify the various functions represented in the shared governance structures.
- Define the four primary principles of shared governance: partnership, equity, accountability, and ownership.
- Discuss the responsibility of the staff nurse in shared governance.

KEY TERMS

accountability willingness to invest in decision making and express ownership in those decisions

board of trustees responsible for overseeing the activities of a nonprofit organization, ranging from huge foundations to small local charities. A board of trustees usually has between 5 and 20 members. Many members of a board of trustees hold other external positions, but the board of trustees may also include senior management of the nonprofit

equity maintains a focus on services, patients, and staff; is the foundation and measure of value; and says that no one role is more important than any other

ownership recognition and acceptance of the importance of everyone's work, and of the fact that an organization's success is bound to how well individual staff members perform their jobs

partnership health care providers and patients along all points in the system; a collaborative relationship among all stakeholders and nursing required for professional empowerment

senior leadership senior management group or team; in many organizations this consists of the head of the organization and his or her direct reports (also called C-suite leaders)

shared governance shared decision making based on the principles of partnership, equity, accountability, and ownership at the point of service. This management process model empowers all members of the health care workforce to have a voice in decision making, thus encouraging diverse and creative input that will help advance the business and health care missions of the organization

Decision making occurs throughout all levels of any organization. Strategic planning initiatives usually occur at the senior leadership level with input from all stakeholders. Organizations are usually designed to facilitate such communication and decision making. Organizational design is a formal, guided process for integrating the people, information, and technology of an organization, and serves as a key structural element that allows corporations to maximize value by matching their corporate design to overall strategy (Burton, DeSanctis, & Obel, 2004).

Health care organizations are a complex mix of stakeholders, such as patients/families, communities, physicians, nurses, other health care disciplines, and so on. The major goal of all organizations is the delivery of effective, efficient care while enhancing the patient experience.

Although many hospitals may differ in framework, particularly between large and small organizations or those with for-profit or nonprofit missions, most follow accepted models of hierarchy well established in the business realm.

A board of directors (board of trustees) is invariably at the top of most organizational structures in health care. This board may be formed by a vote of trustees in a founding organization or by stakeholders in the hospital franchise. Typically it contains more tenured hospital professionals like doctors, nurse members, community members, and researchers, but many are also populated with local lawyers, entrepreneurs, politicians, and even celebrities who might help lend the hospital a competitive edge.

A hospital's president or chief executive officer is usually responsible for answering to the board and carrying out its funding, regulatory oversight, and research initiatives. This chief often serves as an ex officio member as does the chief nurse. Many nonprofit facilities will populate the board in alignment with its particular mission. For instance, the board of a Catholic hospital will often have faith and medical leaders serving, each focused on a different element of the mission.

The senior leadership team is usually the first link in the chain connecting organizational alignment to the strategic goals. The chief nurse is the link for the planning, alignment, and implementation of the nursing strategic plan, as discussed in Chapter 3. The chief nurse is strategically positioned within the organization to effectively influence and communicate with other executive stakeholders, including the board of trustees. Senior level nursing leaders serve at the highest levels of the organization, with the chief nurse typically reporting to the chief executive officer.

Communication between senior leaders and the other stakeholders of the organization is of vital importance to its success. The central roles of the senior leadership include (Porter-O'Grady & Malloch, 2015, p. 146) the following:

- Link between the board and staff
- Inform the board and translate strategy to the system
- Provide good linkage between the various loci of control
- Create a positive context for worker relationships
- Build the infrastructure of decisions and action

The senior leadership is interested in the effectiveness of the system in decision-making actions and outcomes. The actual decisions and actions are usually made at the level of the point of care. A shared governance model forms the basis of decision making throughout most institutions. Shared governance is the vehicle through which nurses at all levels of the organizations make and share decisions.

SHARED GOVERNANCE

Governance is about power, control, authority, and influence. It answers the question in an organization of "Who rules?" Nursing shared governance extends that rule to nurses (Hess, 2004). Nursing shared governance models have always focused on nurses controlling their professional practice. It is a theme that flows consistently through shared governance research and literature. Structure is of vital importance to the success of shared governance. The American Nurses Credentialing Center (ANCC, 2019) states that shared leadership/participative decision making is a model in which nurses are formally organized to make decisions about clinical practice standards, quality improvement, staff and professional development, and research (ANCC, 2019, p. 160). As one of the early Magnet hospitals noted, "unlike participatory management environments, [shared governance structures] ensure that the practicing nurse has not only the right but the power to make practice decisions" (George et al., 2002; Hess, 2004).

This power to make practice decisions characterizes the autonomy of nurses to control nursing practice. Shared governance activities may include participatory scheduling, joint staffing decisions, and/or shared unit responsibilities (e.g., every registered nurse [RN] is trained to be "in charge" of their unit or area, and shares that role with other professional team members, perhaps on a rotating schedule) to achieve the best patient care outcomes. The same control over practice, at the unit level, requires a transition from the historically hierarchical design of health care decision making to a more decentralized decision-making process. To make that happen, employee partnership, equity, accountability, and ownership must occur at the point of service (e.g., on the patient care units).

Partnership

Partnership links health care providers and patients along all points in the system, and is a collaborative relationship among all stakeholders and nursing required for professional empowerment (Batson, 2004). Partnership is essential to building relationships, involves all staff members in decisions and processes, implies that each member has a key role in fulfilling the mission and purpose of the organization, and is critical to the health care system's effectiveness (Porter-O'Grady & Hinshaw, 2005).

Equity

Equity is the best method for integrating staff roles and relationships into structures and processes to achieve positive patient outcomes. Equity maintains a focus on services, patients, and staff; is the foundation and measure of value; and says that no single role is more important than any other. Although equity does not equal equality in terms of scope of practice, knowledge, authority, or responsibility, it does mean that each team member is essential to providing safe and effective care (Porter-O'Grady & Hinshaw, 2005).

Accountability

Accountability is a willingness to invest in decision making and express ownership in those decisions. Accountability is the core of shared governance. It is often used interchangeably with responsibility and allows for evaluation of role performance. It supports partnerships and is secured as staff produce positive outcomes (Porter-O'Grady & Hinshaw, 2005).

Ownership

Ownership is recognition and acceptance of the importance of everyone's work and of the fact that an organization's success is bound to how well individual staff

members perform their jobs. To enable all team members to participate, ownership designates where work is done, and by whom. It requires all staff members to commit to contributing something, to own what they contribute, and to participate in devising purposes for the work (Koloroutis, 2004; Porter-O'Grady & Hinshaw, 2005).

At least 90% of the decisions need to be made at the point of service. Indeed, in matters of practice, quality, and competence, the locus of control in the professional practice environment must shift to practitioners. Only 10% of the unit-level decisions should belong to management (Porter-O'Grady & Hinshaw, 2005). A recent comparative analysis by Kramer and Schmalenburg (2003), who interviewed 279 nurses at 14 Magnet hospitals, found the highest staff nurse ownership of practice issues and outcomes occurred where there were visible, viable, and recognized structures devoted to nursing control over practice.

Box 6.1 shows the differences between the decentralized shared governance interactions and those of the more centralized decision-making structures.

In fact, Florence Nightingale (1992) represented a shared governance model in 1859 with the following quote:

The key provider at point of service, the staff nurse, moves from the bottom to the center of the organization. Nurses are the primary employees who do the work and connect the organization to the recipient of its service. An entirely different sense and set of variables now affect the design of the organization; the only one who matters in a service-based organization is the one who provides its service. All other roles become servant to that role. In this way, the paradigm shifts to a relationship-based, staff-centered, patient-focused professional nursing practice model of care in which nurse managers or supervisors assume the role of servant leaders managing resources and outcomes.

Many structures have evolved over the years to ensure the effectiveness of this nursing decision making.

The most common model is the Councilor Model. In this model, unit-based councils form the decision making and action bodies at the unit or point of service level. Other councils are formed around major initiatives and strategic priorities. Fig. 6.1 shows a schematic of the shared governance councils of The Lahey Clinic with a description of each council's function.

BOX 6.1   Self-Governance Versus Shared Governance

Participatory Management

Goals
Leaders request input from staff to determine goals; use of input is optional.

Use of input
Leader is not required to use staff input.

How decisions are made
Final decision lies with leader, who may accept or reject staff input.

Leadership style
Hierarchical leader

Level at which decisions are made
Centralized decision making

Shared Governance

Goals
Staff are given the responsibility, authority, and accountability to determine what goals to pursue.

Use of input
Staff obtains input from colleagues and others.

How decisions are made
Leaders clearly articulate the guidelines for the decision (e.g., "We have $10,000 to spend on xx.") and staff make autonomous decisions that stay within the guidelines.

Leadership style
Servant leader

Level at which decisions are made
Decentralized decision making
   So just what IS shared governance? Shared governance **IS**
- a model that ensures that decisions are made by the people working at the point of care,
- a leadership development strategy,
- a way to identify future positional leader,
- a tenant of professional practice, or
- a key expression of organizational culture.

Shared governance **IS NOT**
- the replacement or elimination of positional leadership,
- a strategy to support downsizing of leadership,
- self-governance, or
- abdication of leadership responsibilities.

(Adapted from Guanci, G. & Medeiros, M. (2018). *Shared Governance that Works*. Minneapolis, MN: Creative Health Care Management.)

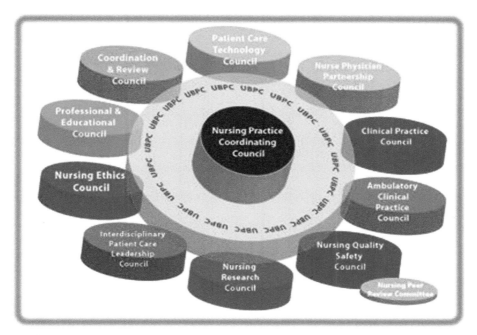

Fig. 6.1 The Lahey Clinic nursing shared governance model. *UBPC,* Unit-Based Practice Council.

Nursing Governance Councils

Unit-Based Councils

The shared governance structure has evolved to include the Unit-Based Practice Councils (UBPCs) that includes the Nurse Practitioner Committee and Certified Registered Nurse Anesthetists. They meet regularly and identify opportunities for improvement in nursing practice in their respective units that enhance excellence in patient care. The UBPC structure is the essential process for staff nurse decision making in operational and professional practice issues at the unit level.

Central Councils

The following is a description of the 11 Shared Governance Central Councils and their functions. These councils include nursing staff from all areas in nursing and focus on processes for relationship building and mutual collaboration, and the development and promotion of policies, guidelines, and standards of practice that enhance professional nursing practice, and promote quality in patient care (Glickman, Baggett, Krubert, Peterson, & Schulman, 2007).

1. *Nursing Practice Coordination Council:* The purpose of this council is to provide a forum for shared decision making in nursing practice and best practice initiatives across the organization by representatives from the UBPCs and central shared governance councils. All councils will share best practices and solve nursing practice problems, creating linkage across ambulatory and tertiary care.

2. *Clinical Practice Council:* The purpose is to review all policies and nursing practice guidelines and ensure that they conform to current standards of care, are evidence based, incorporate research, and reflect interdisciplinary collaboration as appropriate.

3. *Ambulatory Clinical Practice Council:* The purpose of this council is to review all ambulatory policies and practice guidelines and ensure that they conform with current standards of care, are evidence based, incorporate research, and reflect interdisciplinary collaboration as appropriate.

4. *Nurse Physician Partnership Council:* The purpose of this council is to create a partnership between nurses and physicians to jointly manager and problem solve, to provide a forum of shared ideas, discuss issues, and disseminate new information that will enhance patient outcomes.

5. *Nursing Research Council:* This council provides the scientific foundation for nursing practice, dedicated to the support of nursing research and evidence-based practice at Lahey Clinic. The council's objectives include educating staff about the research process and evidence-based practice, providing resources and research consultation that facilitate the conduct of nursing research; disseminating research findings from organization, local, and national meetings; and facilitating the use of research findings to improve patient care.

6. *Nursing Quality Safety Council:* The purpose of this council is to review data related to quality and safety initiatives including National Patient Safety Goals, Core Measures, and Failure Modes and Effects Analysis results. This council makes recommendations that promote and maintain a nursing environment where the best practices in safety and quality are able to be provided for patient care.

7. *Patient Care Technology Council:* This is a multidisciplinary council that facilitates the implementation of departmental and organization objectives related to technology to enhance patient care. This council develops guidelines and protocols for technology initiatives, ensures that clinical applications reflect standards of care and nursing practice, and solicits input and feedback from end users.

8. *Professional and Educational Council:* The purpose of this council is to facilitate a culture where learning is viewed as a life-long process, which is essential to the growth and development of all nurses at Lahey Clinic. This council develops and reviews all staff education materials, the nursing practice guidelines, oversees the process of incorporating evidence-based practice and nursing research into patient care practices, and supports professional development through Pathways to Expertise and Certification.

9. *Coordination and Review Council:* The purpose of this council is to review, revise, and standardize job descriptions; streamline documentation; and approve and revise clinical administrative policies as necessary for accurate nursing functions and process.

10. *Nursing Ethics Council:* As voted by the Nursing Practice Coordinating and Review Council in February 2008, this council is designated as a central council where staff nurses participate in identifying strategies and educational initiatives to improve the staff nurse knowledge on ethical principles and problem-solving processes.

11. *Interdisciplinary Patient Care Leadership Council:* The purpose is collaborative discussion and shared decision making on operational patient care issues and

Continued

Nursing Governance Councils—cont'd

updates on current patient care initiatives, including Joint Commission Readiness and a review of the status of initiatives related to the organization's strategic plan. This council is incorporated in the shared governance structure and allows collaboration with other disciplines who are invited to discuss organizational initiatives and strategies and seek broad nursing input for the most comprehensive approach to address patient care and operational concerns.

(From *Lahey Clinic Shared Governance Structure.* Retrieved January 21, 2014, from <www.lahey.org/For_Healthcare_Professionals/Nursing/Nursing_Governance_Structure/>.)

Another example of shared governance principles and structures follows:

Shared Governance Structure Mount Sinai/Beth Israel Hospital

Unit-Based Practice Councils

Unit-Based Councils represent their own culture while using the organization's shared governance framework and bylaws. They deal with patient care practices and issues rather than business decisions. Issues identified at the point of patient care are initially addressed within the unit by the Unit Practice Council.

These councils are authorized to make decisions that affect their unit. Decisions are made by consensus and supported by evidence-based practice.

Effective communication is an essential strategy at all of the following levels:

Between unit council and staff

Between unit council members

Between unit council and management council

Between unit council and organization-wide councils

Nurse Executive Council

The role of this council is the management of resources as defined in the strategic plan and nursing conceptual framework.

This council examines the delivery of patient care as it is affected by the availability of human, fiscal, material support, and system linkage resources.

Nursing Quality and Patient Safety Council

This council provides a forum to develop and review nursing quality indicators. It defines and measures key processes of patient care, performs product evaluation and reviews for safety, monitors performance through data collection, and designs processes to improve efficiency and effectiveness of patient care.

A representative from this council may be assigned to attend any hospital or system-wide Quality and Patient Safety Committee meetings to represent the discipline of nursing, and to coordinate and enhance communication.

Nursing Professional Standards and Practice Council

This council defines standards, policies, and procedures for clinical practice, and care delivery. It identifies the need for development of new policies or revisions to current policies related to research findings, new technology, and/or practice changes. A representative from this council may be assigned to attend any hospital or system-wide committee meeting that addresses nursing standards and/or practice issues, to represent the discipline of nursing, and to coordinate and enhance communication.

Nursing Staff Development, Education, and Research Council

This council advances the practice of nursing, and fosters the nursing role in patient education through staff development and evidence-based research initiatives.

A representative from this council may be assigned to attend any hospital or system-wide committee meeting that addresses nursing professional development and nursing research, to represent the discipline of nursing, and to coordinate and enhance communication.

Nursing Informatics and Communication Council

In collaboration with members from Information Technology and Nursing Informatics, this council will provide guidance and expertise into the development and implementation of the electronic documentation systems, and nursing information systems. A representative from this council may be assigned to attend any hospital or system-wide committee meeting that addresses nursing informatics and/or affects nursing communication, to represent the discipline of nursing, and to coordinate and enhance communication.

Advanced Practice Nurse Council

This council provides the opportunity for advanced practice nurses (APNs), with support from the chief nursing

Continued

Nursing Governance Councils—cont'd

officer (CNO) and the Director of Ambulatory Services, to identify areas of improvement and to share best practices within this diverse group of clinicians.

A representative from this council may be assigned to attend any unit-based hospital or system-wide committee or council meeting as a clinical resource.

Nursing Strategy and Vision Coordinating Council

This council coordinates the work of all the councils and delivers results from the strategic plan. It also mediates any conflict that arises for the councils. This council stays appraised of regulatory changes, and any new work that

emerges outside the strategic plan, to ensure that the work is assigned to the appropriate councils for action and implementation.

Entity-Based Council

This council serves as a communication link for geographically remote sites within a multicampus system that uses the same shared governance model.

Representatives from the site-specific, entity-based council share information discussed in the house-wide councils to ensure that appropriate changes can be applied properly, or adopted at a particular campus or remote setting.

(From *Shared Governance Structure of Beth Israel.* Retrieved January 21, 2014, from <www.bethisraelnynursing.com/patient-care/shared-governance-structure>.)

Shared governance is much more than a set of committees. The number, titles, and arrangements of committees are not as important as the people who make up the membership. Rather, their expertise and knowledge that guide their actions, what they have power to do, and their commitment to both their profession and the mission of their organization are more likely predictors of success. The meaning of success in terms of shared governance and patient care is the control of practice leading to better patient outcomes (Hess, 2004).

Although definitions, models, structures, and principles of shared governance (or collaborative governance, participatory governance, shared or participatory leadership, staff empowerment, or clinical governance) vary, the outcomes are consistent. The evidence suggests that shared governance processes result in the following:

- Increased nurse satisfaction with shared decision making, related to increased responsibility that is combined with appropriate authority and accountability
- Increased professional autonomy, as higher staff and nurse manager retention
- Greater patient and staff satisfaction

- Improved patient care outcomes
- Better financial states because of cost savings/cost reductions

(Anthony, 2004; Hess, 2004; Wilson, Squires, Widger, Cranely & Tourangeau, 2008)

The first step in participation in shared governance is membership in a unit-based council. This council allows the new nurse to become aware of the major operational and practice issues affecting the unit. It will also allow for the opportunity to contribute to the decisions made affecting the unit. Membership is usually composed of all members of the nursing staff of a particular unit. It is important for nurses to take membership in such councils seriously, and to view them as an opportunity to be empowered to make decisions about their practice and the practice of the entire institution. They must assume accountability, a willingness to invest in decision making, and express ownership in those decisions. Accountability is the core of shared governance and empowerment as a nurse. As the nurse grows professionally, advancement through the decision-making structure is expected.

👤 CLINICAL CORNER

Shared decision making is an essential part of nursing professional practice as it creates a culture of empowerment for everyone, from clinical staff to executive nursing leadership. Shared governance is a vehicle for professional nurse engagement, fostering new ideas, nursing research, and evidence-based practices. Professional nurse engagement is rewarded through clinical ladder

programs, recognition through nursing excellence awards, publications, and conference presentations. The structure we have implemented includes a specific council for each level: directors, APNs, educators, nurse managers, and clinical RNs to assess practice, implement necessary changes, and evaluate through data analyses and professional and patient outcomes. Each council meets monthly

Continued

then moves the policies, projects, and research studies they are working on through all the councils for consideration and input. Nursing Leadership is our highest decision-making council, chaired by the CNO, where all the council chairs, directors, and managers meet to vote.

We value the role of the clinical RN as the health care provider who is positioned closest to the patient and family to make patient care delivery decisions. The Nurse Practice Council is at the heart of shared governance. Each unit sends a RN representative to the monthly meeting as a prescheduled 8-hour business day. The morning session is divided into four core committees: Informatics, Professional Practice, Recruitment & Retention, and Evidence-Based Practice & Research, with each council member participating in two of the four meetings. In the afternoon the entire council comes together for the Performance Improvement Committee and the CNO's State-of-Affairs presentation. Each chair of the four committees then presents the work they are doing to the entire council, eliciting feedback and discussion to make decisions on moving projects forward.

Nurse autonomy and empowerment lead to increased nurse job satisfaction and improved patient outcomes. Shared governance councils also develop skills such as team building, networking, public speaking, and writing proficiency.

A team-building activity used by our Nurse Practice Council was to have each unit create a mosaic using any bits of material found on the unit, such as medication cups, pieces of disposable gloves, needle caps, and so on. The unit staff needed to think of a message or vision that they feel displays the essence of caring. Each person on the unit contributed material and time to put the mosaic together in their break room. Once completed, all the units displayed their creations in an art exhibit in our main lobby before hanging the mosaics in their units.

With each service line unit so busy in their day-to-day work, they are often amazed to hear about the practices, projects, and successes on the other units. The intensive care unit was inspired to replicate the Geriatric Unit's bereavement process of placing a wreath on the door of a patient who died to alert the unit that quiet reflection was needed at this time. This networking encourages nurses to get to know each other as professionals and coworkers, offering an opportunity to develop sharing and caring relationships with each other.

Great work needs to be shared. Publications and presentations are excellent venues to use, but public speaking and writing abstracts, or designing creative posters, are often a deterrent for many nurses. Our council members have mentored and coached each other to accomplish these skills. By starting small, such as presenting to each other, then to the organization, then at state and national levels, our members have experienced professional growth and self-confidence. The previously mentioned mosaics were displayed at the National Magnet Conference's Art Exhibit. Our bereavement programs have been published in nursing journals and original research studies conducted by the staff through the shared governance model.

To truly be successful it takes the commitment of each participating member. Choosing membership is a crucial element and should be done at the unit level by the team. The chosen member should be seen as a representative of that unit, bringing needs and ideas from the unit for practice improvements, and bringing back to the unit the information discussed at council. It is a very rewarding opportunity for nurses to be involved in decision making. An old adage says that if you are not part of the solution you must be part of the problem. Complaining about barriers and problems will not improve the situation. It will take a professional and thoughtful approach within shared governance to identify the opportunities and problem solve using evidence-based practices.

Mary Ann Hozak, MSN, RN, NEA-BC
Magnet Program Director, Director of Nursing Quality
and Innovation
St. Joseph's Regional Medical Center, Paterson, NJ

EVIDENCE-BASED PRACTICE

(From Kutney-Lee, A., Germack, H., Hatfield, L., Kelly, S., Maquire, P., Dierkes, A., Del Guidice, M., & Aiken, L. H. (2016). *The Journal of Nursing Administration, 46*(11), 605–612.)

Organizations that foster employee engagement outperform their counterparts in terms of job satisfaction and retention, profitability, and performance (Harter, Schmidt, & Hayes, 2002). Facing competitive environments, hospitals have a vested interest in promoting a culture of engagement among nurses, who are the largest part of the hospital workforce. One strategy to increase nurse engagement is shared governance, in which staff nurses are active and empowered participants in decision making.

Continued

EVIDENCE-BASED PRACTICE—cont'd

There is little empirical evidence on the effects of shared governance on patient outcomes. The purpose of this cross-sectional study was to examine differences in nurses' levels of engagement in shared governance across 425 hospitals in 4 U.S. states and to study its associations with nurse job outcomes related to retention, nurse-related quality of care and patient safety, and the patient experiences as measured by the Healthcare Common Procedure Coding System (HCPCS) survey.

Forty-two percent of hospitals (n=177) were classified as having the "most engaged" nurses, 36% (n=155) had "moderately engaged" nurses, 19% (n=80) had "somewhat engaged" nurses, and 3% (n=13) were classified as "least engaged." Across these categories, hospitals differed significantly in terms of staffing, teaching, high-technology, nonprofit, and Magnet status. With regard to staffing, "most engaged" hospitals had significantly lower patient-to-nurse ratios than the "least engaged" hospitals (4.8 vs. 6.3, respectively; $P < .001$).

Across HCPCS outcomes, the percentage of patients who provided a favorable response to each item was significantly higher in the "most engaged" compared with "least engaged" hospital. The percentage of patients reporting that they would definitely recommend the hospital was over 14 percentage points higher in the "most engaged" compared with the "least engaged." With regard to quality of care, greater proportions of "least engaged" nurses than the "most engaged" nurses described quality of care on their unit as fair or poor (33% vs. 8%, respectively; $P < .001$) and graded patient safety as poor or failing (15% vs. 2%, respectively; $P < .001$).

Among the nurse job outcomes, the odds of a nurse reporting high burnout were 36% lower for nurses working in the "most engaged" compared with the "moderately engaged" hospitals. By extension, these estimates indicate that the odds of job dissatisfaction and intention to leave are 80% and 71% lower, respectively, in hospitals with the "most engaged" nurses compared with the "least engaged."

Hospitals that provide nurses with greater opportunities to be engaged in shared governance are more likely to provide better patient experiences, superior quality of care, and have more favorable nurse job outcomes compared with hospitals in which nurses are not engaged in organizational decision making. The findings suggest that increasing nurse engagement is a system-level approach to improving nurse, financial, and patient outcomes.

Objective: The objectives of this study were to examine differences in nurse engagement in shared governance across hospitals and to determine the relationship between nurse engagement and patient and nurse outcomes.

Background: There is little empirical evidence examining the relationship between shared governance and patient outcomes.

Methods: A secondary analysis of linked cross-sectional data was conducted using nurse, hospital, and HCPCS survey data.

Results: Engagement varied widely across hospitals. In hospitals with greater levels of engagement, nurses were significantly less likely to report unfavorable job outcomes and poor ratings of quality and safety. Higher levels of nurse engagement were associated with higher HCPCS scores.

Conclusions: A professional practice environment that incorporates shared governance may serve as a valuable intervention for organizations to promote optimal patient and nurse outcomes. Organizations that foster employee engagement outperform their counterparts in terms of job satisfaction and retention, profitability, and performance.

References

Harter, J., Schmidt, F., & Hayes, T. (2002). Business unit level relationship between employee satisfaction, employee engagement, and business outcomes: a meta-analysis. *Journal of Applied Psychology, 87*(2), 268.

NCLEX® EXAMINATION QUESTIONS

1. _____ is shared decision making based on the principles of partnership, equity, accountability, and ownership at the point of service. This management process model empowers all members of the health care workforce to have a voice in decision making, thus encouraging diverse and creative input that will help advance the business and health care missions of the organization.
   A. Partnership
   B. Equity
   C. Accountability
   D. Shared governance

2. Which council's purpose is to provide a forum for shared decision making in nursing practice and best practice initiatives across the organization by representatives from the UBPCs and central shared governance councils?
   A. Clinical Practice Council
   B. Nursing Practice Coordination Council
   C. Ambulatory Clinical Practice Council
   D. Nurse Physician Partnership Council

3. Which council's purpose is to facilitate a culture in which learning is viewed as a lifelong process that is essential to the growth and development of all nurses at Lahey Clinic?
   A. Coordination and Review Council
   B. Professional and Educational Council
   C. Nursing Ethics Council
   D. Interdisciplinary Patient Care Leadership Council

4. Which council examines the delivery of patient care as it is affected by the availability of human, fiscal, material support, and system linkage resources?
   A. Unit-Based Practice Councils
   B. Interdisciplinary Patient Care Leadership Council
   C. Nurse Executive Council
   D. Coordination and Review Council

5. Shared governance processes result in all of the following, except:
   A. Increased nurse satisfaction with shared decision making
   B. Increased responsibility that is combined with appropriate authority and accountability
   C. Greater patient and staff satisfaction
   D. Lower retention

6. According to Burton (2004) _____ is a formal, guided process for integrating the people, information, and technology of an organization, and serves as a key structural element that allows corporations to maximize value by matching their corporate design to overall strategy.
   A. Organizational design
   B. Decision making
   C. Shared governance
   D. Accountability

7. Self-governance _____.
   A. Occurs at the point of care
   B. Is position based
   C. Has high staff input
   D. Integrates equity and accountability

8. Which council provides the opportunity for APNs, with support from the CNO and the Director of Ambulatory Services, to identify areas of improvement and to share best practices within this diverse group of clinicians?
   A. Advanced Practice Nurse Council
   B. Nurse Executive Council
   C. Unit-Based Council
   D. Nursing Informatics and Communication Council

9. Which council is concerned with the management of resources as defined in the strategic plan and nursing conceptual framework?
   A. Nurse Executive Council
   B. Unit-Based Council
   C. Nursing Quality and Patient Safety Council
   D. Advanced Practice Nurse Council

10. Who is responsible for answering to the board of trustees in an institution?
    A. Chief executive officer
    B. Chief nursing officer
    C. Chief financial officer
    D. Safety officer

Answers: 1. D 2. B 3. B 4. C 5. D 6. A 7. B 8. A. 9. A 10. A

REFERENCES

ANCC (2019). *Magnet application manual.* Silver Spring, MD: ANCC.

BIBLIOGRAPHY

Anthony, M. (2004). Shared governance models: the theory, practice, and evidence. *[Manuscript 4] The Online Journal of Issues in Nursing, 9*(1). https://www.nursingworld.org/MainMenuCategories/ANAMarketplace/ANAPeriodicals/OJIN/TableofContents/Volume92004/No1Jan04/Shared-GovernanceModels. (Accessed 18 January 2010).

Batson, V. (2004). Shared governance in an integrated health care system. *AORN Online, 80*(3), 493–514.

www.aornjournal.org/article/S0001-2092(06)60540-1/abstract. (Accessed 20 September 2019).

Burton, R. M., DeSanctis, G., & Obel, B. (2004). *Organizational design: A step-by-step approach*. Cambridge, UK: Cambridge University Press.

George, V., Burke, L. J., Rodgers, B., Duthie, N., Hoffmann, M., Koceja, V., et al. (2002). Developing Staff Nurse Shared Leadership Behavior in Professional Practice. *Nursing Administration Quarterly*, *26*(3), 44–59.

Glickman, S., Baggett, K., Krubert, C., Peterson, E., & Schulman, K. (2007). Promoting quality: The health care organization from a management perspective. *International Journal of Quality Health Care*, *19*(6), 341–348.

Guanci, G., & Medeiros, M. (2018). *Shared governance that works*. Minneapolis, MN: Creative Health Care Management.

Hess, R. (2004). From bedside to boardroom–nursing shared governance. *Online Journal of Issues in Nursing*, *9*(1). www.nursingworld.org/MainMenuCategories/ANA-Marketplace/ANAPeriodicals/OJIN/TableofContents/Volume92004/No1Jan04/FromBedsidetoBoardroom.aspx. (Accessed 21 January 2019).

Koloroutis, M. (Ed.), *Relationship based care: A model for transforming practice*. Minneapolis, MN: Creative Health Care Management.

Kramer, M., & Schmalenburg, C. E. (2003). Magnet hospital nurses describe control over nursing practice. *Western Journal of Nursing Research*, *25*(4), 424–452.

Nightingale, F. (1992). *Notes on nursing: What it is, and what it is not*. Philadelphia: J.B. Lippincott. (Commemorative Edition).

Porter-O'Grady, T., & Hinshaw, A. S. (2005). Introduction: The concept behind shared governance. In D. Swihart (Ed.), *Shared governance: A practical approach to transform professional nursing practice* (pp. 1–12). Danvers, MA: HCPro.

Porter-O'Grady, T., & Malloch, K. (2015). *Quantum leadership*. Burlington, MA: Jones & Bartlett Learning.

Wilson, B., Squires, M., Widger, K., Cranely, L., & Tourangeau, A. (2008). Job satisfaction among a multigenerational nursing workforce. *Journal of Nursing Management*, *16*(6), 716–723.

Professional Decision Making and Advocacy

OBJECTIVES

- Discuss the professional nurse's role as a health care and patient advocate.
- Define the four spheres of political influence in which nurses can effect change.
- Identify various actions that a nurse can take to advocate for health.

- Discuss current issues of importance for nurses in practice.
- Define the various types of policy.
- Describe the processes that exist within a health care organization for policy development.

KEY TERMS

advocacy a political process by an individual or group that aims to influence public policy decisions and resource allocation decisions within political, economic, and social systems and institutions

policy encompasses the choices that a society, segment of a society, or organization makes regarding its priorities and the ways that it allocates resources to attain those goals

In Chapter 6, the role of the nurse in organizational decision making and accountability was discussed. The Institute of Medicine (IOM) report *The Future of Nursing*: Leading Change Advancing Health (IOM, 2011) called for the preparation of nurses to advance health across the nation. Public, private, and governmental health care decision makers at every level should include representation from nursing on boards, on executive management teams, and in other key leadership positions. (ANCC, 2019, p. 6). ANCC in the Magnet criteria calls for nursing's commitment to community involvement and advocacy (ANCC, 2019). Contrary to what many nurses believe, patient and health care is a highly political activity. Nurses are engaged in a continuous competition for scarce resources on behalf of patients. Policy and politics are the ways that nurses can influence the quality, safety, and accessibility of health care in the United States. As the largest single group of health professionals (3.1 million), registered nurses have the ability to be an incredible force by sheer numbers; in addition, policymakers also rely on nurses' expertise.

Policy has been simply defined as "authoritative decision making" (Stimpson & Hanley, 1991, p. 12). There are many types of policy.

- Public policy: Policy formed by governmental bodies such as legislation passed by a state legislature, for example, the regulations about mandatory staffing ratios in California.
- Social policy: Pertains to the policy decisions that promote the welfare of the public, for example, local ordinances that require children to wear helmets while bicycling.
- Health policy: This includes actions to promote the health of individual citizens, such as health promotion reimbursements to vaccinate all children.

- Institutional policy: These policies govern workplaces. They include the administrative and nursing polices within a health care organization. Such policies govern how you would practice within that institution.
- Organizational policies: This includes the positions taken by professional organizations, such as the American Nurses Association (ANA) and specialty organizations. An example would be the position paper calling for the Bachelor of Science in Nursing as the entry level for nursing licensure.

There are four major arenas of political action in nursing: the workplace, the government, professional organizations, and the community. The four spheres are shown in Fig. 7.1. The reasons that nurses act to

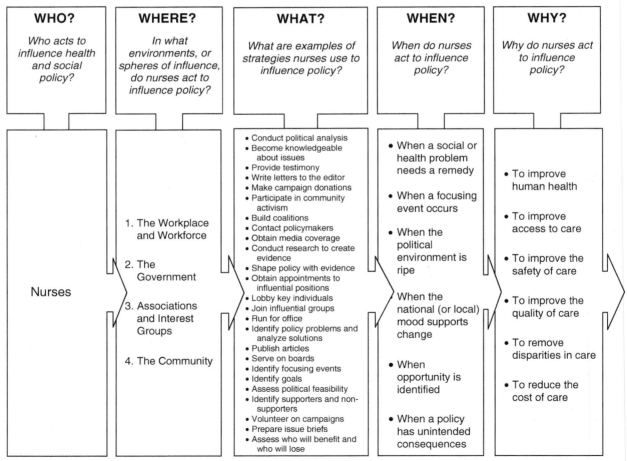

Fig. 7.1 The who, what, where, when, and why of nursing's policy influence. (From Mason, D., Leavitt, J., & Chafee, M. (2016). *Policy and politics in nursing and health care.* St Louis: Elsevier.

influence policy usually relate to attempting to improve health, to improve access to health care, to improve the safety of care, to improve the quality of care, to remove disparities in care, and to reduce the cost of care.

Your workplace will be a major arena for your work with policy development. The Magnet model requires that nurses are involved in decision-making groups throughout the organization and in the community. In Chapter 6 shared governance structures were discussed. One of the common shared governance committees present in most hospitals is the Nursing Practice and Standards Committee. The charge of such a committee usually focuses on the definition of standards, policies, and procedures for clinical practice and care delivery across the institution. The majority of these policies deal with patient care, but there is also policy development on issues of workplace safety, professional development of nurses, staffing, and other issues that affect the delivery of care. Recent examples of issues that have resulted in policy development at the workplace level include:

- High reliability organizations
- Safe patient handling
- Creation of a just culture (discussed in Chapter 9)
- Healthy work environment for nurses
- Prevention of workplace bullying (discussed in Chapter 9)
- Staffing ratios
- Delegation of nonnursing tasks (discussed in Chapter 13)
- Roles of advanced practice registered nurses

Policy evaluation usually occurs on 3-year cycles within organizations. One-third of existing policies are reviewed each year. New policies are developed as needed and come from new practice issues, new professional guidelines, performance outcomes, research, and other areas. They are rated according to current evidence. They can be brought forward by anyone in the institution. Each policy usually has an identified "owner" who is the practice expert; the critical care clinical nurse specialist may be the owner of the unit-specific critical care nursing policies. Table 7.1 demonstrates an algorithm for policy review and decision making.

As a member of the Professional Practice Committee at your institution, a nurse will be asked to review a policy and to make suggestions for changes. This review will include the current practice and a literature review to determine current best evidence. The nurse is responsible for ensuring that the policies that guide your practice are current and based on sound evidence. Nurses will need to keep current through membership in professional organizations, continued professional development, and journal reading.

Another arena for political action will be through a professional organization. As a nurse, it is very important to continue professional development and to belong to a professional organization. Professional organizations play a major role in the continual shaping of nursing practice across the world. They also play a role in the continued upgrading of nursing and health care. Magnet organizations are expected to document that their nurses belong to professional organizations and improve nursing practice because of such participation.

The ANA represents the interests of nurses regarding many issues. Each year they track over 1000 nursing and health care–related bills across all states, examining priority issues and trends. They also release position statements on many issues of importance to nursing and health care in the United States. Issues of importance in 2019 include nurse staffing, workplace safety, health work environment, violence, incivility and bullying, health system reform, care coordination, barriers to practice, nurse fatigue, moral resilience, barriers to practice, and many other issues of importance (ANA, 2019). For a listing of the position statements of the ANA (2019) go to www.nursingworld.org/positionstatements.

The ANA also supports worthy candidates for federal office who have demonstrated their belief in the legislative and regulatory agenda of the ANA through their Political Action Committee (ANA-PAC).

Although nurses represent one of the largest workforces in the nation at 3.1 million, it is estimated that only 5% belong to the ANA. Many nurses belong to a specialty nursing organization, but the estimate is that they only represent 30% of the total nursing workforce. If you, as a nurse, are to have an effect on policy development that affects your workplace and the health of your community, it is imperative you belong to a professional organization.

The third arena of political activity for nurses is the government. Nurses are increasingly entering government at local, state, and federal levels. There are presently six nurses serving in the U.S. Congress. Government plays an enormously important role in nursing and health care. Nursing practice acts are determined through state legislation. Reimbursements for health care are determined at the federal level.

TABLE 7.1   Policy and Procedure Algorithm Steps

Review Steps	Suggested Actions
1. Select the policy for revision	Routine review or changes in practice; this process is also applicable for new policies
2. Search for evidence	Suggested approaches and sites Research-based evidence: • CINAHL and Medline databases • Cochrane Library • American College of Physicians • National Guideline Clearinghouse (www.guideline.gov) • Turning Research Into Practice (www.tripdatabase.com) • Professional Association Guidelines/Standards of Care • University Health Consortium for other academic hospital policies/procedures • Local standards or policies • Expert opinion/clinical expertise • Clinical articles • Web search • Clinical experts
3. Systematic evaluation of the evidence	Critically appraise research evidence • Assign level of evidence: a method of evaluating the strength of the evidence using the Stetler model • Consider a mechanism for organization of evidence, e.g., an evidence table may be constructed
4. Compare evidence to current policy and make a decision	Decision point • Make no changes • Make language more precise or update references • Revise policy to incorporate new evidence • Develop new policy or procedure based on evidence if indicated • Retire or delete policy if no longer effective for quality patient care
5. Policy review by stakeholders/experts	Send revised policy to stakeholders who have reviewed prior versions of the policy or determine who is appropriate to review a new policy
6. Make revisions based on stakeholder/experts' comments	Revise suggested policy
7. Obtain approval signatures	E-mail signature is accepted at UCH
8. Submit policy to Patient Care Policy and Procedure Subcommittee	Final recommendations and approval by the committee
9. Staff education as needed	Present to Nurse Educator Council if needed
10. Web submission	Hospital-wide policies are located on the hospital's intranet

CINAHL, Cumulative Index to Nursing and Allied Health Literature; UCH, University of Colorado Hospital.
(From Oman, K., Duran, C., & Fink, R. (2008). Evidence-based policy and procedures. *Journal of Nursing Administration*, 38(1), 49.)

Issues of importance during the 2019 federal legislative calendar included the following:
• Reducing gun violence
• Nursing shortage
• Appropriate staffing
• Workplace health and safety
• Environmental issues
• Opioid crisis

One final point is that the nurse can have a tremendous impact on the health of the community. Nursing contributions to improve community health have a historical perspective, and they are currently recognized and expected in Magnet organizations. Historically, nurses such as Florence Nightingale improved sanitation services in England, thereby reducing cholera in London. Lillian Wald greatly improved the health care access to services in early 1900s New York through the development of the Henry Street Settlement. Although you may not see yourself in the same league as these iconic nurses, you have the responsibility to work to improve the health of the community. You may be called on to support the agenda of communities that are trying to develop a better place for their citizens to live. Nurses are often asked to serve on local boards of health and boards of education. You may also be asked to serve on local advisory boards/committees such as community planning boards and senior services advisory boards.

The IOM report (IOM, 2011) challenges nurses and society to ensure that nurses are represented in leadership positions in health care, including governing boards. The sparse data that exist indicate that physicians make up more than 20% of the governing board members of hospitals, and less than 5% are nurses. In this era of greater accountability for clinical performance, the role of the nurse in improving processes and accountability of care is paramount. A recent study in New York City documented a slight increase in nurse membership on organizational decision making, with 93% of hospitals reporting physicians on their governing boards compared with 26% with nurses, 7% with dentists, and 4% with social workers or psychologists. The overrepresentation of physicians declined with the other health care organizations. Only 38% of home care agencies had physicians on their governing boards, 29% had nurses, and 24% had social workers. What better representative of the community that an organization serves than the professionally educated nurse? Nurses possess a level of insight into health care issues and policymaking unlike any other health care professional.

What can you as a nurse do to influence policy?

1. *Keep abreast of developments:* Know what is happening both in your community and in the country generally. Keep up-to-date with public issues by attending public meetings and reading newspapers and journals.
2. *Write and publish:* Well-placed articles can help influence opinion. Keep an eye on newsworthy issues that would benefit from a nursing perspective.
3. *Join professional organizations that match your interests and share your positions:* Your contribution might be more effective if channeled through a larger group with an established reputation and credibility.
4. *Know who key players are:* Be aware of key players such as politicians and officials in local, regional, and national government.
5. *Know key nursing positions and networks:* Know key positions and networks that you (or your organization) might work with to have input in policy.
6. *Identify nurses in influential positions outside nursing:* They may be in policy or senior management positions in departments of health or other health organizations. These groups can be useful resources to help you achieve your health policy goals.
7. *Communicate your position through:*
   - Ongoing representation on policymaking
   - Committees or boards
   - Lobbying
   - Making submissions
   - Meeting with people in positions of influence

CLINICAL CORNER

The Importance of a Nurse on a Board of Trustees

I have been privileged enough to serve as a member of various boards of trustees, overseeing the operations of health care facilities. As a nurse, I feel that I bring a unique perspective to the governing board of a health care organization. It seems natural that a nurse should be a member of such governing boards, yet it is often not the case.

The IOM report (IOM 2011) on the future of nursing discusses the importance of nursing leadership on governing boards. The report states that "private, public, and governmental health care decision makers at every level should include representation from nursing on boards, on executive management teams, and on other key leadership positions" (IOM, 2011). Nurses do indeed serve in leadership positions, serving on executive management teams as chief nursing officers, yet only 6% of board positions were held by nurses; 20% are physicians. (AHA, 2018).

It is interesting that nurses are seldom viewed as leaders in the development of health care systems and delivery (Khoury; Blizzard; Moore; Hassmiller, 2011), but nurses are consistently rated as the most ethical profession (Gallup, 2018). Survey reports say that nurses should have more input and impact in policy development

Continued

CLINICAL CORNER—cont'd

The Importance of a Nurse on a Board of Trustees

(Khoury et al., 2011). Respondents from this same survey said that nurses should have more influence in reducing medical errors, increasing the quality of care, and influencing health care efficiency and reducing costs (Hassmiller & Combes, 2012). Who better than a nurse, then, for a leadership position on a board of trustees?

As a board member, I feel that I bring a unique perspective to the operations of the health care facility. The majority of employees in the system are nurses, so I bring a unique understanding of their perspective to the decision making of the board. I also have a knowledge of the current evidence and best practice in nursing and health care that form important decision points in the strategic plan of the organization.

A nurse also brings a unique broad-based skill and knowledge set to the table. We have experienced the various patient care processes that either facilitate or impede patient care. Such knowledge can assist the health care institution in the development of patient care processes that are efficient and patient friendly. A nurse also understands the complicated world of health care reimbursement and its relationship to patient satisfaction and high-quality care. As a nurse, I have an awareness of the job design of care delivery, the actual work systems, the community orientation, and the accountability of patient care outcomes and a documented ability to lead.

I am often asked, "What is the nursing perspective?" And, it is interesting that this perspective at times is different from that of the larger group. One such difference came with the advent of the electronic medical record (EMR) within a health care facility. The initial timeline of implementation for the EMR project dealt with the physician order being set as the first outcome. These order sets were in the very early stages of implementation and would have prolonged the EMR implementation for 18 months. A stronger knowledge of physician ordering patterns was required to fully implement the order sets. The nursing documentation and medication administration system implementation would be able to be implemented within 1 year, and it would be able to provide a wealth of information regarding physician ordering. Along with the nursing executive team, I was able to alter the EMR implementation timeline to allow the organization to learn from the rich data made available from the new EMR. As the physician order sets were evaluated, a wealth of information evaluated against current evidence allowed the organization to integrate best practice more fully with order sets.

Nurse leaders understand the requirements of day-to-day patient care and they understand the constraints on health care quality and outcomes. They have the ability and skills necessary to drive improvement, deal with conflict management, and facilitate decision making, and the compassion and capacity to positively affect patient care across all communities. Who better to be a board member then a NURSE!

Kathleen M. Burke, PhD, RN

EVIDENCE-BASED PRACTICE

(From Graystone, R. (2019). Nurses on boards a national perspective. *Journal of Nursing Administration, 49*(2), 111–112.)

Nurses are a natural fit for board service. They represent the largest segment of the health care workforce and have ranked as the most trusted profession for 18 years. Nurses are leaders in the community and the health care field, yet they are noticeably absent from board positions. The American Nurses Association (ANA) and the American Nurses Foundation are working to change this. The goal is to put 10,000 nurses on boards by 2020. To move this forward, the Foundation is conducting a pilot program in partnership with Magnet-recognized organizations. The purpose of this program is two-fold: to help nursing officers to quantify how many of their nurses are on boards and to identify opportunities to integrate board service into existing programs. Nurses can serve on the boards of professional organizations. The Magnet criteria specifically ask "for improved patient outcomes related to … clinical nurse's participation in professional organizations" (ANCC, 2019).

Senior nursing leaders have stated why they want their nurses to be involved: "We want to develop our nurses as leaders in the community." Nurses bring value to health care facilities and communities and other areas. They bring their value to the local school board, YMCA, or the local environmental center where they can bring their advocacy to health-enhancing changes such as recycling and emissions evaluation.

How can you get involved? To learn about the Foundation's work to increase the representation of nurses on all types of boards of directors, visit www.https://www.nursingworld.org/foundation/programs/nurses-on-boards/. To register in the national databases and have your board service counted toward the goal of 10,000 nurses by 2020, sign up at https://www.nursesonboardscoalition.org/about/.

References

American Nurses Credentialing Center [ANCC]. (2019). Magnet application manual. Silver Spring, MD: ANCC.

NCLEX® EXAMINATION QUESTIONS

1. Which of the following policies includes actions to promote the health of individual citizens, such as health promotion reimbursements to vaccinate all children?
   A. Public
   B. Institutional
   C. Social
   D. Health

2. Which of the following committees focuses on the definition of standards, policies, and procedures for clinical practice and care delivery across the institution?
   A. Practice and standards
   B. Safety
   C. Infection control
   D. Shared governance

3. What are the major arenas of political action in nursing?
   A. Workplace and government
   B. Professional organizations
   C. Community
   D. All are correct

4. The reasons that nurses act to influence policy are usually related to:
   A. Improve health
   B. Improve access to health care
   C. Improve the quality of care
   D. All are correct

5. Professional organizations play a major role in the continual shaping of nursing practice across the world. One example is:
   A. American Nurses Association
   B. Nurse Practitioner Association
   C. National Institute of Safety and Health (NIOSH)
   D. Occupational Safety Health Administration (OSHA)

6. Issues of importance during the 2019 federal legislative calendar include the following:
   A. Reducing gun violence and the opioid crisis
   B. Nursing shortage and environmental issues

   C. Appropriate staffing and workplace health and safety
   D. All of the above

7. With 93% of hospitals reporting physicians on their governing boards, what is the percentage of nurses in attendance?
   A. 26%
   B. 50%
   C. 70%
   D. 80%

8. Which of the following is an organization that has succeeded in avoiding catastrophes in an environment where normal accidents can be expected because of risk factors and complexity?
   A. Just culture
   B. High reliability
   C. Magnet institutions
   D. Institutions with 70% of RNs with a Bachelor of Science in Nursing

9. A political process by an individual or group that aims to influence public policy and resource allocation decisions within political, economic, and social systems and institutions is:
   A. Policy change
   B. Advocacy
   C. Institutional policy
   D. Public policy

10. Which of the following is a policy that pertains to the governing of workplaces?
    A. Social
    B. Health
    C. Organizational
    D. Institutional

Answers: 1. D   2. A   3. D   4. D   5. A   6. D   7. A
8. B   9. B   10. D

REFERENCES

American Hospital Association [AHA]. (2018). *Governance Survey*. Chicago, IL: AHA.

American Nurses Association [ANA]. (2019). *ANA official position statements*. Silver Spring, MD: ANA.https://www.nursingworld.org/positionstatements.

American Nurses Credentialing Center [ANCC]. (2013). *Magnet application manual*. Silver Spring, MD: ANCC.

American Nurses Credentialing Center [ANCC]. (2019). *Magnet application manual*. Silver Spring, MD: ANCC.

Institute of Medicine. (2011). *The future of nursing: Leading change advancing health*. Washington, DC: The National Academies Press.

BIBLIOGRAPHY

American Nurses Association. (2019). Retrieved October 24, 2019 from https://www.nursingworld.org/practice-policy/pro-issues-panel/.

American Hospital Association [AHA]. (2018). *AHA hospital statistics*. Chicago: AHA.

American Nurses Association [ANA]. (2014). *Advocacy*. ANA. Retrieved July 19, 2019, from http://nursingworld.org/MainMenuCategories/Policy-Advocacy.

Gallup Survey. (2018). *Nurses top honesty and ethics list for 17th year*. Retrieved October 24, 2019 from https://www.aha.org/news/insights-and-analysis/2018-0110-nurse-watch-again-top-gallup-poll-trusted-professions

Hassmiller, S., & Combes, J. (2012). Nurse leaders in the boardroom: a fitting choice. *Journal of HealthCare Management*, *57*(1).

International Council of Nurses (ICN). (2005). *National comparison groups and reports: Guidelines for shaping effective health policy*. Retrieved July 2019, from www.icn.ch/images/stories/documents/publications/guidelines/guideline_shaping.pdf.

Khoury, C., Blizzard, R., Moore, L., & Hassmiller, S. (2011). Nursing leadership from bedside to boardroom: a Gallup national survey of opinion leaders. *Journal of Nursing Administration*, *41*(7/8), 299–305.

Lyttle, B. (2011). Politics: a natural step for nurses. *American Journal of Nursing*, *111*(5), 19–20.

Mason, D., Keepnews, D., Homberg, J., & Murray, E. (2013). The representation of health professionals on governing boards of health care organizations in New York City. *Journal of Urban Health*, *90*(5), 888–901.

Mason, D., Leavitt, J., & Chafee, M. (2016). *Policy and politics in nursing and health care*. St Louis: Elsevier.

Oman, K., Duran, C., & Fink, R. (2008). Evidence-based policy and procedures. *Journal of Nursing Administration*, *38*(1), 47–51.

Stimpson, M., & Hanley, B. (1991). Nurse policy analysis. *Nursing and Health Care*, *12*(1), 10–15.

Communication in the Work Environment

OBJECTIVES

- Identify the principles of good communication.
- Discuss the importance of good communication in the management of care.
- Identify various means of communication used in health care.
- Review the components of a change-of-shift report.
- Discuss SBAR (situation, background, assessment, recommendation) communication and its use in health care.

- Discuss TeamSTEPPS (Team Strategies and Tools to Enhance Performance and Patient Safety) and its importance in the safe delivery of care.
- Identify principles of communication when dealing with patients/families and staff members.
- Review communication principles when dealing with conflict resolution.

KEY TERMS

change-of-shift report process by which patient information is shared by nurses who have taken care of the patient for the previous shift, and are reporting to the incoming caregivers
communication process by which information is shared between and among individuals

computerized physician order entry (CPOE) process by which clinician orders are entered through electronic information systems
handoff the transfer of information (along with authority and responsibility) during transitions in care across the continuum; to include an opportunity to ask questions, clarify, and confirm

huddle ad hoc planning to reestablish situation awareness, reinforcing plans already in place, and assessing the need to adjust the plan

SBAR (situation, background, assessment, recommendation) template for communication among professionals that includes communication about situation, background, assessment, and recommendation

Team STEPPS (Team Strategies and Tools to Enhance Performance and Patient Safety) an evidence-based framework to optimize team performance across the health care delivery system

COMMUNICATION

Communication forms the basic principle when managing and coordinating care. Much of what nurses do needs to be communicated to the patient, family, and fellow staff members. Professional communication sets the tone of our management style, and often the tone of the unit in which we work. Communication and the lack of a consistent process for communication of a patient's condition have been cited as variables in the number of medical errors that occur in hospitals. A recommendation of the Institute of Medicine., 1999 calls for hospitals to "develop a working culture in which communication flows freely."

Sullivan and Decker (2009) noted five principles of effective communication:

1. Giving information is not the same as communication, which requires interaction, understanding, and response. For example, if a nurse asks a staff member to do something, but the staff member does not understand, information has been given but communication has not occurred.

2. The sender of the communication is responsible for clarity. Nurses and nurse managers must make sure that their communication is clear; it is not the job of the receiver of the message "to translate." If the receiver of the message has to translate the message, the possibility of error increases. For example, if you expect the unlicensed nursing personnel to report back to you immediately if a patient's temperature increases, you need to specifically say just that.

3. Use simple, exact language. The sender of the message needs to use words that are easily understood by the receiver of the communication. The words need to be precise and unambiguous. For e-mail communication "I" message language is inappropriate; professional e-mail needs to avoid the use of all slang and shortcuts.

4. Communication encourages feedback. Although feedback is not always positive, it is essential for making sure that the receiver understands the message. It is not enough to ask, "Did you understand?" The answer may be an automatic "yes" because the receiver expects that is what you want to hear. Feedback can be verbal ("I do not understand what you said"), or nonverbal (rolling of eyes when asked to do a task).

5. Sender must have credibility. A credible sender is perceived as trustworthy and reliable. Receivers who think the sender is not reliable may ignore the message.

6. Use direct communication channels when possible. Direct communication (person to person, face to face, or in writing) is best because there is less chance of the message being distorted as it passes through senders. Face-to-face communication is preferred as it allows the sender to get immediate feedback about the message.

E-mail

In the new technological age, much of interdepartmental and staff-to-staff communication involves electronic mail, or e-mail. Communication using such technology should follow the principles just stated, but it also needs to follow the basic principles of e-mail netiquette. Tschabitscher (2005) offered 10 rules for e-mail netiquette, which have been adapted as follows:

1. *Use e-mail the way you want everybody to use it:* Do not use it to send nonprofessional concerns.

2. *Take another look before you send the message:* Proofread your comments for appropriateness and confidentiality.

3. *Quote original messages properly in replies:* Make your e-mail replies easy to read by quoting in a useful manner.

4. *Avoid irony, sarcasm, and emotional tones in e-mail:* Keep the message objective.

5. *Clean up e-mails before forwarding them:* Forwarding e-mails is a great way of keeping track of a concern, but make sure that the original idea is not lost.

6. *Send plain text e-mails:* Avoid fancy formatting of e-mails. Cutesy pictures are for personal, not professional, communication.

7. *Writing in all capital letters is shouting:* Capital letters are also difficult to read.

8. *Ask before you send large attachments:* Large attachments may clog e-mail systems.

9. *The use of "smileys" raises an alarm:* Avoid the use of emoticons, instant messaging (IM) language, texting shortcuts, and Internet slang.

10. *Avoid "me too" messages:* Content needs to be specific and complete.

11. *Do not "reply to all":* Unless that is the intent of the message.

(Adapted from *Top 26 Most Important Rules of E-mail Etiquette.* Copyright 2009 by Heinz Tschabitscher. Retrieved September 19, 2019, from http://email.about.com/od/email-netiquette/tp/core_netiquette.htm. Used with permission.)

COMMUNICATION WITH PATIENTS AND STAFF

Nurses and nurse leaders also communicate with families and staff. Difficult situations often involve patients and staff, and disagreements, or complaints about the delivery of, or assignments of care. According to Sullivan and Decker (2009), nurse leaders need to keep the following in mind when dealing with patient or staff issues:

- Patients and their families are customers and should be communicated to with honesty and respect. Even if the communication involves dealing with a complaint, the customer needs to receive prompt and tactful assistance. The same philosophy is appropriate for an employee; he or she is a stakeholder in the work environment and also requires honesty and respect in communication.

- Nurses need to find a balance between avoiding medical jargon that is too complex, and using terms that are too simple and condescending. Paying attention to both verbal and nonverbal feedback will help nurse managers negotiate this challenge.

- Provide angry, or upset customers, or staff members a private, neutral place for communicating their concerns.

- When possible, if customers or stakeholders are not native speakers, and/or are not fluent in English, try to provide interpreter service. For patients, professional interpreters and language lines (including those for American Sign Language) should be used. Unless it is an emergency, do not use family members, as the practice is a potential violation of patient privacy. Family members also may have an agenda that will bias their communication with the patient. Each hospital has specific regulations about patient translation and privacy regulations. When communicating to fellow employees with limited language skills, make sure that the message is clear and understood.

- Learn about cultural issues to be able to recognize communication issues with both patients and staff members that are culturally based. Culturally competent responses to patients and fellow staff greatly enhance communication.

There are many modes of communication in the health care organization. One mode is used to communicate with the patient and family. Much of the nursing curricula have been spent on the theories and principles of professional and therapeutic communication. The Joint Commission (2014) also has some very specific regulations dealing with patient/family communication and the necessity of open and honest communication. It is crucial that patients and families understand the communication that is directed toward them. Cultural competence in communication is a vital skill of every nurse.

Another mode of communication deals with communication about the patient. Hospitals are institutions that are operational on a 24/7 basis and, therefore, require communication processes that are sound and reliable and can communicate vital patient information. The communication processes also need to follow Health Insurance Portability and Accountability Act (HIPAA) guidelines (see Chapter 17). Processes that are used in the communication of patient care include transcription of orders, change-of-shift reports, SBAR (situation, background, assessment, recommendation) reporting reporting, and TeamSTEPPS (Team Strategies and Tools to Enhance Performance and Patient Safety) communication methods.

Communication among health care professionals remains one of the most challenging concerns reported by the professionals. There are many reasons for inadequate communication, but there are approaches that

TABLE 8.1   Barriers to Communication with Suggested Strategies

Barriers	Tools and Strategies	Outcomes
Inconsistency in team membership	Brief Huddle Debrief	Shared mental model Adaptability
Lack of time	Team STEPP	Team orientation
Lack of information sharing	Cross-monitoring	Mutual trust
Hierarchy	Feedback	Team performance
Defensiveness	Advocacy and assertion	*Patient Safety!!*
Conventional thinking	Two-challenge rule	
Complacency	CUS	
Varying communication styles	DESC script Collaboration	
Conflict	SBAR	
Lack of coordination and follow-up with coworkers	Call-out Check-back Handoff	
Distractions		
Fatigue		
Workload		
Misinterpretation of cues		
Lack of role clarity		

CUS, Concerned, uncomfortable, safety of the resident is at risk; *DESC,* describe, express, specify, consequences; *SBAR,* situation, background, assessment, recommendation; *Team STEPP,* strategies and tools to enhance performance and patient safety. (From *Agency for Health care Research and Quality (AHRQ). Team STEPPS.* (2014). Retrieved July 30, 2017, from <www.ahrq.gov/professionals/education/curriculum-tools/teamstepps/instructor/essentials/pocketguide.html.>)

TABLE 8.2   Key Principles

Team Structure
Delineates fundamentals such as team size, membership, leadership, composition, identification, and distribution.

Leadership
Ability to coordinate the activities of team members by ensuring team actions are understood, changes in information are shared, and that team members have the necessary resources.

Situation Monitoring
Process of actively scanning and assessing situational elements to gain information and understanding or maintain awareness to support functioning of the team.

Mutual Support
Ability to anticipate and support other team members' needs through accurate knowledge about their responsibilities and workload.

Communication
Process by which information is clearly and accurately exchanged among team members.

(From Agency for *Health care Research and Quality (AHRQ). TeamSTEPPS.* (2014). Retrieved July 30, 2017, from <www.ahrq.gov/professionals/education/curriculum-tools/teamstepps/instructor/essentials/pocketguide.html>.

have been found to improve patient safety, and to make interprofessional communication more consistent. Table 8.1 reviews some of the barriers reported by health care team members and potential strategies to improve communication.

TeamSTEPPS is an important communication method when working in team situations. The majority of care is delivered in an interdisciplinary manner, and communication among all team members needs to be open, honest, and reliable. The principles of TeamSTEPPS culture are listed in Table 8.2. The team, whose responsibility it will be to care for the patient over

the next 8 to 12 hours, forms during the change of shift. The communication that will occur among this team is a vital process for ensuring patient safety.

An Effective Team Leader Will:
- Organize the team
- Articulate clear goals
- Make decisions through collective input of members
- Empower members to speak up and challenge when appropriate
- Actively promote and facilitate good teamwork
- Be skillful at conflict resolution

Team Events that will Occur During the Shift Include:

Planning
- *Brief:* Short session before start of shift to discuss team formation; assign essential roles; establish expectations and climate; and anticipate outcomes and likely contingencies.

Problem Solving

- *Huddle:* Ad hoc planning to reestablish situation awareness; reinforce plans already in place; and assess the need to adjust the plan. Huddles also occur after unexpected events such as patient falls, and for evaluation of the safety of the situation.

Process Improvement

- *Debrief:* Informal information exchange session designed to improve team performance and effectiveness; after action review. This is important in the culture of continual improvement; a team always needs to consider how to improve their performance.

BRIEF CHECKLIST

During the brief, the team should address the following questions:

____ Who is on the team?
____ Do all members understand and agree on goals?
____ Are roles and responsibilities understood?
____ What is our plan of care?
____ What is staff and provider availability throughout the shift?
____ What is the workload among team members?
____ What is the availability of resources?

(Agency for Healthcare Research and Quality AHRQ, 2014)

DEBRIEF CHECKLIST

The team should address the following questions during a debrief:

____ Communication clear?
____ Roles and responsibilities understood?
____ Situation awareness maintained?
____ Workload distribution equitable?
____ Task assistance requested or offered?
____ Were errors made or avoided? Availability of resources?
____ What went well, what should change, what should improve?

The feedback loop is very important in the improvement of care (Agency for Healthcare Research and Quality AHRQ, 2014). Feedback should be a routine component of daily patient care. Feedback is information provided for the purpose of improving team performance.

Feedback should be:

Timely: Given soon after the target behavior has occurred

Respectful: Focus on behaviors, not personal attributes
Specific: Be specific about what behaviors need correcting
Directed toward improvement: Provide directions for future improvement
Considerate: Consider a team member's feelings and deliver negative information with fairness and respect

Communication About the Patients: Transcription of Orders

The creation of physicians' and nursing orders in patient care forms the basis of the therapeutic regimen for the patient. This was often divided into two processes: the transcription of the physician's orders and the creation of the nursing care plan. Both of these documents need to be communicated effectively to all members of the health care team. Historically, the nurse has been responsible and accountable for the transcription process. This accountability was, and remains, documented by the nurse "signing off" the order as it is transcribed. With the increasing use of computerized physician order entry (CPOE), the role of the nurse in the transcription process is changing (Box 8.1). The order is transmitted directly by the physician or practitioner to the specific

---

BOX 8.1 Impact of Computerized Physician Order Entry

Handwritten orders have become a thing of the past for patients and their caregivers in the John Dempsey Hospital (UConn Health Center, Farmington, CT) intensive care and cardiac step-down units, where an electronic system for entering physicians' orders was recently adopted. The system, introduced on a pilot basis on one of the surgical floors last spring, is designed to improve patient safety and reduce medical errors.

"The electronic physician order entry system not only eliminates handwriting and transcription errors, it provides many online alerts and warnings for clinical caregivers, and distributes orders as they are written directly and immediately to ancillary units," says Roberta Luby, Assistant Vice President for Information Technology Strategic Projects, who supervised the rollout. The process is much safer and more streamlined."

When a physician orders a medication for a patient with the new electronic system, the order goes to the pharmacy with no manual intervention.

Goodnough, K. (2007). Electronic system for physician orders improves patient safety. *UConn Advance*, 25(29).

patient department, and it is automatically placed on the order sheets. A new order alert is highlighted on the computer system when a new order is entered. These orders are then integrated with the existing therapeutic regimen that is part of the computerized record.

In agencies where there is no CPOE, it will be important to follow the policy for transcription of orders. Each institution has specific guidelines dealing with the transcription of orders, and one must be familiar with the institution's guidelines. A sample policy for the transcription of orders is shown in Fig. 8.1.

Examples of communication about orders are also seen in the verbalization of orders with actions, such as in the following examples.

Call-Out: Strategy used to communicate important or critical information.

- Informs all team members simultaneously during emergent situations
- Helps team members anticipate next steps
- Directs responsibility to a specific individual responsible for carrying out the task

Example during an incoming trauma:

Leader: "Airway status?"
Resident: "Airway clear"
Leader: "Breath sounds?"
Resident: "Breath sounds decreased on right"
Leader: "Blood pressure?"
Nurse: "BP is 96/62"

Check-Back: Process of using closed-loop communication to ensure that information conveyed by the sender is understood by the receiver as intended. (Agency for Healthcare Research and Quality AHRQ, 2014)

The steps include the following:

Sender initiates the message

Receiver accepts the message and provides feedback

Sender double-checks to ensure that the message was received

EXAMPLE

Doctor: "Give 25 mg Benadryl IV push"
Nurse: "25 mg Benadryl IV push"
Doctor: "That's correct"

The communication of these orders to all caregivers is the responsibility of the nurse. The order needs to be communicated directly to others as it was entered. The manner in which these orders are communicated varies, but many institutions use a nursing care plan, medication/therapeutic orders, and nursing flow sheet to communicate the plan of care. These plans are also communicated via the change-of-shift report.

Communication About the Patients: Changes in Condition

Nurses are also expected to communicate changes in patient conditions to the team caring for the patient. This communication may be made to the physician to receive a new set of medical orders, to members of the health care team to update them on a patient's condition, or to a rapid response team. SBAR is a communication mechanism useful for framing any conversation, especially those requiring a rapid response from a clinician (Institute for Healthcare Improvement, 2007). Fig. 8.2 shows a template for an SBAR report to a physician that can be used in a number of situations requiring communication about a patient's condition.

The following guidelines need to be followed:

1. Before calling the physician, follow these steps:
- Have I seen and assessed the patient myself before calling?
- Has the situation been discussed with the nursing coordinator?
- Review the chart for the appropriate physician to call.
- Know the admitting diagnosis and date of admission.
- Have I read the most recent physician's progress notes, and notes from the nurse who worked the shift before me?
- Have available the following when speaking with the physician:
  - Patient's chart
  - List of current medications, allergies, intravenous fluids, and labs
  - Most recent vital signs
  - Reporting lab results: provide the date and time test was done and results of previous tests for comparison
  - Code status
2. When calling the physician, follow the SBAR process:

(S) Situation: What is the situation you are calling about?
- Identify self, unit, patient, and room number
- Briefly state the problem, what it is, when it happened or started, and the severity

(B) Background: Pertinent background information related to the situation could include the following:
- Admitting diagnosis and date of admission

**TEXAS TECH UNIVERSITY
HEALTH SCIENCES CENTER.**

Ambulatory Clinic Policy and Procedure

Title:	**Orders, Receiving and Noting**	Policy Number:	**3.04**
		Version Number	**4**
Regulation Reference:	**Joint Commission, Current Nursing Skills Test**	Effective Date:	**6/2011**
		Original Approval:	**4/2002**

POLICY STATEMENT:

It is the policy of TTUHSC Ambulatory Clinics to accurately transcribe orders and to implement the orders correctly and efficiently. Orders transcription may be done by an RN or LVN.

SCOPE:

This policy applies to all TTUHSC ambulatory clinic operations conducted through its Schools of Medicine and School of Nursing.

PROCEDURE:

1. **Who May Give or Write Orders** – Only licensed providers (attending physician, consultant, fellow, resident, physician assistant or nurse practitioner) may give or write orders. Orders written by students, authorized as part of their education program, will not be honored by the nursing staff or ancillary personnel unless validated/countersigned by a licensed physician.

2. **Verbal and Telephone Orders** – Verbal orders, except telephone orders, will be accepted in emergencies or when it is not practical for the physician to write the order. Orders must be given to an RN or LVN.

   a. The RN or LVN should record the order directly onto a clinic progress note, labeled "T.O" or "V.O."

   b. The RN or LVN should read back what has been written to the ordering physician, validating the accuracy of the order.

   c. The verbal order and documentation should include:

      1) Date and time received

      2) Patient name, age, weight (when appropriate)

      3) Drug name

      4) Dosage form

      5) Exact strength or concentration

      6) Dose frequency and route

      7) Purpose indication (as appropriate)

3. **Registered Nurse or Licensed Vocational Nurse**

   a. Reviews orders and identifies those needing immediate attention.

   b. Documents final validation or orders by signing first initial, last name, title, date, and time (as appropriate to clinic documentation).

   c. The order should be signed by the physician or practitioner as soon as possible.

CERTIFICATION:

This policy was approved by the Deans for the Schools of Medicine and Nursing June 2011.

Fig. 8.1 Sample policy for transcription of orders. (*From Texas Tech University Health Sciences Center. Orders, receiving and noting. Policy No. 3.04.* [2007]. Retrieved July 30, 2010, from http://www.ttuhsc.edu/provost/clinic/policies/ACPolicy3.04.pdf.)

S	**Situation**
	I am calling about <u><patient name and location></u>
	The patient's code status is <u><code status></u>
	The problem I am calling about is_____
	      I am afraid the patient is going to arrest
	
	I have just assessed the patient personally:
	
	Vital signs are: Blood pressure_____/_____Pulse_____Respiration_____Temperature_____
	
	I am concerned about the:
	      Blood pressure because it is over 200 or less than 100 or 30 mmHg below usual
	      Pulse because it is over 140 or less than 50
	      Respiration because it is less than 5 or over 40
	      Temperature because it is less than 96 or over 104

B	**Background**
	The patient's mental status is:
	      Alert and oriented to person, place, and time
	      Confused and cooperative or noncooperative
	      Agitated or combative
	      Lethargic but conversant and able to swallow
	      Comatose, eyes closed, not responding to stimulation
	The skin is:
	      Warm and dry
	      Pale
	      Mottled
	      Diaphoretic
	      Extremities are cold
	      Extremities are warm
	The patient is not or is on oxygen
	      The patient has been on _____ (l/min) or (percent) oxygen for _____ minutes (hours)

A	**Assessment**
	      This is what I think the problem is: <u><say what you think is the problem></u>
	      The problem seems to be cardiac infection neurologic respiratory
	      I am not sure what the problem is, but the patient is deteriorating
	      The patient seems to be unstable and may get worse, we need to do something

R	**Recommendation**
	I suggest or request that you <u><say what you would like to see done></u>
	      Transfer the patient to critical care
	      Come to see the patient at this time
	      Talk to the patient or family about code status
	      Ask the on-call family practice resident to see the patient now
	      Ask for a consultant to see the patient now
	Are any tests needed:
	      Do you need any tests like CXR ABG EKG CBC or BMP?
	      Others?
	If a change in treatment is ordered then ask:
	      How often do you want vital signs?
	      How long do you expect this problem will last?
	      If the patient does not get better, when would you want us to call again?

Fig. 8.2 This SBAR (situation, background, assessment, recommendation) tool was developed by Kaiser Permanente. (Used with permission from the *Institute for Healthcare Improvement. SBAR technique for communication: A situational briefing model.* [2007]. Retrieved July 30, 2010, from <www.ihi.org/IHI/ Topics/PatientSafety/SafetyGeneral/Tools/SBARTechniqueforCommunicationASituationalBriefingModel.htm>)

- List of current medications, allergies, intravenous fluids, and labs
- Most recent vital signs
- Lab results: provide the date and time test was done and results of previous tests for comparison
- Other clinical information
- Code status

(A) Assessment: What is the nurse's assessment of the situation?

(R) Recommendation: What is the nurse's recommendation, or what does he or she want?

Examples:

- Notification that patient has been admitted
- Patient needs to be seen now
- Order change

3. Document the change in the patient's condition and physician notification.

Communication About the Patients: Change of Shift

Change-of-shift reports vary across institutions. The purposes of the report are to exchange information that is necessary for future patient care, and to discuss the present status of the patient. These reports occur during the overlapping time between shifts. They occur in a variety of ways, with the most common being (1) change-of-shift meetings in which the outgoing and the incoming nurses meet face to face for a review of the pertinent information, (2) tape-recorded reports in which the outgoing nurse "reports" all pertinent information to the incoming nurse, and (3) "walking" reports in which the incoming and the outgoing nurses "walk" to the patient's room and report the pertinent information while observing the patient.

There are advantages and disadvantages to each form of change-of-shift report. The face-to-face meetings and walking reports allow for questions to be exchanged between the nurses. The walking report also has the added advantages of both nurses assessing the patient's situation, and of patient participation. Both of these face-to-face reports, however, can be costly if they are not completed in a timely manner. The taped report can be a more efficient way to impart the necessary information, but there is little opportunity for questioning and sharing of information, which may be important to the plan of care.

Regardless of the type of change-of-shift report, there are some pointers that may assist the incoming nurse.

- *Report vital information:* Allergies, code status, diagnosis, critical laboratory values, and family and medical team information.
- *Review current status and therapeutics of the patient:* This may be done in a systems approach (head to toe) or using an organization-specific report document.
- *Discuss upcoming plans:* This is important so the incoming nurse can prepare for events, such as a patient who is going for an examination and needs to have nothing by mouth (NPO).
- Review discharge plan as appropriate.
- *Discuss any other information pertinent to the patient's care:* This may include family responses to care and results of multidisciplinary team meetings.

The report is a vital link in the communication of patient status and needs. It is a crucial time to communicate accurate information about the patient status and the plan of care. One of the most frequent errors in shift report is the omission of critically important safety information. A change-of-shift report may be given orally in person, by audiotape recording, or during walking-planning rounds at the patient's bedside. Many hospitals are moving toward the use of walking reports (in the patient room) at the end of shifts. This type of change-of-shift reporting allows the incoming nurse to assess the patient situation and to ask questions of the outgoing nurse based on the assessment. It also allows the patient to participate and to confirm the information the outgoing nurse is communicating.

There are several options for organizing the information that one passes on in the handoff to the next shift. Some hospitals have templates for the report that are used by all staff members. SBAR is used in some institutions. Some institutions organize the report according to body systems; the report is presented based on the patient's body systems. Some organize the report on a "head-to-toe" assessment. Some report by exception, focusing solely on variances or patient problems. No matter what style of report is used, it should be done professionally using the guidelines given in Table 8.3, which compares the do's and don'ts of change-of-shift reports. Another example is "I Pass the Baton" for handoff reporting. This is part of the TeamSTEPPS method of teamwork and communication.

STEP

A tool for monitoring situations in the delivery of health care. The leader of the care delivery team and all members of the team are tasked with situation

TABLE 8.3   Comparison of Do's and Don'ts of Change-of-Shift Report

Do's	Don'ts
Provide only essential background information about the client (name, age, sex, physician's diagnosis, medical history, allergies)	Review all routine care procedures or tasks (e.g., bathing, scheduled changes)
Identify the client's nursing diagnosis or health care problems and their related causes	Review all biographic information already available in written form
Describe objective measurements or observations about the client's condition and response to health problem; emphasize recent changes	Use critical comments about a client's behavior, such as "Mrs. Willis is so demanding"
Share significant information about family members as it relates to client's problems	Make assumptions about relationships between family members
Continually review ongoing discharge plan (e.g., need for resources, client's level of preparation to go home)	Engage in idle gossip
Relay to staff significant changes in the way therapies are given (e.g., different position for pain relief, new medication)	Describe the basic steps of a procedure
Describe instructions given in teaching plans and the client's response	Explain detailed content unless staff members ask for clarification
Evaluate results of nursing or medical care measures (e.g., effect of back rub or analgesic administration)	Simply describe results as "good" or "poor"; be specific
Be clear about priorities to which incoming shift must attend	Force incoming staff to guess what to do first

(Adapted from Potter, P. A., & Perry, A G. (2008). *Fundamentals of nursing* (7th ed). St. Louis: Mosby.)

TABLE 8.4   Handoff

Strategy Designed to Enhance Information Exchange During Transitions in Care

__ Human resources
__ Triage acuity
__ Equipment

Assess Progress toward goal
__ Status of team's patient(s)?
__ Established goals of team?
__ Tasks/Actions of team?
__ Plan still appropriate?

(From *AHRQ. Team*STEPPS. (2014). Retrieved July 30, 2018, from <www.ahrq.gov/professionals/education/curriculum-tools/teamstepps/instructor/essentials/pocketguide.html>)

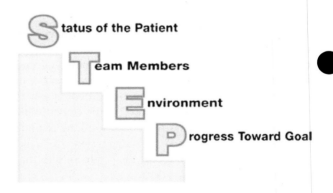

monitoring. Components of situation monitoring are as follows (Agency for Healthcare Research and Quality AHRQ, 2014):

Assess Status of Patient
__ Patient history
__ Vital signs
__ Medications
__ Physical exam
__ Plan of care
__ Psychosocial

Assess Team Members' levels
__ Fatigue
__ Workload
__ Task performance
__ Skill
__ Stress

Assess Environment
__ Facility information
__ Administrative information

CONFLICT RESOLUTION

Conflict resolution among staff members or patients and families is a challenging part of the profession. The resolution process includes using the principles of negotiation, which can result in one group winning, or both groups winning. In situations in which the outcome is a win/win result for both sides, collaboration and negotiation are required.

In dealing with conflict resolution, the following communication principles apply (adapted from Jones, 2007, p. 214):

- Identify who is involved in or who is the source of the conflict
- Identify interests and clarify issues
- Build mutual trust
- Separate the individuals from the conflict
- Stay in the present; avoid dwelling in the past
- Avoid placing blame
- Remain focused on the identified issues
- Discover options
- Develop outcomes
- Come to a consensus

In the TeamSTEPPS model, the following communication method is used (AHRQ, 2014).

DESC Script is a constructive approach for managing and resolving conflict.

From AHRQ, 2014. www.ahrq.gov/professionals/education/curriculum-tools/teamstepps/instructor/essentials/pocketguide.html.)

D: Describe the specific situation or behavior; provide concrete data

E: Express how the situation makes you feel/what your concerns are

S: Suggest other alternatives and seek agreement

C: Consequences should be stated in terms of impact on established team goals; strive for consensus

There are times when staff members need to evaluate the progress of the team as it progresses through the day. One such method is cross-monitoring. This is an error reduction strategy that involves:

- Monitoring actions of other team members
- Providing a safety net within the team
- Ensuring mistakes or oversights are caught quickly and easily
- "Watching each other's back"

Team members also need to advocate for patient safety and at times will need to communicate concerns. Ways of doing this include:

Advocating for the patient.

- Invoking when team members' viewpoints do not coincide with that of the decision maker; asserting a corrective action in a firm and respectful manner
- Making an opening
- Stating the concern
- Offering a solution
- Obtaining an agreement

Two-Challenge Rule:

When an initial assertion is ignored:

- It is your responsibility to assertively voice concern at least *two times* to ensure it has been heard
- The team member being challenged must acknowledge

If the outcome is still not acceptable:

- Take a stronger course of action
- Use supervisor or chain of command

Empowers all team members to "stop the line" if they sense or discover an essential safety breach.

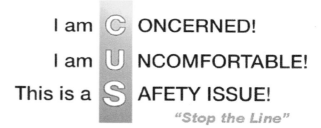

I am CONCERNED!
I am UNCOMFORTABLE!
This is a SAFETY ISSUE!
"Stop the Line"

Remember that as a nurse you will communicate information about patients to staff and to families so that all team members can make appropriate decisions about patient care. It is important that all forms of communication are timely, accurate, and relevant.

ORGANIZATION-WIDE COMMUNICATION

The last type of communication is organization-wide communication. Organization-wide communication occurs in many formats. Formal communication about changes in practice, policy, and other important institution-wide activities often occurs formally through newsletters, intranet communication, formal education, or other methods of structured communication. Such formal communication usually is governed by the organizational culture and is defined by a specific flow. That is, the communication is directed to the specific individuals and groups that need the communication. A change in nursing policy is communicated from the nursing practice council to the care unit and then to the individual nurses. This top-to-bottom communication often follows defined distribution channels. Formal communication also occurs from the bottom up. Health care organizations have methods of collecting information from point-of-care workers that are delivered up the chain of command. It is important for all employees to know and respect the chain of command. For example, if a staff nurse has a concern, he or she is to communicate it to the person who is next in the chain of command, the immediate supervisor. The supervisor then takes the communication up the chain of command. The chain of command follows the organizational structure of the organization. Some of this formal information may take the form of data collection through the use of employee surveys, customer complaints, budget requests, or strategic planning information. This information is further discussed in Chapter 3.

Informal communication also occurs in all institutions and in many situations, but it often occurs with individuals who are not part of the organizational hierarchy. Nurses often talk during breaks about patient conditions, suggestions for plans of care, and policies and procedures. The content may be perceived as formal, but the actual communication occurs in a nonstructured setting. Another type of informal communication is the "grapevine." Communication via the grapevine occurs outside of the traditional formal structures. A challenge with grapevine communication is that it is often altered as it moves across the grapevine. Another concern about informal communication is its lack of defined lines of communication. Information communicated via an informal network may not reach all parties. Therefore, it is vital that information about the patient, staff policies and rules, and any information that is necessary for practice be communicated via a formal structure so that receipt of the information can be validated.

SUMMARY

Good communication is essential to the operations of all patient care activities. Communication occurs among staff, patients, and families; from staff to staff; and among departments. Professional communication forms the basis for the delivery of patient care from shift to shift and from staff member to staff member. The communication needs to be timely, efficient, correct, and respectful, and it needs to be delivered to all in need of the information, and understood by those who receive it.

CLINICAL CORNER

TeamSTEPPS (Team Strategies and Tools to Enhance Performance and Patient Safety) is an evidence-based patient safety system that aims to optimize patient outcomes by improving communication and teamwork skills among members of the health care team. This program has been adapted from Crew Resource Management, which has its roots in the aviation industry. A major learning point in TeamSTEPPS is that the entire health care team is responsible for patient safety, not just the physician in charge, and that every member of the team plays a role. Health care institutions, where TeamSTEPPS is a part of the culture, encourage and expect all members of the team to "speak up when something is wrong." Through the use of root cause analysis it has been shown that the majority of patient safety issues in health care can be traced back to poor communication. TeamSTEPPS provides the health care team with the tools and resources they need to foster teamwork and improve overall patient safety. Using interdisciplinary education facilitates breaking down the hierarchy of medicine. Often TeamSTEPPS education sessions are the first time that all members of the health care team from all disciplines are learning and training together. There are multisite, ongoing research projects to measure the effectiveness of this training.

The Valley Hospital has begun to ingrain TeamSTEPPS philosophy into its culture. It is part of the larger "just culture" of the institution. Through the use of simulation, the patient care units have begun to weave TeamSTEPPS into interdisciplinary education. The main concepts of teamwork, communication, and speaking up when you see something that is not right, or "stopping the line" are the concepts that have been embraced at this institution. The expectation is that all members of the health care team will report and act on anything that is wrong or

CLINICAL CORNER—Cont'd

concerning. It is hoped that this concerted effort among all of us will further increase our already strong safety results. They will continue to adapt these concepts and many others from TeamSTEPPS to improve patient safety and optimize communication among the team members.

Beth McGovern, MSN, RNC-OB
Clinical Practice Specialist, Women and Children's Services, The Valley Hospital, Ridgewood, NJ

EVIDENCE-BASED PRACTICE

(From McAllen, E. R., Stephens, K., Swanson-Biearman, B., Kerr, K., & Whiteman, K. (2018). Moving shift report to the bedside: an evidence-based quality improvement project. *Online Journal of Issues in Nursing, 23*(2).)

A Midwestern, 532-bed, acute care, tertiary, Magnet designated teaching hospital identified concerns about fall rates and patient and nurse satisfaction scores. Research has shown that the implementation of bedside report has increased patient safety and patient and nurse satisfaction. An evidence-based practice change incorporating bedside report into standard nursing care was implemented and evaluated over a 4-month time period on three nursing units. Fall rates, Hospital Consumer Assessment of Healthcare Providers and Systems (HCAHPS) and Press Ganey scores, and nurses' response to a satisfaction survey were measured before and after the project implementation.

- Hospital leaders and health care organizations are making concentrated efforts to change their environments to assure patient safety and patient and nurse satisfaction.
- Bedside shift report (BSR) enables accurate and timely communication between nurses; includes the patient in care; and is paramount to the delivery of safe, high-quality care. Report, when completed at the patient bedside, allows the nurse to visualize and assess the patient and the environment, and communicate with and involve the patient in the plan of care.
- A team of nursing administrators, directors, staff nurses, and a patient representative was assembled to review the literature and make recommendations for practice changes.
- Patient participation in the report is paramount to delivery of safe, high-quality care.
- The team completed a gap analysis to determine evidence-based practices for shift report compared with the current practice.

- The team incorporated fictitious patient information that aligned with typical patient conditions from each area. Fig. 8.1 Medical Unit Nurse Script.
ISBARQ: Introduction, Situation, Background, Assessment, Recommendation, Questions
INTRODUCTION:
Off-going nurse introduce the oncoming nurse
SITUATION:
Patient name
Reason for admission
Code status
BACKGROUND:
Pertinent history
Laboratory and x-ray results
Other testing results
Consults
ASSESSMENT:
Assessment to include pertinent findings for assigned patient population
Medications and treatments
Pending tests
White board update
Safety and Environmental Check
IVs, Drains, Pain
Mobility
Environmental scan: clutter, side rails, visual assessment of room safety
RECOMMENDATION:
Pertinent information from Plan of Care
Follow-up tests to be completed
QUESTIONS:
Thank the patient and ask if he/she has any questions.
- The BSR began with the outgoing nurse introducing the oncoming nurse to the patient, followed by an assessment of the patient and environment.

Continued

EVIDENCE-BASED PRACTICE—Cont'd

An example of the audit report is illustrated in Fig. 2.

Fig. 8.2 BSR Shift Report Time Audit Tool.

BSR Process Audit Tool	Number of Nurses/ Shift	Time	Report Shift/ Date/ Time
Nursing Unit:			
Number of Nurses/Shift			
Report Start Time			
Report End Time			
Total Time			
Census			
Auditor			
Satisfaction Surveys			

("Press Ganey Survey," 2015) and two questions from HCAHPS (HCAHPS Survey, 2015).

TABLE 8.1   Patient Satisfaction Survey Questions

Press Ganey Questions

1. Friendliness/courtesy of the nurses 2. Prompt response to call light 3. Nurse attitude toward requests 4. Nurses kept you informed 5. Instructions for care at home 6. Staff addressed emotional needs 7. Response to concerns or complaints 8. Staff worked together to care for you

HCAHPS Questions

1. During this hospital stay, how often did nurses explain things in a way you could understand? 2. During this hospital stay, how often did nurses listen carefully to you?

Results

Patient falls decreased by 24% in the 4 months after BSR implementation compared with preimplementation falls. The orthopedic unit experienced the greatest reduction in the number of falls at 55.6%, followed by the neuroscience unit at 16.9%, and the general surgery unit at a 6.9% reduction.

Fig. 3 Nursing Unit Falls Per 1000 Patient Days

TABLE 8.1   Patient Satisfaction Survey Questions—Cont'd

Improvement in patient satisfaction as measured by Press Ganey scores occured as a result of BSR Only the general surgery unit had statistically significant ($p = .03$) improvement in patient satisfaction after implementation of BSR with the average Press Ganey score for the eight questions producing a result that increased from average score 87.7% to 91.6%. HCAHPS showed improvement, but the changes were not statistically significant.

Fig. 4. Press Ganey Eight Question Average Score *BSR*, Beside shift report; HC*AHPS*, Healthcare Common Procedure Coding System.

TABLE 8.2   Nursing Survey Results

Discussion

Despite the perception that report took longer, many nurses commented that the extra time was worth it because they recognized the value of BSR for patient care.

- Earlier identification and correction of potential errors during BSR may have improved the quality of patient care.

Implications for Nursing Management

BSR is a significant change to the current shift report practice and culture of most organizations, but it is associated with both improved patient safety and patient and nurse satisfaction.

- Future projects should consider measuring communication and teamwork improvements related to BSR
- Sharing success stories helps to encourage continued participation in BSR

BSR, Bedside shift report.

NCLEX® EXAMINATION QUESTIONS

1. As a nurse, you are aware of the importance of giving report to a nurse that is receiving the patient. During this transition the nurse has the opportunity to ask questions and clarify information. This is referred to as:
   A. Change-of-shift report
   B. Physician order entry
   C. Communications
   D. Handoff

2. When a nurse is working as a team, which of the following is an effective tool to use?
   A. Situation monitoring
   B. Huddle
   C. STEP
   D. TeamSTEPPS

3. The electronic physician order entry system:
   A. Prevents all medication orders
   B. Decreases medication errors, which can occur when the physician writes the order illegibly
   C. Is an issue when the system goes down
   D. Is up to the physician if it is used

4. When calling the health care provider and using the SBAR form of communication, what should be under the situation criteria?
   A. Identify the patient's ethnicity and religious affiliation
   B. Briefly state the problem, time it started, and its severity
   C. Describe the patient's mental status
   D. Inform the physician if the family visits

5. In the new technological age, much of interdepartmental and staff-to-staff communication involves electronic mail, or e-mail. Which of the following is not proper etiquette when sending an e-mail?
   A. Using all caps
   B. Making sure you want your reply to go to all recipients of your response

   C. Rereading e-mail prior to sending
   D. Clarifying what the sender meant, if not understood

6. Nurse leaders need to keep the following in mind when dealing with patient issues:
   A. Provide a quiet room to discuss issues
   B. Allow family to vent in the hallway
   C. Tell the patient there is a shortage of staff
   D. Discuss an incident report will be completed

7. As a nurse you need to have proper communication with patients/families. You are admitting a new patient who speaks Arabic. Which of the following is the first step to be sure the patient/family understand the education provided during the admission process?
   A. Have the 6-year-old son translate
   B. Call translator via phone that the facility uses for communication
   C. Check the facility list for employees who act as translators
   D. Both B and C are correct

8. An effective team leader will:
   A. Organize the team
   B. Articulate clear goals
   C. Make decisions through collective input of members
   D. All are correct

9. A_____occurs after unexpected events such as patient falls and for evaluation of the safety of the situation.
   A. Huddle
   B. Brief
   C. Debrief
   D. Feedback loop

Answers: 1. D 2. D 3. B 4. B 5. A 6. A 7. D 8. D 9. D

BIBLIOGRAPHY

Agency for Healthcare Research and Quality (AHRQ). (2014) *TeamSTEPPS*. Retrieved July 30, 2017, from www.ahrq.gov/professionals/education/curriculum-tools/team-stepps/instructor/essentials/pocketguidehtml.

Goodnough, K. (2007). Electronic system for physician orders improves patient safety. *UConn Advance, 25*(29).Retrieved July 30, 2017, from http://advance.uconn.edu/2007/070423/07042311.htm.

Institute for Healthcare Improvement. (2007) *SBAR technique for communication: A situational briefing model*. Retrieved July 30, 2017, from www.ihi.org/IHI/Topics/PatientSafety/SafetyGeneral/Tools/SBARTechniqueforCommunication-ASituationalBriefingModel.htm.

Institute of Medicine. (1999). *To err is human*. Washington, DC: IOM.

Jones, R. (2007). *Nursing leadership and management*. Philadelphia: F. A. Davis.

Potter, P. A., & Perry, A. G. (2008). *Fundamentals of nursing* (7th ed.). St. Louis: Mosby.

Sullivan, E., & Decker, P. (2009). *Effective management in nursing* (3rd ed.). Redwood City, CA: Addison-Wesley Publishing.

Texas Tech University Health Sciences Center. (2007). *Physician's orders, receiving and noting*. [Policy No. 3.04.] Retrieved July 30, 2017, from www.ttuhsc.edu/som/clinic/policies/CPolicy3.04.pdf.

The Joint Commission. (2014) *Comprehensive accreditation manual: The official handbook*. [Update 2]. Oakbrook Terrace, Illinois: TJC.

Tschabitscher H. (2005). *Top 10 most important rules of e-mail netiquette*. Retrieved July 30, 2017, from http://email.about.com/cs/netiquettetips/tp/core_netiquette.htm.

Tschabitscher, H. (2009). *Top 26 most important rules of email etiquette*. Retrieved July 30, 2017, from http://email.about.com/od/emailnetiquette/tp/core_netiquette.htm.

9

Personnel Policies and Programs in the Workplace

OUTLINE

OBJECTIVES

- Discuss employment law as it relates to health care.
- Differentiate between workplace safety and patient safety.
- Explain why violence in the workplace is of particular concern for nurses.
- Differentiate between abuse and assault.
- Compare and contrast lateral and vertical violence.
- Identify legal issues concerning workplace violence.
- Identify issues of importance for safety in the workplace.

- Discuss potential safety hazards in the workplace.
- Review measures to protect the employee.
- Identify interventions designed to deal with workplace violence.
- Identify signs and symptoms of impaired practice.
- Discuss the role of the nurse and nurse manager in dealing with impaired colleagues.
- Explain the role of the employee assistance program.

KEY TERMS

employee assistance program (EAP) confidential, short-term counseling service for employees with personal problems that affect their work performance
equal employment opportunity same employment opportunities must exist in an institution for all individuals regardless of race, color, national origin, religion, sex, age, or disability

horizontal violence coworker act of assault, verbal abuse, threats, battery, manslaughter, or homicide
impaired practice professional working while under the influence of a mind-altering chemical such as alcohol or drugs

sexual harassment unwelcome sexual advances, request for sexual favors, or other verbal or physical conduct of a sexual nature, when this conduct explicitly or implicitly affects an individual's employment, unreasonably interferes with an individual's work performance, or creates an intimidating, hostile, or offensive work environment

workplace violence any violent act, including physical assaults and threats of assault, directed toward persons at work or on duty

This chapter deals with multiple issues of importance within the nursing workplace. The first section deals with the hiring and interviewing processes, and their importance to entering the workplace. The later section deals with the personnel policies and programs that effect the safe working environment for nursing staff.

EMPLOYEE LAW

There are a number of federal and state laws that play a major role in the employment of staff. It is very important to have an understanding of these laws and any local or institution-specific regulations affecting the human resource function of your job. Understanding these laws will decrease your exposure to liability in your hiring practices.

Equal Employment Opportunity Laws

Several laws have been implemented to ensure there are equal employment opportunities for all individuals regardless of race, color, national origin, religion, sex, age, or disability. These laws are enforced by the U.S. Equal Employment Opportunity Commission.

The federal laws prohibiting job discrimination are as follows (www.eeoc.gov/abouteeo/overview_laws.html):

- *Title VII of the Civil Rights Act of 1964 (Title VII):* Prohibits employment discrimination based on race, color, religion, sex, or national origin.
- *The Equal Pay Act of 1963 (EPA):* Protects men and women who perform substantially equal work in the same establishment from sex-based wage discrimination.
- *The Age Discrimination in Employment Act of 1967 (ADEA):* Protects individuals who are 40 years of age or older.
- *Title I and Title V of the Americans with Disabilities Act of 1990 (ADA):* Prohibit employment discrimination against qualified individuals with disabilities in the private sector, and in state and local governments.

- *Sections 501 and 505 of the Rehabilitation Act of 1973:* Prohibit discrimination against qualified individuals with disabilities who work in the federal government.
- *The Civil Rights Act of 1991:* Among other things, provides monetary damages in cases of intentional employment discrimination.

Included in these laws are laws that prohibit sexual harassment in the workplace. It is the responsibility of the organization to have human resource policies and procedures in place that are in compliance with the requirements of these laws (Table 9.1).

Many of these regulations relate to the hiring process (see Chapter 20), whereas some relate to the work environment. In addition to the employment laws and regulations, many institutions are unionized. Some organizations have differing unions for different sets of employees. The nurses may be unionized under a nurses union, the environmental care employees may be represented by another union, and the licensed practical nurses may belong to a different union again. In such a multiunion environment, it is important for you to know the provisions of the union agreement(s). The union agreement(s) will affect everything from the hiring process (see Chapter 20) to the delivery of patient care. If you join a unionized environment, as a new employee you will receive orientation materials from the union in addition to its benefits and contract requirements. The new manager in a unionized environment will also receive information regarding all of the union rules that affect the management of the unit.

WORKPLACE VIOLENCE

In a national survey of registered nurses (RNs) conducted by the American Nurses Association (ANA) in 2001, 88% of working nurses reported that health and safety concerns influence their decisions to continue working in the field of nursing, and also the kind of nursing work they choose to perform. Hospitals are

TABLE 9.1   Selected Federal Labor Legislation

Year	Legislation	Primary Purpose of the Legislation
1935	Wagner Act; National Labor Relations Act	Unions, National Labor Relations Board established
1947	Taft-Hartley Act	Equal balance of power between unions and management
1962	Executive Order 10988	Public employees could join unions
1963	Equal Pay Act	Became illegal to pay lower wages based on gender
1964	Civil Rights Act	Protected against discrimination based on race, color, creed, national origin, etc.
1967	Age Discrimination in Employment Act	Protected against discrimination based on age
1970	Occupational Safety and Health Act	Ensured healthy and safe working conditions
1974	Wagner Amendments	Allowed nonprofit organizations to unionize
1990	Americans with Disabilities Act	Barred discrimination against workers with disabilities
1991	Civil Rights Act	Addressed sexual harassment in the workplace
1993	Family and Medical Leave Act	Allowed work leaves based on family and medical needs

perceived as places of safe haven, but in reality they are potential breeding grounds for many types of incidents, ranging from disruptive staff, patients, and families, to chemical and infection exposure. Nurses have a right to a safe workplace.

Approximately 15% of all nonfatal violence occurs in the workplace (U.S. Department of Justice, 2011). In fact, a safe workplace is necessary for the provision of patient care (ANA, Department of Government Affairs, 2007). This chapter deals with issues of concern for the nurse dealing with potentially explosive workplace situations.

Workplace violence ranges from offensive or threatening language, to homicide. The National Institute for Occupational Safety and Health (NIOSH) defines workplace violence as violent acts (including physical assaults and threats of assaults) directed toward persons at work or on duty. Workplace violence can be divided into four categories: violence by strangers, clients (patients), coworkers, and personal relations (American Association of Critical Care Nurses AACN., 2004).

More than 5 million U.S. hospital workers from many occupations perform a wide variety of duties. They are exposed to many safety and health hazards, including violence. Recent data indicate that hospital workers are at high risk for experiencing violence in the workplace.

Statistics for workplace violence in nursing indicate the following:

• In 2009 more than 50% of emergency center nurses experienced violence by patients on the job. There were 2050 assaults and violent acts reported by RNs requiring an average of 4 days away from work. Of these acts, 1830 were inflicted with injuries by patients or residents (Emergency Nurses Association, 2009).

• From 2003 to 2009, eight registered nurses were fatally injured at work [Bureau of Labor Statistics BLS, 2011].

• A study of student nurses reported that 53% had been put down by a staff nurse (Longo, 2007); 52% reported having been threatened, or experienced verbal violence at work (American Association of Critical Care Nurses AACN., 2004; retrieved from www.nursingworld.org/Bullying-Workplace-Violence).

Employee assaults may originate from patients, families, and coworkers. Assault can range from minor to major assaults. Outbursts of violence can affect the employee causing disability, psychological trauma, or death. Several risk factors may lead to violence in the health care setting (Tomey, 2004) including:

• People under the influence of alcohol or drugs
• Working understaffed
• Long waiting times
• Overcrowded waiting rooms
• Working alone
• Unlimited public access
• Poorly lit corridors, rooms, parking lots
• Contact with public
• Exchange of money
• Working in community-based settings
• Hospitalized prisoners
• Isolated work with patients during exams and treatments

Hospitals are microcosms of society and, as such, are socialized to violence.

Workplace violence is a multifaceted event with the potential to increase in frequency and scope (Ehrmann & Zuzelo, 2007). As a nurse and manager, you need to have a basic understanding of the risk for workplace violence to intervene in effective, efficient, and meaningful ways. You have already learned about potentially violent patients and how to handle them, but you need to be able to transfer some of this knowledge to the potentially violent employee. Boxes 9.1 and 9.2 provide warning signs of physical violence.

Although there is no universal strategy to prevent workplace violence, all hospitals have developed security plans to protect the employee from an unsafe workplace. The risk factors vary from hospital to hospital and from unit to unit. You have learned many ways of assessing individuals for altered levels of dealing with stress

---

BOX 9.1   Warning Signs of Violence

- Attendance problems
- Carelessness at work
- History of physical violence
- Performance problems
- Personality changes
- Poor hygiene
- Substance abuse
- Social isolation

(From Tomey, A. M. (2004). *Guide to nursing management and leadership* (7th ed., p. 162). St. Louis: Mosby.)

BOX 9.2   Signs of Impending Physical Violence

- Clenched jaws or fists
- Increased movement
- Increased respirations
- Pacing
- Shouting threats
- Staring or pointing
- Use of profanity

(From Gates, D. M., & Kroeger, F. (2003). Violence against nurses: the silent epidemic. *ISNA Bulletin, 29, 25–29*; National Institute for Occupational Safety and Health (NIOSH). *Occupational violence*. (2002a). DHHS (NIOSH) publication No. 2002-101. <www.cdc.gov/niosh/topics/violence/> Accessed July 2019.)

---

and intervening in such situations. These are important to remember.

Maintain behavior that helps diffuse anger:
- Present a calm, caring attitude
- Do not match the threats
- Do not give orders
- Acknowledge the person's feelings (e.g., "I know you are frustrated.")
- Avoid any behavior that may be interpreted as aggressive (e.g., moving rapidly, getting too close, touching, or speaking loudly)

Be alert:
- Evaluate each situation for potential violence when you enter a room or begin to relate to a staff member, patient, or visitor.
- Be vigilant throughout the encounter.
- Do not isolate yourself with a potentially violent person.
- Always keep an open path for exiting; do not let the potentially violent person stand between you and the door.

Take these steps if you cannot defuse the situation quickly:
- Remove yourself from the situation.
- Call security for help.
- Report any violent incidents to your management.

When you are dealing with potential staff violence or patient and family violence, it is important to maintain the safety of the patient care situation. If possible, remove the potentially violent individual from the patient care area.

CONFLICT MANAGEMENT

In managing the conflict, you will need to determine the cause of the conflict. First, determine the basis of the conflict. Is there difficulty between two shifts (intergroup), or two individuals (interpersonal)? Often there is conflict between shifts that spills over to stressful situations. Some of these conflicts may relate to perceptions of work left undone by one shift, or other work-related concerns. Second, you will need to analyze the source of the conflict. Conflict management techniques stress the importance of open and honest communication, and assertive dialogue. During conflict situations the nurse manager should view the total situation and use positive communication. Conflict resolution techniques are described in a variety of ways by a variety of authors

(Tomey, 2004; Yoder-Wise & Kowalski, 2006). The following is a list of strategies for conflict resolution, which is the third step of conflict management (Huber, 2013).

- *Avoiding:* If you avoid the problem, you can trick yourself into believing that there is no problem.
- *Withholding or withdrawing:* In this situation, parties remove themselves from participation in a solution; this does not resolve a conflict.
- *Reassuring:* Parties do not withdraw, but try to make everyone feel good. In this situation, reassuring strategies are used to diffuse strong conflicts; this may be a way of hindering open communication.
- *Accommodating:* This is often used in vertical conflict when there is a power differential. It may also be used when one individual has a vested interest in a solution that may be relatively unimportant to the other individual.
- *Competing:* This is an assertive strategy in which one individual's needs are satisfied at another's expense.
- *Compromising:* This strategy is used when both individuals play a part in the decision. It is a basis of conflict management.
- *Confronting:* Individuals will speak for themselves in a way that the other individual hears the concern.
- *Collaborating:* Parties work together to find a mutually beneficial solution.
- *Bargaining and negotiating:* This involves both parties in a back-and-forth discussion to reach a level of agreement.
- *Problem solving:* The goal is to find a workable solution for all parties.

The following strategies will help the nurse manager resolve conflict before it escalates into a serious situation.

- *Recognize conflict early:* Recognizing the early warning signs of conflict is the first step toward resolution. Pay attention to body language and be cognizant of the moods of the staff.
- *Be proactive:* Address the issue of concern at an early stage. Avoiding the conflict may cause frustration and escalate the problem.
- *Actively listen:* Focus your attention on the speaker. Try to understand, interpret, and evaluate what's being said. The ability to listen actively can improve interpersonal relationships, reduce conflicts, foster understanding, and improve cooperation.
- *Remain calm:* Keep responses under control and emotions in check. Do not react to volatile comments.

Your calmness will help set the tone for the parties involved.

- *Define the problem:* Clearly identify and define the problem. A clear understanding of the issues will help minimize miscommunication and facilitate resolution.
- *Seek a solution:* Manage the conflict in a way that successfully meets the goal of reaching an acceptable solution for both parties (Johansen, 2012).

Box 9.3 provides a model for managing conflict.

BOX 9.3   Model for Managing Conflict

Determine the Basis of the Conflict
Intrapersonal
Interpersonal
Group
Intergroup
Organizational

Analyze the Sources of the Conflict
Cultural differences
Different facts
Separate pieces of information
Different perceptions of the event
Defining the problem differently
Divergent views of power and authority
Role conflicts
Number of organizational levels
Degree of association
Parties dependent on others
Competition for scarce resources
Ambiguous jurisdictions
Need for consensus
Communication barriers
Separation in time and space
Accumulation of unresolved conflict

Consider Alternative Approaches to Conflict Management
Avoiding
Accommodating
Compromising
Collaborating
Competing

Choose the Most Appropriate Approach
Implement the conflict management strategy
Evaluate the results

(From Tomey, A. M. (2004). *Guide to nursing management and leadership* (7th ed., p. 144). St. Louis: Mosby.)

HORIZONTAL VIOLENCE IN THE WORKPLACE

Many of the issues that interfere with workplace safety arise from the interactions routinely occurring between staff members. In times of stress, there is often miscommunication among colleagues. Most of these conflicts can be resolved with open communication. However, there is a growing concern among health employees about horizontal violence between staff members. Horizontal violence is an act of aggression toward another colleague (Box 9.4). It may range from verbal or emotional abuse, or extend to physical abuse. Subtle acts of horizontal abuse may include belittling a fellow staff member, withholding information, or freezing a colleague out of group activities. As a nurse the challenge will be to identify behaviors that could be considered horizontally violent. Some of this behavior occurs between physicians and nurses. Two-thirds of nurses say that they have experienced such abuse at the hands of physicians (Cook, Green, & Topp, 2001; Rosenstein, 2002; The Joint Commission, 2008).

BOX 9.4   Horizontal Violence in the Workplace

Nonverbal behaviors such as the raising of eyebrows or making faces in response to comments by the victim

Verbal remarks that could be characterized as being snide or abrupt responses to questions raised by the victim

Activities that undermine the victim's ability to perform professionally, including either refusing or not being available to give assistance

The withholding of information about a practice or patient that will undermine a victim's ability to perform professionally

Acts of sabotage that deliberately set up victims for negative situations in their work environment

Group in-fighting and establishment of cliques designed to exclude some staff members

Failure to resolve conflicts directly with the individual involved, choosing instead to complain to others about an individual's behavior

Failure to respect the privacy of others

Broken confidences

(From Longo, J., & Sherman, R. (2007). Leveling horizontal violence. *Nursing Management*, 38(3), 35.)

Horizontal conflict is based on differences between colleagues. Vertical conflict relates to differences between managers and staff associates. These differences are often related to inadequate communication, opposing interests, and lack of shared attitudes. If staff members continue with horizontally violent behavior, the outcome is low morale and stress (Rosenstein, 2002). As a new nurse leader, it will be your responsibility to stop such behavior. The following steps are recommended to stop the cycle (Longo & Sherman, 2007, p. 36):

- Analyze the culture of your work unit by observing for verbal and nonverbal cues in the behavior of your staff.
- Name the problem when you see it, and use the term "horizontal violence."
- Raise the issue at staff meetings and educate your staff about horizontal violence to help break the silence.
- Allow staff members to tell their stories if horizontal violence is part of the culture of the unit.
- Ensure there is a process for dealing with this issue if it occurs in your unit and be responsive when issues are brought to your attention.
- Engage in self-awareness activities and reflective practice to ensure that your leadership style does not support horizontal violence.
- Provide your nursing staff members with training about conflict management skills, and empower them to defend themselves against bullying behavior.

Although there is no federal standard that requires workplace violence protections, effective January 1, 2009, The Joint Commission created a new standard in the "Leadership" chapter (LD.03.01.01) that addresses disruptive and inappropriate behaviors. Some states have sought legislative solutions including mandatory establishment of a comprehensive prevention program for health care employers, in addition to increased penalties for those convicted of assaults of a nurse and/or other health care personnel. These states include AL, AK, AR, AZ, CA, CO, CT, FL, HI, ID, IL, IA, KS, LA, MI, MS, MT, NE, NV, NJ, NM, NY, NC, OH, OK, RI, TN, VT, VA, WV, and WY (Retrieved from <www.nursingworld.org/Bullying-Workplace-Violence> July 2019).

SEXUAL HARASSMENT

Some instances of abuse may be forms of sexual harassment. Sexual harassment can result from collegial interpersonal conflict. Sexual harassment is a form of sex discrimination that violates Title VII of the Civil Rights Act of 1964. It is defined as unwelcomed sexual advances, request for sexual favors, or other verbal, or physical conduct of a sexual nature, when this conduct explicitly or implicitly affects an individual's employment, unreasonably interferes with an individual's work performance, or creates an intimidating, hostile, or offensive work environment (U.S. Equal Employment Opportunity Commission, 2015).

All employment agencies are required to have sexual harassment policies and reporting procedures. This will be part of your new hire and mandatory annual education. When exposed to an incident of sexual harassment, remember that it needs to be confronted immediately. Confront the harasser with a statement such as, "I need you to know that I do not want you telling me sexual jokes." If the behavior continues, inform your immediate supervisor.

Incidences of interpersonal conflict are inevitable in any workplace. It is the responsibility of both staff and leadership to recognize concerns and then intervene appropriately if the workplace is to be conducive to a satisfying and professional workplace.

As a nurse and nurse manager, you must do the following (American Association of Critical Care Nurses AACN., 2004, p. 2):

- Actively develop a culture where violence is not tolerated, incidents are promptly addressed and managed, and comprehensive support for coworkers who experience violence is provided
- Advocate for enforceable violence management policies in the workplace, and hold others accountable for their behavior
- Participate in educational training on violence awareness and prevention.
- Mentor colleagues on how to respond when incidents occur

VIOLENCE: OCCUPATIONAL HAZARDS IN HOSPITALS

As a nurse manager, you may be involved in the development of a comprehensive violence prevention program. No universal strategy exists to prevent violence. The risk factors vary from hospital to hospital and from unit to unit. The goal of the violence prevention program is to identify risk factors in specific work scenarios, and to

develop strategies for reducing them (NIOSH, 2002a, 2002b).

Occupational Safety and Health Administration (OSHA) has identified eight essential components for a violence prevention plan.

1. Management commitment
2. Employee involvement
3. Work site analysis
4. Prevention of hazards
5. Training and education
6. Prompt recognition, control, and monitoring
7. Record keeping
8. Evaluation

This follows a model that is similar to the work of the hospital-wide safety committee.

The safety committee has the responsibility for developing and implementing the environmental controls within a hospital setting. This committee is also responsible for documenting that physical rounds are made in the facility and outside of the facility to maintain the hospital's environmental and administrative controls for violence prevention (Box 9.5).

BOX 9.5 Hospital's Environmental and Administrative Controls for Violence Prevention

Environmental Controls
- Install emergency alarms
- Install monitoring systems (cameras)
- Install metal detectors
- Provide security escorts to parking lots/decks
- Provide adequate waiting areas to prevent overcrowding
- Provide staff members with secure, lockable bathrooms
- Provide adequate lighting
- Replace lights immediately if defective
- Provide video for high-risk areas

Administrative Controls
- Establish liaison with local police and fire departments
- Report incidents of violence
- Require employees to report assaults and/or threats
- Provide a trained response team
- Distribute visitor passes
- Maintain proper reports of incidents
- Develop and implement hospital-wide safety plan
- Enforce all safety and security policies and procedures
- Distribute staff identification badges (enforce use of same)

BOX 9.6 **Employee Education**

- Workplace violence prevention policy and procedure
- Early recognition of escalating behavior
- Early reaction response plan of violent behavior
- Cultural and ethnic diversity awareness plan
- Location and activation of emergency alarms
- Awareness of emergency exits
- Awareness of employee roles in the event of workplace violence

All hospitals are required to have a new employee/volunteer/student orientation program and an annual employee/volunteer program that must be clearly documented. The human resources department of the hospital is required to maintain these records. The state board of health and/or The Joint Commission usually requests these documents on an inspection or a survey. Required employee education is documented in Box 9.6.

Precise record keeping is required in the event of an incident. The hospital will have either a policy and procedure for a written incident report or a computer-based program. Whether your hospital uses the written form or the computer-based program, the exact date, time, and occurrence must be properly documented. The follow-up of the event is also clearly documented for future reference. The documents are used for impending court cases, review of types of employee and/or visitor injuries, needlestick injuries, or bodily harm.

WORKPLACE VIOLENCE CHECKLIST

As a new nurse contemplating working within a facility, the checklist in Box 9.7 can serve as an assessment of the personal safety of the facility.

IMPAIRED PRACTICE

Sometimes issues of staff conflict are symptomatic of other personal issues that may be impairing a staff member. Such issues may be stress at home, financial difficulties, or actual impairment from drugs and/or alcohol. Although all staff members will have personal issues that affect the workplace at various times, it is important for you to know when these personal issues interfere with workplace and/or patient safety.

The ANA estimated that 7% to 10% of nurses in the United States are impaired by alcohol or drugs. Some of this addictive behavior is accentuated by the constant availability of mind-altering drugs, and some nurses come to the workplace with addictive difficulties.

Boxes 9.8 and 9.9 provide signs and physical symptoms of alcohol or drug dependency.

Marquis and Huston (2014) discussed the profile of the impaired nurse and group characteristics into three primary areas: personality/behavior changes, job performance changes, and time and attendance changes.

Common Personality/Behavior Changes of the Chemically Impaired Employee

- Increased irritability with patients and colleagues; often followed by extreme calm
- Social isolation, eats alone, avoids unit social functions
- Extreme and rapid mood swings
- Euphoric recall of events or elaborate excuses for behaviors
- Unusually strong interest in narcotics, or the narcotic cabinet
- Sudden, dramatic change in personal grooming or any other area
- Forgetfulness, ranging from simple short-term memory loss to blackouts
- Change in physical appearance, which may include weight loss, flushed face, red or bleary eyes, unsteady gait, slurred speech, tremors, restlessness, diaphoresis, bruises, cigarette burns, jaundice, and ascites
- Extreme defensiveness regarding medication errors

Common Job Performance Changes of the Chemically Impaired Employee

- Difficulty meeting schedules and deadlines
- Illogical or sloppy charting
- High frequency of medication errors, or errors in judgment affecting patient care
- Frequently volunteers to be medication nurse
- Has a high number of assigned patients who complain that their pain medication is ineffective in relieving their pain
- Consistently meeting work performance requirements at minimal levels, or doing the minimum amount of work necessary
- Judgment errors
- Sleeping or dozing on duty

BOX 9.7 Workplace Violence Checklist

This checklist helps identify present or potential workplace violence problems. Employers may be aware of other serious hazards not listed here.

Periodic inspections for security hazards include identifying and evaluating potential workplace security hazards and changes in employee work practices, which may lead to compromising security. Please use the following checklist to identify and evaluate workplace security hazards. **TRUE** notations indicate a potential risk for serious security hazards.

____T____F This industry frequently confronts violent behavior and assaults of staff.

____T____F Violence has occurred on the premises or in conducting business.

____T____F Customers, clients, or coworkers assault, threaten, yell, push, or verbally abuse employees, or use racial or sexual remarks.

____T____F Employees are NOT required to report incidents or threats of violence to employer, regardless of injury or severity.

____T____F Employees have NOT been trained by the employer to recognize and handle threatening, aggressive, or violent behavior.

____T____F Violence is accepted as "part of the job" by some managers, supervisors, and/or employees.

____T____F Access and freedom of movement within the workplace are NOT restricted to those persons who have a legitimate reason for being there.

____T____F The workplace security system is inadequate (e.g., door locks malfunction, windows are not secure, and there are no physical barriers or containment systems).

____T____F Employees or staff members have been assaulted, threatened, or verbally abused by clients and patients.

____T____F Medical and counseling services have NOT been offered to employees who have been assaulted.

____T____F Alarm systems such as panic alarm buttons, silent alarms, or personal electronic alarm systems are NOT being used for prompt security assistance.

____T____F There is no regular training provided on correct response to alarm sounding.

____T____F Alarm systems are NOT tested on a monthly basis to ensure correct function.

____T____F Security guards are NOT employed at the workplace.

____T____F Closed circuit cameras and mirrors are NOT used to monitor dangerous areas.

____T____F Metal detectors are NOT available or NOT used in the facility.

____T____F Employees have NOT been trained to recognize and control hostile and escalating aggressive behaviors and to manage assaultive behavior.

____T____F Employees CANNOT adjust work schedules to use the "buddy system" for visits to clients in areas where they feel threatened.

____T____F Cellular phones or other communication devices are NOT made available to field staff to enable them to request aid.

____T____F Vehicles are NOT maintained on a regular basis to ensure reliability and safety.

____T____F Employees work in areas where assistance is NOT readily available.

(From Occupational Safety and Health Administration (OSHA). (2003). *Guidelines for preventing workplace violence for health care and social service workers* (rev. 2003). Washington, DC: OSHA, U.S. Department of Labor. <www.osha.gov/SLTC/etools/hospital/hazards/workplaceviolence/checklist.html.> Accessed July 2019; Huber, D. L. (2013). *Leadership and nursing care management* (3rd ed., p. 681). Philadelphia: Elsevier.)

BOX 9.8 Signs of Nursing Drug Diversion

- Arriving early, staying late, and coming to work on scheduled days off
- Excessive wasting of drugs
- Regularly signing out large quantities of controlled drugs
- Volunteering often to give medication to other nurses' patients
- Taking frequent bathroom breaks

- Patients reporting unrelieved pain despite adequate prescription of pain medication
- Discrepancies in the documentation of controlled substance administration
- Medications being signed out for patients who have been discharged or transferred, or who are off the unit for procedures or tests

(From Maher-Brisen. (2011). Addiction: an occupational hazard in nursing. *American Journal of Nursing*, 107(8), 778–779.)

BOX 9.9   Physical Symptoms of Alcohol or Drug Dependency

- Shakiness, tremors of hands, jitteriness
- Slurred speech
- Watery eyes, dilated or constricted pupils
- Diaphoresis
- Unsteady gait
- Runny nose
- Nausea, vomiting, diarrhea
- Weight loss or gain
- Blackouts (memory losses while conscious)
- Wears long-sleeved clothing continuously

(From Sullivan, E., Bissel, L., Williams, E. (1988). *Chemical dependency in nursing: the deadly diversion.* Menlo Park, CA: Addison-Wesley Nursing.)

BOX 9.10   Examples of New Jersey Board of Nursing Level I Mandatory Reporting

- Suspected drug diversion
- Misappropriation
- Theft
- Physical and verbal abuse
- Sexual abuse or exploitation
- Intoxication on duty
- Failing to account for wastage of controlled medication

- Complaints from other staff members about the quality and quantity of the employee's work

Common Time and Attendance Changes of the Chemically Impaired Employee

- Increasingly absent from work without adequate explanation or notification; most frequently absent on a Monday or Friday
- Long lunch hours
- Excessive use of sick leave, or requests for sick leave after days off
- Frequently calling in to request compensatory time
- Arriving at work early, or staying late for no apparent reason
- Consistent lateness
- Frequent disappearances from the unit without explanation

It is your responsibility as a nurse and nurse manager to report any issues of coworker behaviors. You should be alert to any signs and symptoms (see Box 9.4) of a coworker under the influence and be aware of methods of reporting. You should report the health care worker to your immediate supervisor. It is the supervisor's responsibility to take further action. In keeping with the institution's policies and procedures, the human resources department should be alerted to assist the supervisor or nurse manager with confronting the employee. Reporting laws and consequences vary in each state. Clear documentation regarding the employee must be kept. Documentation should include tardiness, absenteeism, patient or coworker complaints, records of controlled substances on the unit, and physical signs and symptoms both observed and reported. (see section "Employee Assistance Programs" in this chapter.)

Health care workers who abuse drugs or alcohol place both the patient and their fellow staff at considerable risk. It is important for you to know your responsibilities when dealing with an impaired nurse. The safety of the patient is paramount. Many state boards of nursing have adopted mandatory reporting of suspected impairment. Look to the rules and regulations in your state to determine your responsibility.

An example is the New Jersey Board of Nursing Level I mandatory reporting, which always requires the following to be reported (Box 9.10):

- Conduct that clearly violates expected standards of care and may result in various degrees of harm.
- Conduct that demonstrates a pattern of poor judgment or skill.

AMERICAN NURSES ASSOCIATION CODE OF ETHICS

The ANA Code of Ethics for nurses does not distinguish the cause from the effect. In a situation where a nurse suspects another practitioner may be impaired, the nurse's duty is to take action designed both to protect patients and to ensure that the impaired individual receives assistance in regaining optimal function. This advocacy role does not stop once the impairment is identified. Nurses in all roles should advocate for colleagues whose job performance may be impaired to ensure they receive appropriate assistance, treatment, and access to fair institutional and legal processes. This includes supporting the return to practice of the individual who has sought assistance and is ready to resume professional duties (American Nurses Association ANA, 1991).

Many boards of nursing have set up advocacy programs for impaired nurses to provide them with the assistance necessary to overcome the addiction. Information about these programs is available on state board websites.

But what do you do immediately when you suspect a coworker is coming to work impaired? You call your immediate supervisor. Different hospitals have differing procedures on handling such situations, and it is important to follow the procedure. What you do not do is nothing. Many state boards of nursing have investigatory units that will assist the agency in uncovering suspected drug diversion or unsafe practice. In these situations, the health care agency refers the complaint to the state board, which then investigates and determines final action. In such a situation, if the complaint is found to be valid, the state board will have the nurse surrender his or her license to practice. The nurse is then referred to assistance and is monitored by the state board. Reinstatement of the license can occur depending on the rules and regulations of the state board. Nurses can also voluntarily surrender their license if they think that they are in need of assistance.

In the late 1970s, the ANA began efforts to secure assistance for chemically and mentally impaired nurses (Haack & Yocum, 2002). The assistance is in the form of diversion programs, intervention, or peer assistance programs. It is a voluntary, confidential program for RNs whose practice may be impaired because of chemical dependency or mental illness.

EMPLOYEE ASSISTANCE PROGRAMS

All of the issues dealt with in this chapter may be supported by the use of employee assistance programs (EAPs). The majority of health care employers across the United States have created EAPs. An EAP is a confidential, short-term counseling service for employees with personal problems that affect their work performance. EAPs grew out of industrial alcoholism programs of the 1940s. They should be part of a larger company plan to promote wellness that involves written policies, supervisor and employee training, and an approved drug testing program (Canadian Centre for Occupational Health and Safety, 2015).

These programs allow employees to confidentially deal with concerns that may be causing problems in their personal or professional life. As a nurse manager you may refer staff members to this program. An example of an employee issue would be continual patterns of lateness and/or attendance. More serious issues may be for a drug or alcohol abuse problem. A referral can also be a self-referral. EAPs always protect the employee's privacy, and assist employees in getting the help that they need without fear of a break of confidentiality. Family members may also use the EAP in some institutions. Exact steps for the referral process should be in the hospital's policy and procedure manual.

EAP services provide counseling to employees and their families in an attempt to help the employee and his or her family return to a functional unit. EAPs may provide assistance in dealing with the following issues:

- Personal issues
- Job stress
- Relationship issues
- Eldercare, childcare, parenting issues
- Harassment
- Substance abuse
- Separation and loss
- Balancing work and family
- Financial or legal
- Family violence

Some EAP providers are also able to offer other services including retirement or layoff assistance and wellness/health promotion and fitness (e.g., weight control, nutrition, exercise, or smoking). Others may offer advice on long-term illnesses, disability issues, counseling for crisis situations (e.g., death at work), or advice specifically for managers/supervisors in dealing with difficult situations (Canadian Centre for Occupational Health and Safety, 2015).

SUMMARY

The nursing workplace is a complicated environment.

After employment, the nurse needs to be aware of the professional policies and programs that ensure a safe practice workplace. The nurse within a shared governance environment is expected to take a leadership role in the continued development of a safe workplace and to continually advocate for a safe workplace.

CLINICAL CORNER

Lateral Violence: Can She Take It and Can She Make It?

New graduate nurses are among the most vulnerable to becoming a victim of lateral violence. Some experienced nurses seem to believe it is their "duty" to make sure the new graduate has what it takes to make it in their unit. Successful assimilation of the new graduate into the nursing staff is a key responsibility of the preceptor, charge nurse, and nurse manager, as illustrated by the following vignette.

A new graduate nurse is in the second week of her orientation in the surgical intensive care unit (ICU) of an academic teaching hospital. Because this new grad had successfully worked as a tech on the unit while in nursing school, the nurse manager hired her, knowing that some of the nurses oppose hiring any new grads. The preceptor assigned to orient this new graduate is an experienced ICU nurse and an excellent teacher who is committed to seeing that this new nurse succeeds. However, she has been assigned to teach a basic life support course during the morning today, and the charge nurse has been asked to act as preceptor to the new grad. This charge nurse's opinion that new grads do not belong in the ICU setting is well known, but on this busy day there is no other preceptor available. During the interdisciplinary rounds on a very complex patient assigned to the new grad, the charge nurse grills her about aspects of the patient's medical condition that even experienced nurses may not know. Although embarrassed for the new grad, none of the nurses, physicians, or other team members speak up to help the

new grad. Two of the charge nurse's closest friends are heard in the background laughing and saying, "Get her!"

This is an example of sabotage where the new graduate is set up to fail and to look bad in front of the team. It is also an example of the negative behaviors that often drive new graduates out of a unit—and sometimes out of nursing altogether.

How can this negative situation be reversed for the vulnerable new graduate?

1. *Individual intervention* by the preceptor to provide support and encouragement and education to the new graduate to repair the damage done to her self-confidence; this includes suggestions of what the new graduate can say if a similar situation occurs
2. *Private discussion* between preceptor and charge nurse confronting the negative charge nurse's behavior
3. *Group meeting* with nurse manager, all preceptors, and all charge nurses to develop a plan for teaching new graduates and other new staff in a way that is supportive rather than unfair "testing"
4. *Educational offering* about lateral violence in nursing that teaches all staff how to manage episodes of lateral violence and includes them in developing an action plan to eliminate lateral violence from their unit
5. *Intervention with staff* that illustrates how lateral violence behaviors among staff members compromises the care and safety of patients

Karen M. Stanley

EVIDENCE-BASED PRACTICE

Bautistan, J., Lauria, P., Contreras, M., Maranion, M., Villaneuva, H., Sumaguingsing, R., & Abeleda, R. (2019). Specific stressors relate to nurses' job satisfaction, perceived quality of care, and turnover intention. *International Journal of Nursing Practice, 26*(1), e12774.

Nursing is recognized as one of the most stressful occupations. A recent survey found that it is the second most stressful job in the United States (Herbert, 2017). Currently, scholars have shown that stress in nursing practice can lead to poor nursing outcomes, such as job satisfaction (Hayes, Douglas, & Bonner, 2015). Stress is also shown to be related to poor quality of care (Stalpers, Van Der Linden, Kaljouw, & Schuurmans, 2017). Although previous works have demonstrated that stress can lead to poor outcomes, it is unclear which stressors tend to

affect such outcomes. This cross-sectional and descriptive correlational study has the following research questions:

- Which stressor has the highest occurrence?
- Which stressor is related to job satisfaction, perceived quality of care, and turnover intention?

Four hundred and twenty-seven staff nurses working in a 522-bed tertiary care hospital participated. The 34-item Nursing Stress Scale was used to measure stress. The three dependent variables of job satisfaction, perceived quality of care, and turnover intention were measured by items from various reliable scales.

Based on the results, respondents reported that stress caused by workload had the highest mean score (M = 1.70, standard deviation [SD] = .71). A close inspection of the items regarding workload shows that stress caused by

Continued

EVIDENCE-BASED PRACTICE—cont'd

having "too many non-bedside nursing tasks" (M = 1.95, SD = 89) had the highest mean score. This was followed by other workload items such as "not enough staff to adequately cover the unit" (M = 1.86, SD = .99) and "breakdown of the computer" (M = 1.78, SD = .91). Conversely, the stressor that had the lowest occurrence was work uncertainty (M = .83, SD = .66).

Among various stressors, only workload (B = −.32, B = −.42, $p < .001$) was negatively related to job satisfaction. This indicates that a high workload is likely to reduce nurses' job satisfaction. Similarly, only workload was negatively related to perceived quality of care (B = −.27, B = −.26, $p < .001$). This indicates that a high workload reduces nurses' perceived quality of care that they render to patients.

Finally, workload (B = .30, B = .27, $p < .001$) and conflict with nurses (B = .41, B = .28, $p = .004$) were positively related with turnover intention. This indicates that a high workload and conflicts with nurses increases nurses' intention to resign. It was also found that younger nurses (B = −.04, B = −21, $p = .004$) and those assigned to specialty areas (B = −.25, B = −.16, $p = .004$) were more likely to report greater turnover intention.

The results have several implications for nursing management. First, it is crucial for nurse managers to have an open line of communication with their staff. Previous research shows that conflicts often arise and remain unresolved because of poor communication between staff nurses and their superiors (Wagner et al., 2015). Stress can be mitigated when there is an open line of communication between staff nurses and their superiors. Second, the results also reiterate the importance of resolving workload issues. The utilization of workforce date analytics needs to be further explored.

References

Hayes, B., Douglas, C., & Bonner, A. (2015). Work environment, job satisfaction, stress and burnout among hemodialysis nurses. *Journal of Nursing Management, 23*(5), 588–598.

Herbert, T. Have you got one of the most stressful jobs? (2017). <https://metro.co.uk/2017/11/08/have-you-got-one-of-the-most-stressful-jobs-7063089/> Accessed July 2019.

Stalpers, D., Van Der Linden, D., Kaljouw, M., & Schuurmans, M. (2017). Nurse-perceived quality of care in intensive care units and associations with work environment characteristics: a multicentre survey study. *Journal of Advanced Nursing, 73*(6), 1482–1490.

Wagner, J., Bezuidenhout, M.C., & Roos, J.H. (2015). Communication Satisfaction of professional nurses working in public hospitals. *Journal of Nursing management, 23*(8), 974–982. https://doi.org/10.1111/jonm.12243.

NCLEX® EXAMINATION QUESTIONS

1. Several laws have been implemented to ensure that there are equal employment opportunities for all individuals regardless of race, color, national origin, religion, sex, age, or disability. As a nurse you should:
   A. Be aware of the different acts to protect employees
   B. Not need to be involved with this
   C. Be aware that human resources takes care of this issue
   D. Know that once the nurse is hired, you can ask questions about race, religion

2. The list of strategies for conflict resolution according to Huber (2013) includes avoiding, withholding, and commending. As a new nurse you may be in a situation of conflict. What would you do?
   A. Inform my preceptor
   B. Inform the nurse manager
   C. Inform human resources
   D. Keep it to yourself to prevent further conflict

3. You have overheard an individual speak for themselves in a way that you can hear, this concern is called:
   A. Confronting
   B. Collaborating
   C. Problem solving
   D. Competing

4. You have witnessed another nurse using an assertive strategy in which one individual's needs are satisfied at another's expense, this is called competing. What would you do as a new nurse still on probation?
   A. Do not discuss this with anyone
   B. Mention this behavior to your preceptor
   C. Wait and see if it happens again before doing anything
   D. Tell the human resource director because it is a human resource issue

5. You have been assigned to work the 7 a.m. to 7 p.m. shift. There is a culture on this shift of not working as a team and having issues with assignments. In managing conflict, what is the first step?
   A. Determine the cause of the conflict
   B. Determine who is right and who is wrong
   C. Determine the punishment for the people in conflict
   D. Determine who was the aggressive person

6. You have witnessed a nurse that seems to have anger issues. You are the charge nurse and have asked this nurse to come into the nurse managers' office. Which of the following does not maintain behavior that helps diffuse anger?
   A. Do not match threats
   B. Avoid any behavior that may be interpreted as aggressive
   C. Yell louder at the individual who is shouting at you
   D. Do not give orders

7. Which of the following is not considered a risk factor for violence in the health care setting?
   A. Isolated work with patients during exams and treatments
   B. Unlimited public access
   C. Overcrowded waiting rooms
   D. Security guard appointed to walk employee to car

8. You have witnessed workplace violence, a nurse and a patient care technician speaking loudly near a patient room. Which agency regulates violent acts (including physical assaults and threats of assaults) directed toward persons at work or on duty?
   A. U.S. Department of Justice
   B. National Institute for Occupational Safety and Health (NIOSH)
   C. Occupational Safety and Health Administration (OSHA)
   D. American Nurses Association (ANA)

9. As a nurse you should be aware of the different agencies that monitor cases of intentional employment discrimination. Which agency has an act in place to protect the employee?
   A. The Civil Rights Act of 1991
   B. Title I and Title V Act of 1990
   C. Title VII of the Civil Rights Act of 1964
   D. The Equal Pay Act (EPA) of 1963

10. Once you have evaluated the unit you were assigned to as a new nurse, the unit seems to have issues of horizontal violence. Which of the following is not an act of horizontal violence?
    A. A nursing assistant tells the nurse she should not bother her or she will hurt her
    B. Two nurses are speaking loudly and one nurse pulls the arm of the individual
    C. One nursing assistant tells her coworker, another nursing assistant, that she will hurt her when the shift is over
    D. Two employees are speaking to each other about the assignment and speak with the charge nurse about it

Answers: 1. A   2. B   3. A   4. C   5. A   6. C   7. D
8. B   9. A   10. D

REFERENCES

American Association of Critical Care Nurses [AACN]. (2004). *Position statement: Workplace violence prevention*. Aliso Viejo, CA: Author.

American Nurses Association [ANA]. (1991). ANA position statement on abuse of prescription drugs. <www.nursingworld.org/MainMenuCategories/Policy-Advocacy/Positions-and-Resolutions/ANAPositionStatements/Position-Statements-Alphabetically/Abuse-of-Prescription-Drugs.html> Accessed July 2019.

American Nurses Association, Department of Government Affairs. (2007). Health care worker safety. <www.anapoliticalpower.org> Accessed July 2019.

Bureau of Labor Statistics (BLS). (2011). *Workplace injuries and illnesses-2011*. Washington, DC: US Department of Labor.

Canadian Centre for Occupational Health and Safety. (2015). Employee assistance programs (EAP). <www.ccohs.ca/oshanswers/hsprograms/eap.html> Accessed July 2019.

Cook, J., Green, M., & Topp, R. (2001). Exploring the impact of physician verbal abuse on perioperative nurses. *AORN Journal, 74*(3), 317–320, 322–327, 329–331.

Ehrmann, G., Zuzelo P.R. (2007). Conference abstracts: 2007. Presented at the National Association of Clinical Nurse Specialists (NACNS) National Conference, February 28–March 3, 2007: Phoenix, AZ.

Emergency Nurses Association (2009). *Workplace Violence*. www.ena.org. Accessed July 2019.

Haack, M. R., & Yocum, C. J. (2002). State policies and nurses with substance abuse disorders. *Journal of Nursing Scholarship, 34*(1), 89–94.

Huber, D. L. (2013). *Leadership and nursing care management* (5th ed.). Philadelphia: Elsevier.

Johansen, M. (2012, February). Keeping the peace: Conflict management strategies for nurse managers. *Nursing Management, 43*(2), 50–54.

Longo, J. (2007). Horizontal violence among nursing students. *Archives of Psychiatric Nursing, 21*(3), 177–178.

Longo, J., & Sherman, R. (2007). Leveling horizontal violence. *Nursing Management*, 38(3), 34–37, 50–51.

Marquis, B., & Huston, C. (2014). *Leadership roles and management functions in nursing: theory and application* (5th ed.). Philadelphia: Lippincott Williams & Wilkins.

National Institute for Occupational Safety and Health [NIOSH]. (2002a). Occupational violence. DHHS (NIOSH) publication No. 2002–2101. www.cdc.gov/niosh/docs/2002-101/.

National Institute for Occupational Safety and Health [NIOSH]. (2002b). Workplace violence. DHHS (NIOSH) publication No. 2002–2101. www.cdc.gov/niosh/docs/2002-101/.

Rosenstein, A. (2002). Nurse-physician relationships: impact on nurse satisfaction and retention. *American Journal of Nursing*, 102, 26–34.

The Joint Commission. (2008). Sentinel event alert: Behaviors that undermine a culture of safety. <www.jointcommission.org/assets/1/18/SEA_40> Accessed July 2019.

The U.S. Equal Employment Opportunity Commission. (2015) Sexual harassment. www.eeoc.gov/laws/types/sexual_harassment.cfm.

Tomey, A. M. (2004). *Guide to nursing management and leadership* (7th ed.). St. Louis: Mosby.

U.S. Department of Justice. (2011). "State" Bill "The Violence Prevention in Health Care Facility Act." <www.nursingworld.org/MainMenuCategories/Policy-Advocacy/State/Legislative-Agenda-Reports/State-WorkplaceViolence/ModelWorkplaceViolenceBill.pdf> Accessed July 2019.

Yoder-Wise, P. S., & Kowalski, K. E. (2006). *Beyond leading and managing: Nursing administration for the future*. St. Louis: Elsevier.

BIBILOGRAPHY

American Nurses Association [ANA]. (2012). *Bullying in the workplace: reversing a culture*. Silver Spring, MD: ANA.

Becher, J., & Visovsky, C. (2012). Horizontal violence in nursing. *Medical Surgical Nursing*, 21(4), 210–213.

Erikson, L., & Williams-Evans, S. (2000). Attitudes of emergency nurses regarding patient assaults. *Journal of Emergency Nursing*, 26(3), 210–215.

Gates, D.M., & Kroeger, F. (2003). Violence against nurses: The silent epidemic. *ISNA Bulletin*, 29, 25–29.

Jones, R. A. (2007). *Nursing leadership and management: theories, processes and practice*. Philadelphia: F. A. Davis.

Longo, J., Dean, A., Norris, S. D., Wexner, S. W., & Kent, L. N. (2011). It starts with a conversation: A community approach to creating healthy work environments. *Journal of Continuing Education in Nursing*, 42(1), 27–35.

Maher-Brisen, P. (2011). Addiction: an occupational hazard in nursing. *American Journal of Nursing*, 107(8), 778–779.

Occupational Safety and Health Administration [OSHA], U.S. Department of Labor. (2003). *Guidelines for preventing workplace violence for health care and social service workers*. Washington, DC: OSHA. OSHA publication 3148 (rev. 2003).

Roche, M., Diers, D., Duffield, C., & Catling-Paull, C. (2010). Violence toward nurses, the work environment, and patient outcomes. *Journal of Nursing Scholarship*, 42(1), 13–22.

Sullivan, E., Bissel, L., & Williams, E. (1988). *Chemical dependency in nursing: The deadly diversion*. Menlo Park, CA: Addison-Wesley Nursing.

Thomas, C., & Siela, D. (2011). The impaired nurse: would you know what to do if you suspected substance abuse? *American Nurse Today*, 6(8).

Case Scenario: An advanced practice nurse (APN) is hired by a Magnet health care organization that implements specific councils for each level of decision making. The new APN is hired to help guide the organization in reassessing structure to ensure the administration's desired policy of self-governance. However, there has been a lot of conflict within the organization between individuals desiring more empowerment of nurses and those who understand those desires but found their experiences in more hierarchical structures to be "efficient and time-tested." The new APN's first decision, then, is to have an all-inconclusive workshop in which participants will share their understanding of effective governance and decision making in the hopes of helping everyone come to an understanding and thus begin to move forward with a consensual goal.

ITEM TYPE: CLOZE

1. **Choose the *most likely* options to complete the statement below** (Chapter 6).

   In helping each side establish their viewpoint, the APN points out that it is the ____1____ who provide a forum for shared decision making in nursing practice and best practice initiatives across the organization by representatives from the UBCs and central shared governance councils, while the ____2____ is concerned with the management of resources as defined in the strategic plan and nursing conceptual framework.

Options for 1	Options for 2
A. Nurse Executive Council	E. Nurse Executive Council
B. Advanced Practice Nurse Council	F. Advanced Practice Nurse Council
C. Nurse Practice Coordination Council	G. Nurse Practice Coordination Council
D. Clinical Practice Council	H. Clinical Practice Council

ITEM TYPE: EXTENDED MULTIPLE RESPONSE

2. The APN overhears one small group arguing over an ongoing unit conflict between staff members. Their unit leader looks to the APN for help. Once the basis and cause of this conflict is determined, which of the following strategies should the APN advise their unit leader to use to move toward a positive outcome? (Chapter 6)

CHECK ALL THAT APPLY

___A. Avoiding for de-escalation
___B. Confronting
___C. Encouraging withdrawal
___D. Taking a wait-and-see approach
___E. Compromising
___F. Reassuring

ANSWERS

1. C, E—The Nurse Practice Coordination Council provides a forum for shared decision making in nursing practice and best practice initiatives across the organization by representatives from the UBCs and central shared governance councils, while the Nurse Executive Council is concerned with the management of resources as defined in the strategic plan and nursing conceptual framework.
2. B, E

SECTION 3

Exemplary Professional Practice

SECTION OUTLINE

127

10

Professional Development

OBJECTIVES

- Discuss professional development opportunities of the nurse.
- Analyze the nurse's responsibility in individual professional development.
- Analyze the progression of nursing clinical competence.
- Discuss the importance of professional organizations in professional development.
- Identify the steps and progression of the staff registered nurse (RN) in a clinical ladder program.
- Review the various certifications available for the nurse.

KEY TERMS

certification recognition by a professional organization of nursing knowledge in a particular specialty

competencies areas in which employees are to be determined to be qualified to perform

clinical ladder process whereby the employee is developed for progression within a position category

organizational learning development of new knowledge and skills within an organization; such learning is achieved through research, development, evaluation, and improvement cycles

professional organizations the commitment to professional development is a hallmark of a Magnet organization and any organization with a focus on excellence. Magnet-recognized organizations use multiple strategies to support a lifelong learning culture that promotes continued role development, academic achievement, and career advancement

BENNER FIVE STAGES

As the new nurse enters the workforce, it is important to realize that this is just the beginning of the professional journey. Benner (1984) posits that the nurse moves through five stages of clinical competence: novice, advanced beginner, competent, proficient, and expert nurse (Box 10.1).

These different levels reflect changes in three general aspects of skilled performance:

1. The first is a movement from reliance on abstract principles to the use of past concrete experience as paradigms.
2. The second is a change in the learner's perception of the demand situation, in which the situation is seen less as a compilation of equally relevant bits and more as a complete whole, in which only certain parts are relevant.
3. The third is a passage from detached observation to involved performer. The performer no longer stands outside the situation but is now truly engaged in the situation.

BOX 10.1 Five Stages of Transition from Novice to Competent Practitioner

Stage I
The nurse is overwhelmed by the number of potentially relevant details that pertain to a patient's care.

Stage II
The new nurse may suffer exhaustion while trying to manage patients within the confines of the unit guidelines and protocols.

Stage III
Successfully embracing policy and protocol enables feelings of confidence and serves as a critical marker of readiness.

Stage IV
A period of transition in the preceptee–preceptor relationship. The preceptor serves as a resource, frequently retreating from the forefront of patient care.

Stage V
The "comfort zone" of a preceptor is withdrawn as orientation is successfully completed.

(From Reddish, M., & Kaplan, L. (2007). When are new graduates competent in the critical care unit? *Critical Care Quarterly, 30*(3),199–205.)

As you read this content, think of your own areas of experience in nursing. Decide where you think you fit.

Stage 1: Novice

Beginners have not had experience in any of the situations that they are expected to deal with as professional nurses. Novices are taught rules to help them perform their duties. The rules are context-free and independent of specific cases; hence, the rules tend to be applied universally. The rule-governed behavior typical of the novice is extremely limited and inflexible. As such, novices have no "life experience" in the application of rules.

"Just tell me what I need to do and I'll do it."

Stage 2: Advanced Beginner

Advanced beginners are those who can demonstrate marginally acceptable performance of their nursing duties, or those who have coped with enough real situations to note (or to have pointed out to them by a mentor) the recurring meaningful situational components. These components require prior experience in actual situations for recognition. Principles to guide actions begin to be formulated. The principles are based on experience.

Stage 3: Competent

Nurses who have been on the job in the same or similar situations for 2 or 3 years develop competence and begin to see their actions in terms of long-range goals or plans of which they are consciously aware. For the competent nurse, a plan establishes a perspective, and the plan is based on considerable conscious, abstract, analytic contemplation of the problem. The conscious, deliberate planning that is characteristic of this skill level helps achieve efficiency and organization. The competent nurse lacks the speed and flexibility of the proficient nurse but does have a feeling of mastery and the ability to cope with and manage the many contingencies of clinical nursing. The competent person does not yet have enough experience to recognize a situation in terms of an overall picture or in terms of which aspects are most salient and most important.

Stage 4: Proficient

The proficient performer perceives a situation as a whole rather than as chopped-up parts or aspects, and performance is guided by maxims. Proficient nurses understand a situation as a whole because they perceive its meaning in terms of long-term goals. The proficient nurse learns from experience what typical events to expect in a given situation and how plans need to be modified in response to these events. The proficient nurse can now recognize when the expected normal picture does not materialize. This holistic understanding improves the proficient nurse's decision making; it becomes less labored because the nurse now has a perspective about which of the many existing attributes and aspects in the present situation are the important ones. The proficient nurse uses maxims as guides, which reflect what would appear to the competent or novice performer as unintelligible nuances of the situation; maxims can mean one thing at one time and quite another thing later. Once one has a deep understanding of the situation overall, however, the maxim provides direction as to what must be taken into account. Maxims reflect nuances of the situation.

Stage 5: The Expert

The expert performer no longer relies on an analytic principle (rule, guideline, and maxim) to connect an understanding of the situation to an appropriate action. The expert nurse, with an enormous background of experience, now has an intuitive grasp of each situation and zeroes in on the accurate region of the problem without wasteful consideration of a large range of unfruitful, alternative diagnoses and solutions. The expert operates from a deep understanding of the total situation. For instance the chess master, when asked why he or she made a particularly masterful move, will just say, "Because it felt right. It looked good." The performer is no longer aware of features and rules; his or her performance becomes fluid and flexible and highly proficient. This is not to say that the expert never uses analytic tools. Highly skilled analytic ability is necessary for those situations with which the nurse has had no previous experience. Analytic tools are also necessary for those times when the expert gets a wrong grasp of the situation and then finds that events and behaviors are not occurring as expected. When alternative perspectives are not available to the clinician, the only way out of a wrong grasp of the problem is by using analytic problem solving (Benner, 1984, pp. 13–34).

You do progress in professional competence as you work. Self-assessment of your current level of performance is an important function in nursing. Much of your progression will also greatly depend on the work environment. The organization provides the environment for the clinical progression of all staff, both for organizational needs and for the personal development of the nurse. Such professional work environments are evidenced in the various health care organizations that have achieved Magnet status (American Nurses Credentialing Center ANCC, 2019).

STAFF COMPETENCY

The Joint Commission states that a hospital must provide the right number of competent staff to meet the needs of the patients (2019). Competent staff are qualified and able to perform the work according to professional standards. Staffing is discussed in Chapter 12. To meet the goal of providing adequate competent staff, the hospital must carry out the following processes and activities:

- Providing competent staff either through traditional employer-employee arrangements or through contractual arrangements with other entities or persons.
- Orienting, training, and educating staff (Box 10.2).
- Providing ongoing in-service and other education and training to increase staff knowledge of specific work-related issues.
- Assessing, maintaining, and improving staff competence.
- Ongoing, periodic assessing of competence to evaluate staff members' continuing abilities to perform throughout their association with the organization.
- Promoting self-development and learning. Staff is encouraged to pursue ongoing professional development goals and provide feedback about the work environment (The Joint Commission, 2019).

BOX 10.2 New Employee Orientation: Mandatory Content

- Mission and governance
- Service excellence requirements
- Code of conduct
- Fire safety
- Safe environment
- Culture of safety
- Age-specific patient content
- Infection control
- Blood-borne pathogens
- Process improvement
- Corporate compliance
- Just workplace
- Health Insurance Portability and Accountability Act (HIPAA)
- Benefits

American Nurses Credentialing Center ANCC, 2019 in the Magnet model calls for the continuous professional development of the nurse as evidenced by advancing degree completion and professional certification. They also call for nurses to participate in professional development activities designed to improve their knowledge, skills, and practice in the workplace. These professional practice activities are designed to improve the practice of nursing and patient outcomes. Both the American Nurses Credentialing Center ANCC, 2019 and the IOM (2010) in the *Future of Nursing* report call for the facilitation of the effective transition of nurses and advanced practice nurses (APNs) into the work environment. This occurs through residency programs at all levels (new graduates, experienced nurses moving to a new specialty, new APN graduates, and APNs moving to new areas of practice).

The nurse's initial step in professional development occurs through an organizational orientation, which is discussed in Chapter 14.

CONTINUED EMPLOYEE DEVELOPMENT

As nurses progress from novice to expert, many health care facilities have a system that allows for promotion of nurses along clinical ladders. Education and benefits for progression in clinical competence form the basis for such ladders.

CLINICAL LADDERS

Clinical ladders are programs that reward nurses for their advancement in nursing. It permits horizontal advancement, allowing excellent clinicians to remain in their role at the bedside. Nurses advance through a determined number of levels within a position category based on predetermined criteria. When a level is reached, there are additional advantages for the nurse. When the highest level for a particular position has been reached, advancement requires additional education in nursing.

Clinical ladders were developed in organizations in reaction to Benner's concept of *From Novice to Expert* (1984). They were developed as a means to promote an individual's growth as a professional nurse on the path to expert status. Using organizationally established criteria in conjunction with an interview, health care organizations decide on the merits of individual clinical advancement. The process for professional-clinical

career ladder progression is usually both clinically and academically based.

Sentara RMH Medical Center supports an environment that promotes professionalism and excellence in nursing care. The following are some areas of clinical practice and professional excellence that are recognized in this clinical ladder program:

- Professional nursing service
- Clinical nursing competence
- Leadership skills
- Continuing education
- Evidence-based practice in nursing
- Nursing career plans
- Volunteer nursing/health service outside of hospital
- Customer service and hospital-wide initiatives for excellence
- National certification in nursing specialty area
- Shared governance participation on hospital or unit committees
- Health education for staff, patients, and others

Objectives

- Promote, recognize, and reward excellence in clinical practice and professionalism of RMH nursing staff
- Promote exceptional bedside nursing patient care and clinical performance by participation in the areas of leadership and continuing education and through evidence-based practice participation
- Provide clear delineation of nursing competence levels
- Use nurses who have been educationally prepared for a variety of levels of practice
- Encourage excellence in practice to ensure quality care of patients
- Champion recruitment and retention of qualified RNs
- Commit to customer service and RMH excellence standards
- Promote participation in volunteer community and health nursing service

Automatic Advancement Levels I and II

- Clinical Nurse I: Clinical ladder entry level for a new graduate bedside RN. After successful completion of department orientation, a nurse will automatically advance to a Clinical Nurse I.
- Description: A new bedside RN developing nursing skills, expanding knowledge, and assuming job responsibilities.
- Clinical Nurse II: After completion of a year of employment, and receiving a satisfactory evaluation, a

bedside RN will automatically advance to Clinical Nurse II level. A newly hired, experienced RN (with at least 1 year of recent nursing experience) will be placed at a Clinical Nurse II level. After successful completion of department orientation and first successful evaluation, the nurse may advance to higher clinical ladder levels following all program requirements. All RNs will remain at Clinical Nurse II level if they do not choose to advance to higher levels.

- Description: An experienced bedside RN capable of independent patient care. Actively developing more advanced nursing skills and knowledge through education and involvement in nursing activities beyond basic job requirements and responsibilities.

Automatic Advancement Levels III, IV, and V

- Clinical Nurse III: Requires annual portfolio submission and complying with all clinical ladder program requirements. Advancement to this level requires self-paced and self-motivated participation.
- Description: A bedside RN highly skilled in patient care. Demonstrates leadership and mentorship abilities. Active involvement in continuing education and in nursing activities beyond the basic job requirements and responsibilities.
- Clinical Nurse IV: Requires annual portfolio submission and compliance with all clinical ladder program requirements. Advancement to this level requires highly self-paced and self-motivated participation.
- Description: A bedside RN who has a broad base of advanced nursing experience. Recognized for professional nursing leadership and knowledge. Leadership extends to education and development of others. Involvement in multiple nursing activities beyond basic job requirements and responsibilities. Acquiring research skills by participating in evaluation of clinical outcomes to improve nursing through evidence-based practice.
- Clinical Nurse V: Requires annual portfolio submission and compliance with all clinical ladder program requirements. Advancement to this highest level on the clinical ladders requires extraordinary and exceptional self-paced and self-motivated participation. (Must be nationally certified in nursing specialty.)
- Description: A bedside registered nurse who has exceptional advanced nursing experience. Recognized

for expert professional nursing leadership and knowledge. Leadership is recognized at a role-model level. Involvement in multiple nursing activities beyond the basic job requirements and responsibilities. Active and ongoing professional involvement in improving nursing through evidenced-based practice, such as research activities, writing a published nursing article, etc. All submitted evidence-based practice submissions and research materials must be presented in a professional format with extensive information such as charts, graphs, studies, stats, outcomes, etc.

(Clinical ladders developed by Rockingham Memorial Hospital. www.rmhonline.org/rmh_human_resources/pages/RMH_clinical_ladders.html.)

As nurses move up the clinical ladder, the educational progression of the nurse becomes more specific. The organization-wide specific education goes beyond the requirements mandated by regulators to those that are specific to the needs and current performance of the organization. Organizations are required to perform annual needs assessments to determine the educational needs of the staff. These assessments need to go beyond what the staff "wants" to learn and need to move toward an outcomes-based model, where the "need to know" education is planned (Fig. 10.1).

Such an educational needs assessment must occur at all levels of the organization so that the educational needs of all levels of nurses (administrators, APN, staff nurses, managers, etc.) can be planned. The nurse's role here is to be self-aware of the current levels of performance outcomes in his or her area and the educational needs based on current evidence-based practice changes.

Not all continuing professional development will be provided by the organization. It is the responsibility of nurses to search out continuing education opportunities and match them to their professional goals. Nurses are expected to set practice and professional goals that align with those of the organization on an annual basis. These goals are set during the annual performance review process (Chapter 15). They most always include professional growth goals.

Large amounts of professional continuing education occur through the professional organizations and certifying organizations within nursing. Box 10.3 lists the varying professional organizations within nursing.

(The Ultimate List of Professional Associations for Nurses [2014]. https://nurse.org/orgs.shtml.)

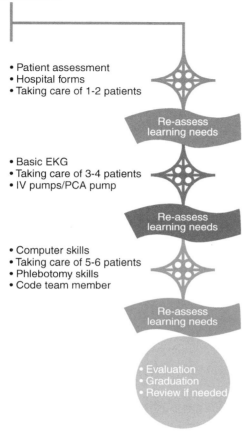

- Start orientation
- Review policy/procedures
- Hospital vision/mission

- Patient assessment
- Hospital forms
- Taking care of 1-2 patients

Re-assess learning needs

- Basic EKG
- Taking care of 3-4 patients
- IV pumps/PCA pump

Re-assess learning needs

- Computer skills
- Taking care of 5-6 patients
- Phlebotomy skills
- Code team member

Re-assess learning needs

- Evaluation
- Graduation
- Review if needed

Fig. 10.1 A sample training roadmap. (Harris, 2007).

BOX 10.3 Sampling of Professional Nursing Organizations

- Academy of Medical-Surgical Nurses
- Academy of Neonatal Nursing
- Air & Surface Transport Nurses Association
- American Academy of Ambulatory Care Nursing
- American Academy of Nurse Practitioners
- American Assembly for Men in Nursing
- American Assisted Living Nurses Association
- American Association of Colleges of Nursing
- American Association of Critical-Care Nurses
- American Association of Diabetes Educators
- American Association of Heart Failure Nurses
- American Association of the History of Nursing
- American Association of Legal Nurse Consultants
- American Association of Managed Care Nurses
- American Association of Neuroscience Nurses
- American Association of Nurse Anesthetists
- American Association of Nurse Assessment Coordinators
- The American Association of Nurse Attorneys
- American Association of Nurse Life Care Planners
- American Association of Occupational Health Nurses
- American College of Cardiovascular Nurses
- American College of Nurse-Midwives
- American College of Nurse Practitioners
- American Holistic Nurses Association
- American Nephrology Nurses Association
- American Nurses Association
- American Nursing Informatics Association
- American Organization of Nurse Executives
- American Pediatric Surgical Nurses Association
- American Psychiatric Nurses Association
- American Society of Ophthalmic Registered Nurses
- American Society for Pain Management Nursing
- American Society of PeriAnesthesia Nurses
- American Society of Plastic Surgical Nurses
- Army Nurse Corps Association
- Asian American/Pacific Islander Nurses Association
- Association of Camp Nurses
- Association of Child and Adolescent Psychiatric Nurses
- Association of Child Neurology Nurses
- Association of Community Health Nursing Educators
- Association of Faculties of Pediatric Nurse Practitioners
- Association of Nurses in AIDS Care
- Association of periOperative Registered Nurses
- Association of Rehabilitation Nurses
- Association of Women's Health, Obstetric and Neonatal Nurses
- Dermatology Nurses' Association
- Emergency Nurses Association
- Endocrine Nurses Society
- Federal Nurses Association
- Home Healthcare Nurses Association
- Hospice and Palliative Nurses Association
- Infusion Nurses Society
- International Association of Forensic Nurses
- International Council of Nurses
- International Nurses Society on Addictions
- International Society of Nurses in Genetics
- International Society of Psychiatric-Mental Health Nurses
- National Alaska Native American Indian Nurses Association
- National Association of Bariatric Nurses

- National Association of Directors of Nursing Administration of Long-Term Care
- National Association of Clinical Nurse Specialists
- National Association of Hispanic Nurses
- National Association of Indian Nurses of America
- National Association of Neonatal Nurses
- National Association of Nurse Massage Therapists
- National Association of Nurse Practitioners in Women's Health
- National Association of Orthopaedic Nurses
- National Association of Pediatric Nurse Practitioners
- National Association for Practical Nurse Education and Service
- National Association of Registered Nurse First Assistants
- National Association of School Nurses
- National Association of State School Nurse Consultants
- National Black Nurses Association
- National Federation of Licensed Practical Nurses
- National Gerontological Nursing Association
- National League for Nursing
- National Nurses in Business Association
- National Nursing Staff Development Organization
- National Organization for Associate Degree Nursing
- National Organization of Nurse Practitioner Faculties
- National Private Duty Association
- National Student Nurses' Association
- Navy Nurse Corps Association
- Nurses Organization of Veterans Affairs
- Oncology Nursing Society
- Pediatric Endocrinology Nursing Society
- Respiratory Nursing Society
- Rural Nurse Organization
- Philippine Nurses Association of America
- Sigma Theta Tau International Honor Society of Nursing
- Society of Gastroenterology Nurses and Associates
- Society of Otorhinolaryngology and Head-Neck Nurses
- Society of Pediatric Nursing
- Society of Trauma Nurses
- Society of Urologic Nurses and Associates
- Society for Vascular Nursing
- Transcultural Nursing Society
- Visiting Nurse Associations of America
- Wound, Ostomy, and Continence Nurses Society

Nursing organizations can be beneficial to all nurses because they help complete the circle between clinical practice and the outside factors that influence nursing. Nursing membership in a professional organization is of vital importance to the future of nursing. Membership in such an organization will assist you in keeping current with up-to-date evidence-based practice and research in addition to providing you a networking base with fellow nursing professionals. It will also allow you access to some of the most current conferences and education within your specialty (Nock, 2017).

One of the first questions a nurse ending the second year of employment needs to ask is, "Do I need to pursue a professional practice certification?" The answer is "yes," especially if you work in a Magnet institution. Certification signifies that the nurse possesses expert knowledge in a practice area. Magnet organizations are expected to have increasing numbers of certified nurses in the future. According to the American Association of Colleges of Nursing, in 2013 there were 62,818 nurses certified at the specialty (not advanced practice) level; health care organizations are strategically planning to increase these numbers. These certifications only reflect those certifications from the American Association of Colleges of Nursing, not other specialty organizations. There are 310 recognized certifications in nursing. Box 10.4 provides a complete list.

BOX 10.4   Titles of Various Nursing Certifications

- Accredited Case Manager
- Acute Care Nurse Practitioner
- Adult Clinical Nurse Specialist
- Adult Nurse Practitioner
- Adult Psychiatric & Mental Health Clinical Nurse Specialist
- Adult Psychiatric & Mental Health Nurse Practitioner
- Adult-Gerontology Acute Care Nurse Practitioner
- Adult-Gerontology Primary Care Nurse Practitioner
- Advance Certified Hospice and Palliative Nurse
- Advanced Certified Hyperbaric Registered Nurse
- Advanced Critical Care Clinical Nurse Specialist: Adult-Gerontology
- Advanced Diabetes Management for Clinical Nurse Specialist & Nurse Practitioner
- Advanced Health & Fitness Specialist
- Advanced Holistic Nurse Board Certified
- Advanced Neurovascular Practitioner
- Advanced Oncology Certified Clinical Nurse Specialist
- Advanced Oncology Certified Nurse
- Advanced Oncology Certified Nurse Practitioner
- Advanced Practice Nurse in Genetics
- Advanced Public Health Nurse (Public/Community Health Clinical Nurse Specialist [PHCNS], BC before 2008)
- Advanced Public Health Nursing

- AIDS Certified Registered Nurse
- Ambulatory Care Nursing
- Bone Marrow Transplant Certified Nurse
- Cardiac Medicine (Subspecialty) Certification
- Cardiac Rehabilitation Nurse
- Cardiac Surgery (Subspecialty) Certification
- Cardiac/Vascular Nurse
- Cardiovascular (Cath Lab, Intervention IF RCIS-certified)
- Cardiovascular (CCU/CVICU and Cath lab)
- Cardiovascular (Ed, telemetry, & stepdown)
- Cardiovascular Educator
- Cardiovascular Nurse Practitioner
- Cardiovascular Nurse Specialist
- Care Manager Certified
- Case Management Nurse
- Certificate for OASIS Specialist – Clinical
- Certification in Hyperbaric Technology
- Certification in Transcultural Nursing – Advanced
- Certification Specialist in Healthcare Accreditation
- Certified Addictions Registered Nurse
- Certified Administrator Surgery Center
- Certified Aesthetic Nurse Specialist
- Certified Alcohol & Drug Counselor
- Certified Ambulatory Perianesthesia Nurse
- Certified Anesthesia Technician
- Certified Anesthesia Technologist
- Certified Anticoagulation Care Provider
- Certified Assisted Living Administrator
- Certified Asthma Educator
- Certified Athletic Trainer
- Certified Bariatric Nurse
- Certified Brain Injury Specialist
- Certified Brain Injury Specialist Trainer
- Certified Breast Care Nurse
- Certified Breast Patient Navigator – Cancer
- Certified Breast Patient Navigator – Imaging
- Certified Breastfeeding Counselor
- Certified Cardiac Device Specialist
- Certified Cardiographic Technician
- Certified Cardiothoracic Nurse (within Cardiac Surgery Subspecialty)
- Certified Case Manager
- Certified Chemical Dependency Counselor
- Certified Childbirth Educator
- Certified Clinical Documentation Specialist
- Certified Clinical Hemodialysis Technician
- Certified Clinical Research Coordinator
- Certified Clinical Research Professional
- Certified Clinical Transplant Coordinator
- Certified Clinical Transplant Nurse
- Certified Coding Associate
- Certified Coding Specialist

- Certified Continence Care Nurse
- Certified Correctional Health Professional
- Certified Corrections Nurse
- Certified Diabetes Educator
- Certified Diabetes Educator Certification
- Certified Dialysis Nurse
- Certified Director of Nursing in Long Term Care
- Certified Disability Management Specialist
- Certified Emergency Nurse
- Certified Enterostomal Therapy Nurse (C) Canada
- Certified EP Specialist
- Certified Flight Registered Nurse
- Certified Foot Care Nurse (new)
- Certified Forensic Nurse
- Certified Gastrointestinal Registered Nurse
- Certified General Nursing Practice
- Certified Health Care Compliance
- Certified Health Care Recruiter
- Certified Health Education Specialist
- Certified Healthcare Emergency Professionals
- Certified Healthcare Executive
- Certified Healthcare Quality Management
- Certified Healthcare Simulation Educator
- Certified Heart Failure Nurse
- Certified Hematopoetic Transport Coordinator
- Certified Hemodialysis Nurse
- Certified Home/Hospice Care Executive
- Certified Hospice and Palliative Nurse
- Certified Hospice and Palliative Pediatric Nurse
- Certified Hyperbaric Registered Nurse
- Certified Hyperbaric Registered Nurse Clinician
- Certified in Cardiovascular Nursing (C) Canada
- Certified in Cardiovascular Perfusion
- Certified in Community Health Nursing (C) Canada
- Certified in Executive Nursing Practice
- Certified in Gastroenterology Nursing (C) Canada
- Certified in Healthcare Research Compliance
- Certified in Hospice Palliative Care Nursing (C) Canada
- Certified in Infection Control
- Certified in Medical-Surgical Nursing (C) Canada
- Certified in Nephrology (C) Canada
- Certified in Neuroscience Nursing (C) Canada
- Certified in Occupational Health Nursing (C) Canada
- Certified in Oncology Nursing (C) Canada
- Certified in Perinatal Loss Care
- Certified in Perioperative Nursing (C) Canada
- Certified in Psychiatric and Mental Health Nursing (C) Canada
- Certified in Rehabilitation Nursing (C) Canada
- Certified in Thanatology: Death, Dying and Bereavement
- Certified Infant Massage Instructor/Educator
- Certified Institutional Review Board (IRB) Professional

- Certified Joint Commission Professional
- Certified Labor Support Doula
- Certified Managed Care Nurse
- Certified Materials & Resource Professional
- Certified Medical Audit Specialist
- Certified Medical Office Manager
- Certified Medical-Surgical Registered Nurse
- Certified Nephrology Nurse – Nurse Practitioner
- Certified Nephrology Nurse
- Certified Neuroscience Registered Nurse
- Certified Nurse Educator
- Certified Nurse in Critical Care (C) Canada
- Certified Nurse in Critical Care Pediatrics (C) Canada
- Certified Nurse Life Care Planner
- Certified Nurse Manager and Leader
- Certified Nurse Midwife
- Certified Nurse Operating Room
- Certified Nursing Home Administrators
- Certified Nutrition Support Clinician
- Certified Nutrition Support Nurse
- Certified Occupational Health Nurse
- Certified Occupational Health Nurse, Case Management
- Certified Occupational Health Nurse, Safety Manager
- Certified Occupational Health Nurse, Safety Manager with CM
- Certified Occupational Health Nurse-Specialist
- Certified Ostomy Care Nurse
- Certified Otorhinolaryngology Nurse
- Certified Pediatric Emergency Nurse
- Certified Pediatric Hematology Oncology Nurse
- Certified Pediatric Nurse
- Certified Pediatric Nurse Practitioner – Acute Care
- Certified Pediatric Nurse Practitioner – Primary Care
- Certified Pediatric Oncology Nurse
- Certified Peritoneal Dialysis Nurse
- Certified Personal Trainer; Exercise Specialist; Clinical Exercise Specialist; Health/Fitness Instructor; Registered Clinical Exercise Physiologist
- Certified Plastic Surgery Nurse
- Certified Post Anesthesia Nurse
- Certified Prenatal/Postnatal Fitness Instructor
- Certified Procurement Transplant Coordinator
- Certified Professional Coder-Hospital
- Certified Professional in Healthcare Information and Management Systems
- Certified Professional in Healthcare Management
- Certified Professional in Healthcare Quality
- Certified Professional in Healthcare Risk Management
- Certified Professional in Learning and Performance
- Certified Professional in Patient Safety
- Certified Radiology Nurse
- Certified Registered Nurse Anesthetist

- Certified Registered Nurse First Assistant
- Certified Registered Nurse Infusion
- Certified Registered Nurse Ophthalmology
- Certified Rehabilitation Registered Nurse
- Certified Renal Lithotripsy Specialist
- Certified Respiratory Therapist
- Certified Safe Patient Handling Professional
- Certified Specialist in Poison Information
- Certified Stroke Registered Nurse
- Certified Surgical First Assistant
- Certified Surgical Technologist
- Certified Transcultural Nurse – Basic
- Certified Transplant Preservationist
- Certified Transport Emergency Nurse
- Certified Urologic Clinical Nurse Specialist
- Certified Urologic Nurse Practitioner
- Certified Urology Registered Nurse
- Certified Vascular Nurse
- Certified Wound Associate
- Certified Wound Care Nurse
- Certified Wound Ostomy Continence Nurse Advance Practice
- Certified Wound Ostomy Nurse
- Certified Wound Specialist
- Certified Wound, Ostomy, Continence Nurse
- Certified Addictions Registered Nurse – Advance Practice
- Child & Adolescent Clinical Nurse Specialist
- Clinical Breast Examiner
- Clinical Documentation Improvement Professional
- Clinical Genetic Nurse
- Clinical Nurse Leader
- Clinical Nurse Specialist Child & Adolescent
- Clinical Nurse Specialist in Home Health Nursing
- Clinical Nurse Specialist Public Community Health
- Clinical Nurse Specialist, Core
- Clinical Research Associate
- College Health Nurse
- Community Health Nurse
- Credentialed Member, American Academy of Medical Administrators
- Critical Care Clinical Nurse Specialist (Adult, Neonatal, Pediatric Acute)
- Critical Care Paramedic – Certified
- Critical Care Registered Nurse (Adult, Neonatal, and Pediatric Acute)
- Critical Care RN with Cardiac Medicine Subspecialty
- Critical Care RN with Cardiac Surgery Subspecialty
- Critical Care RN with Tele-ICU specialty
- Dermatology Certified Nurse Practitioner
- Dermatology Nurse Certified
- Developmental Disabilities Nursing Certification
- Dietetic Technician, Registered

- Diplomate of Acupuncture
- Diplomate of Asian Bodywork Therapy
- Diplomate of Chinese Herbology
- Diplomate of Oriental Medicine
- Electronic Fetal Monitoring
- Emergency Nurse Certified (C) Canada
- Evidence-Based Design Accreditation and Certification
- Family Nurse Practitioner
- Family Psychiatric & Mental Health Nurse Practitioner
- Flight Paramedic – Certified
- Gerontological Clinical Nurse Specialist
- Gerontological Nurse
- Gerontological Nurse Certified (C) Canada
- Gerontological Nurse Practitioner
- Global Professional in Human Resources
- Group Fitness Instructor Certification
- Health and Wellness Nurse Coach Board Certified
- Healthcare Accreditation Certification Program
- Hemapheresis Practitioner Certification
- High-Risk Perinatal Nurse
- Holistic Baccalaureate Nurse, Board Certified
- Holistic Nurse Board Certified
- Home Care Clinical Specialist: OASIS
- Home Care Coding Specialist: Diagnosis
- Home Health Nurse
- Informatics Nurse
- Inpatient Obstetric Nursing
- International Board Certified Lactation Consultant
- Lamaze Certified Childbirth Educator
- Legal Nurse Consultant Certified
- Lifestyle & Weight Management Consultant
- Low Risk Neonatal Nursing
- Master Addiction Counselor
- Master Certified Health Education Specialist
- Maternal Child Nursing
- Maternal Newborn Nursing
- Medical-Surgical Registered Nurse
- MS Nurse
- National Certified Addictions Counselor
- National Certified Counselor
- National Certified School Nurse
- National Registry of Emergency Medical Technicians-First Responder
- National Registry of Emergency Medical Technicians-Intermediate
- National Registry of Emergency Medical Technicians-Paramedic
- National Registry of Emergency Medical Technicians-Basic (Med Tech) (EMT)
- Neonatal Intensive Care Nursing
- Neonatal Nurse Practitioner
- Neonatal Pediatric Transport

- Neurovascular Nurse (RN)
- Nurse Coach Board Certified
- Nurse Executive (Certified Nurse Administration [CNA], BC before 2008)
- Nurse Executive, Advanced (Certified Nurse Administration [CNAA], BC before 2008)
- Nursing Professional Development
- Obstetric, Gynecologic, and Neonatal Nursing
- Oncology Certified Nurse
- Orthopaedic Nurse Practitioner – Certified
- Orthopaedic Nursing Certified (C) Canada
- Orthopedic Clinical Nurse Specialist – Certified
- Orthopedic Nurse Certified
- Pain Management Nurse
- Pediatric Clinical Nurse Specialist
- Pediatric Nurse
- Pediatric Nurse Practitioner
- Pediatric Primary Care Mental Health Specialist
- PeriAnesthesia Nurse Certified (C) Canada
- Perinatal Nurse
- Perinatal Nurse Certified (C) Canada
- Personal Trainer Certification
- Physician Assistant
- Professional in Human Resources
- Progressive Care Certified Nurse
- Progressive Care Certified Nurse with Cardiac Medicine Subspecialty
- Psychiatric & Mental Health Nurse
- Qualified Professional Case Manager
- Quality Auditor
- Registered Cardiac Electrophysiology Specialist
- Registered Cardiac Sonographer
- Registered Cardiovascular Invasive Specialist
- Registered Diagnostic Cardiac Sonographer
- Registered Diagnostic Medical Sonographer
- Registered Dietitian
- Registered Radiology Assistant
- Registered Respiratory Therapist
- Registered Vascular Specialist
- Registered Vascular Technologist
- Reproductive Endocrinology/Infertility Nurse
- RN-Coder
- School Nurse
- School Nurse Practitioner
- Senior Professional in Human Resources
- Sexual Assault Nurse Examiner: Adult
- Sexual Assault Nurse Examiner: Pediatric
- Six Sigma Black Belt
- Telephone Nursing Practice
- Vascular Access-Board Certified
- Women's Health Care Nurse Practitioner
- Wound Care Certified

As you can see, there is a professional organization and certification for all levels of nurses. There is no excuse for a lack of professional growth.

Another decision for the continued professional development of the nurse is whether to continue academic education. The IOM (2010), in the *Future of Nursing*, called for 80% of all nurses in the United States to have a Bachelor of Science in Nursing (BSN) by 2020. There are a number of state-wide initiatives working to move the nursing workforce in this direction. Magnet organizations are also calling for organizations to have plans in place to meet this goal. So if you do not have the BSN, the time is now!

Other degrees in nursing include the Master of Science in Nursing, which focuses on advanced preparation in nursing. A master's degree in nursing is required to become an APN or advanced practice registered nurse and to qualify for an advanced practice certification. The nurse practitioner (NP) tracks (adult NP, family NP, midwifery, certified nurse anesthetist, etc.) require a minimum of a Masters of Science in Nursing. Some states are moving toward a doctorate in nursing practice as the minimum requirement to practice as a NP.

There are three types of doctorates in nursing: a Doctor of Nursing Practice (DNP), which focuses on the clinical aspects of nursing; a Doctor of Nursing Science (DNSc, also a DSN or DNS); and the PhD and EdD, which focus on nursing theory, research, and education. The latter two types are the more common choice for those who wish to be professors at nursing programs or researchers. It is not uncommon to see some doctoral-prepared nurses remaining at the bedside at Magnet organizations.

SUMMARY

Nurses progress on a continuum of competency from novice to expert during their careers according to the work of Benner (1984). This continuum forms the basis for many career development opportunities available to the nurse. The strategic plan of the organization will have human resource objectives with outcomes specifying the academic and professional role progression of its staff. As a nurse, it is your personal and professional responsibility to continually advance your professional knowledge and expertise.

CLINICAL CORNER

Why Pursue a Doctor of Nursing Practice (DNP) Degree?

Today's Doctor of Nursing Practice (DNP) professionals are better adapted than ever to meet the new challenges facing the health care system. The constantly evolving demands of America's diverse and varied health care environment are increasing, requiring nurses who serve in specialized positions to possess new levels of insight, particularly in scientific knowledge and medical practice expertise. These standards have resulted from both an increased complexity of medical illness states and the widely documented links between higher levels of nursing education and improved patient outcomes.

In 2003, the Institute of Medicine (IOM) stated that the attainment of the DNP provides a logical extension of nursing education, focused on safe, effective patient-centered care. The IOM report *Health Professions Education: A Bridge to Quality* stated that nurses must increase their knowledge and skills if they are to deliver enhanced clinical care across services and sights.

The DNP is, therefore, the ultimate practice-focused degree awarded to nurses who want to achieve the highest level of proficiency in the delivery of complex care over the lifespan of the patient. For those nurses who want to positively influence health care in nonpractice-driven roles, the focus is on aggregate, systems, or organizations that will enable the DNP graduate opportunities as administrators, executive leaders, informaticists, health policy specialists, public health specialists, and educators. Prior to the DNP, there was no way for advanced practice nurses to expand their expertise in the practice environment to the doctoral level since PhDs were the domain of researchers and academicians, and the EdD was the primary domain of academia. Today the DNP establishes a higher level of credibility for nurses with aspirations of translating evidence-based care into practice, improving systems of care, and measuring outcomes of groups of patients and communities. The DNP graduates are

Continued

prepared to effect change in organizational and systems leadership and acquire high-level roles in health systems, academia, and policymaking.

As we look to a future that involves increasing the availability of care for all while working and managing care within a fragmented health care system, the global health issues influencing disease and illness states, and a large percentage of the American population nearing or in retirement, one thing becomes certain: the DNP-prepared provider is able to fill the void of an unprecedented need to serve as flexible leaders, independent health care providers, and autonomous decision makers.

I would like to share my personal path that led me to decide to pursue a DNP degree. As a practicing advanced practice nurse, I developed confidence in my ability to manage acute and chronic illnesses. I saw patients in a variety of settings such as private office, emergency room, trauma, and critical care. The dysfunctions in the health care system were becoming more and more frustrating, and I was not able to provide the absolute best care for the patients I served. I found that I was not able to use the latest proven evidence in managing acute and chronic illnesses. This was the impetus forcing me to answer the most important question regarding pursuing a terminal degree: Is the DNP right for me? As I reflected on my options of PhD, EdD, and DNP, I felt that with the attainment of the DNP degree I would gain the best possible outcome and diversity needed to continue professional growth in my career. Therefore, my answer to the question was a resounding "yes." Upon graduation, I thought of an old saying: "It is better to be lucky than good." True or not, there is certainly a lot of serendipity in life. But I also remembered that Louis Pasteur had a different take. He said, "Chance favors the prepared mind." I was reminded of this often as I forged new paths in the health care arena. The DNP degree has enabled me to join an elite group of professionals that possess the tools and training to improve the lives of so many, whether that is through research, clinical practice, leadership, or public service. What I do will matter.

In today's changing demands of the health care environment, the highest level of scientific knowledge and practice expertise is required to assure quality outcomes. The DNP degree prepares the graduate in both leadership and clinical roles to provide the most advanced level of care to individuals, families, and communities. The many factors supporting the momentum for change in education include the rapid expansion of knowledge underlining practice, increased complexity of patient care, and

national concerns about the quality of care and patient safety. The DNP-prepared nurse is the leader in developing the multidisciplinary teams necessary to manage the complexities of diseases in the health care environment. The acquisition of the DNP has made me a more adaptive clinician. I am better able to view my patients and their health concerns, as well as the health care environment, from a different perspective. I see the same patients with their acute or chronic illnesses, but what has changed is my management and treatment of diseases and illnesses that are patient-centered and evidence-based. It is easier to just take care of patients' health issues, addressing only the chief complaint at the time of the encounter. This approach enables providers to have quantity but not necessarily quality of care. I view patients as multidimensional in that they never just present as an illness or a disease. In addition, differences in pathophysiology, culture, and societal and health beliefs are brought with the patient to every encounter. The key is being able to navigate these complex intertwined systems and design the best care for that patient at that encounter.

I have utilized the expert leadership skills acquired in my DNP program in serving for 5 years in the administrative role of vice president for advanced practice providers in my organization. While in this role, the number of advanced practice providers increased from 5 to 45 within the organization and physician network. I continue to maintain my position in academia as faculty for medical students, as well as assistant professor/coordinator of the adult gerontology nurse practitioner track. My clinical expertise enabled me to lead medical missions to Hospital Sacre Coeur in Milot, Haiti, where programs have developed for heart failure and peripartum cardiacmyopathy in concert with population health to improve access, quality, and cost-effective care to the populations in a developing country. These programs were needed to arrest the progression of disease and enhance quality of life. I have also developed the nursing curriculum for the first United States-based nurse training program at Hospital Sacre Coeur to improve the clinical skills and critical thinking of the nurses for improved patient outcomes. Lastly, my clinical and leadership expertise enabled me to develop a business plan that opened the first nurse practitioner–run primary care practice in Bergen County, New Jersey. I am sharing my story because when I was in nursing school, I had no idea that I would end up in any of these roles or career paths. I have realized that the future holds many opportunities, especially with continued learning and the attainment of my terminal degree.

CLINICAL CORNER—cont'd

It is important to understand that the chosen path will be neither obvious nor easy, nor without risk. I always remain open to new opportunities, wherever and however I find them. I let chance favor my prepared mind and translate my ideas and opportunities into real-world actions, even when the path is difficult. I resolve to never stop learning, never stop asking questions, and never forget that health care delivery is an art as well as a science practiced by providers and researchers who bring to the bedside not only technology and training but also humanity, caring, and concern for those in need.

Patients do not put their trust in machines or devices; patients put their trust in caring, qualified providers. I have spent the last 15 years doing research and managing individuals with acute and chronic illness states. However, I made it a point to always remember that the more skilled I became, the more specialized I became, and the more dependent on technology I became, the easier it could be to lose one's humanity, forget one's compassion, and ignore one's instincts. The most important piece I would never lose was my moral compass.

Over the many years in primary care practice, I have experienced challenging situations in my life such as 9/11, a bioterrorist attack, a flu pandemic, the worst recession since the 1930s, a widening gap between rich and poor, unsustainable growth in health care costs, an aging population, growing conflict in many parts of the world, newly emerging biologic threats both naturally occurring and deliberately caused, and global warming. With each challenging time, I took advantage to strengthen my moral compass by directing my energies and talents to doing good, not just doing well. I combined the knowledge and skills I have gained through continuing my education and achieving my terminal degree with the courage of my convictions to be a great provider, leader, educator, and researcher. I resolved to always speak for those in need or underserved, to advance science in the service of humanity, and to hand the next generation an even more innovative, responsive, curative, and preventative health care system than the one that was handed to me. My satisfaction in practicing primary care is the ongoing deep contentment with the decision I made to attain my DNP degree.

Judith Kutzleb, DNP, RN, CCRN, CCA, NP-C
Holy Name Medical Center
Holy Name Medical Partners
Teaneck, New Jersey

EVIDENCE-BASED PRACTICE

Chapter 10 EBP

In the current health care environment, in which organizations are dealing with reimbursement challenges and value-added payment, nursing professional development practitioners must increasingly demonstrate that the time and resources dedicated to educational activities are worth the impact that they have on outcomes. The purpose of this project was to review the return-on-investment literature for professional activities.

The standard educational program evaluation methodology is the Kirkpatrick and Kirkpatrick (2009) model. Kirkpatrick's level of education consists of four hierarchal levels of evaluation: reaction, learning, behavior, and results. In level 1, reaction, the focus is on the learner's perception of the training. This level often uses surveys, questionnaires, or other rating scales for measurement. The next level, learning, measures the increase in knowledge, skill, or capacity due to the learning event. This level uses posttests, checklists, or return demonstration for measurement. Level 3, behavior, considers the extent of behavior change and the improvement achieved by the application of the educational content. This level may be measured through observation of behavior, chart audits, or self-report of learners at a later date, after the content of the learning has had an opportunity to be applied in the work setting. Finally, the highest level of evaluation, results, considers the effect on the business or environment based on performance. Applying this evaluation model builds a compelling chain of evidence for the value relationship between the learning activity and the organization's bottom line (Kirkpatrick & Kirkpatrick, 2007).

Paramoure (2013) presents a model of measurable instructional design to facilitate measurement of return on investment of education. The model begins with the key performance metric (KPM) that is the target of the educational activity. Specific skills associated with the KPM are delineated and lead to the development of measurable performance outcomes. Teaching methods are created to align with the objectives and lead to the evaluation of the learner's achievement of the objectives. Finally, application of new behaviors in the work setting is evaluated along with the impact on the KPM. Return of investment is subsequently measured by quantifying the cost of education and the monetary value of the changes to the KPM.

Continued

EVIDENCE-BASED PRACTICE—cont'd

The review of the literature found 11 studies between 2002 and 2013 that evaluated financial impact of educational interventions. The educational interventions identified in these studies included computer modules (1), newly licensed nurse residency programs (4), customized orientation plan (1), blended learning approach orientation (1), and multifaceted programs (4). The content of the educational interventions included such topics as medication safety, ventilator associated pneumonia, pressure ulcer prevention, ergonomics, and a wellness program.

In the 11 studies, the measurement of the financial impact of professional activities varied, including comparing cost of educational activities to the following:
- Cost of preventing an error resulting in litigation
- Cost of avoiding expenses from error
- Cost of employee turnover
- Previous educational costs and outcomes
- Payments for injuries, personal days, and workers compensation
- Expense of employing agency nurses

Dennison (2007) calculated the cost savings including per error impact, length of stay, and litigation and concluded that the minor expense of education was worth the investment. Hillman and Foster (2011) calculated significant turnover cost savings over 4 years resulting from the implementation of a new nurse residency program. Nelson, Matz, Chen, Siddharthan, Lloyd, and Fragala (2006) described benefit-cost comparisons by calculating injury prevention education and capital equipment costs, then comparing it to treatment expenses, payments for injuries, personal days, and workers compensation savings (annualized savings of $204,599/year).

The outcomes measured and "costed out" included:
- Absenteeism
- Attrition
- Competence and self-confidence
- Expense for agency nurses
- Injury rates
- Job satisfaction
- Lost work days
- Modified work days
- Number of infusion pump alerts
- Number of pressure ulcers
- Patient acceptance
- Rate of ventilator-associated pneumonia
- Reduced time for orientation
- Reported errors
- Retention
- Safety climate
- Turnover
- Turnover intent
- Vacant full-time equivalents

In the current health care environment, the "value-added" of education is an important evaluation of the effectiveness of the education delivered.

References

Opperman, C., Liebig, C., Bowling, J., Johnson, C., & Harper, M. (2016). Measuring return on investment for professional development activities: a review of the evidence. *Journal for Nurses in Professional Development*, 32(3 May/June), 122–129.

Dennison, R. (2007). Medication safety program to reduce risk of harm caused by medication errors. *Journal of Continuing Education in Nursing*, 38(4), 176–184.

Hillman, L., & Foster, R. (2011). The impact of a nursing transitions program on retention and cost savings. *Journal of Nursing Management*, 19(1), 50–56.

Kirkpatick, D., & Kirkpatrick, J. (2007). *Implementing Four Levels: A Practical Guide for Effective Evaluation of Training Programs*. San Francisco: Berrett-Koehler Publisher.

Nelson, A., Matz, M., Chen, F., Siddharthan, K., Lloyd, J., & Fragala, G. (2006). Development and evaluation of multi-faceted ergonomics program to prevent injuries associated with patient handling tasks. *International Journal of Nursing Studies*, 43(6), 717–733.

Paramoure, L. (2013). *ROI by design: Unlock Training's Impact Through Measurable Instruction Design*. Lexington, KY: Author.

NCLEX® EXAMINATION QUESTIONS

1. Benner states there are five stages of nursing competence. They are novice, advanced beginner, competent, proficient, expert. Which category describes the new RN?
   A. Competent
   B. Proficient
   C. Expert
   D. Novice

2. Which stage would describe an APN?
   A. Expert
   B. Proficient
   C. Competent
   D. Novice

3. The Joint Commission states that a hospital must provide the right number of competent staff to meet the needs of the patients (2019).

A. Competent staff are qualified.

B. Competent staff members are able to perform the work according to professional standards.

C. Competent staff members meet the goals.

D. All of the above are correct.

4. Magnet status health care facilities:

A. Are responsible for orienting, training, and educating staff

B. Require that BSN-prepared RNs must fill 50% of the nurses

C. Utilize as many patient care technicians as possible

D. Pay for all travel expenses when a BSN nurse attends seminars

5. Programs that reward nurses for their advancement in nursing are referred to as:

A. Educational seminars

B. Clinical ladders

C. Present at conferences

D. Does not keep the nurses' at the bedside

6. Professional nursing service, leadership skills, and national certification in nursing specialty areas are ways to move up in the clinical ladder. Other means of proving one is eligible to move up in the clinical ladder include:

A. Orienting new nurses

B. Presenting in field of expertise

C. Having a rotating schedule of different shifts

D. Both A and B are correct

7. After completion of a year of employment and receiving a satisfactory evaluation, a bedside RN will automatically advance to:

A. Levels I and II

B. Levels II and III

C. Levels III and IV

D. Level V

8. The nurse that is just ending the _____ year of employment can sit for the specialty certification.

A. First

B. Second

C. Third

D. Fourth

9. When does a newly hired nurse receive information such as fire safety code of conduct, infection control, and culture of safety?

A. Upon hire and annually

B. 2 months after hire

C. 4 months after hire

D. 6 months after hire

10. Nurses should expect that their nursing career will lead them to lifelong learning. This means that nurses:

A. Attend seminars in their area of expertise and receive contact hours

B. Meet the criteria for the Board of Nursing protocol every year

C. Renew their license every year

D. Renew their license every 3 years

REFERENCES

American Nurses Credentialing Center [ANCC]. (2019). *2019 Magnet application manual.* Silver Spring: MD: ANCC.

Benner, P. (1984). *From novice to expert: Excellence and power in clinical nursing practice.* Menlo Park, CA: Addison-Wesley.

Goode, C. J., Lynn, M. R., Krsek, C., et al. (2009). Nurse residency programs: an essential requirement for nursing. *Nursing Economics, 27*(3), 142–159.

Hardy, R., & Smith, R. (2001). Enhancing staff development with a structured preceptor program. *Journal of Nursing Care Quality, 15*(2), 9–17.

Institute of Medicine (2010). *The Future of Nursing: Leading Change, Advancing Health.* Washington D.C.: The National Academies Press.

Krugman, M., Bretscneider, J., Horn, P. B., et al. (2006). The National Post-Baccalaureate Graduate Nurse Residency Program. *Journal for Nurses in Staff Development, 22*(4), 196–205.

Miller, C., I, Wagenberg, C., Loney, E., Porinchak, M.P., & Ramrup, N. (2020). Creating and implementing a nurse mentoring program: a team approach. *Journal of Nursing Administration, 50*(6), 343–348.

Neuman, J., Brady-Schluttner, K., McKay, A., Roslien, J., Tweedell, D., & James, K. (2004). Centralizing a registered nurse preceptor program at the institutional level. *Journal for Nurses in Staff Development, 20*(1), 17–24.

Lee, V., Harris T. (2007). Mentoring new nursing graduates. Retrieved July 8, 2014, from www.minoritynurse.com/features/other/080207d.html.

Nock, B. (2017). 3 Reasons to Join a Professional Nursing Organization. Retrieved October 27, 2019, from https://www.gebaurer.com/blog/reasons-to-join-professional-nursing-organzation.

Sullivan, E. J., & Decker, F. J. (2013). *Effective leadership and management in nursing* (5th ed.). Upper Saddle River, NJ: Prentice-Hall.

The Joint Commission. (2019). *Hospital accreditation standards.* Oakbrook Terrace, IL: Author.

Williams, C. A., Goode, C. J., Krsek, C., et al. (2007). Post-baccalaureate nurse residency 1-year outcomes. *Journal of Nursing Administration, 37*(7/8), 357–365.

11

Professional Practice and Care Delivery Models and Emerging Practice Models

OUTLINE

OBJECTIVES

- Differentiate between the traditional function care delivery models and professional care delivery models.
- Discuss the pros and cons of each of the delivery systems.
- Determine the responsibility of the nurse in the professional practice model.

- Identify outcome measures of professional practice and care delivery models.
- Differentiate between a professional practice model and a care delivery system.
- Identify the opportunities for nurses related to the emerging models of practice and care delivery.

KEY TERMS

Accountable Care Organization (ACO) a collaboration among primary care clinicians, a hospital, specialists, and other health professionals who accept joint responsibility for the quality and cost of care provided to its patients

care delivery system a system for the delivery of care that delineates the nurses' authority and accountability for clinical decision making and outcomes; it is integrated with the professional practice model and promotes continuous, consistent, efficient, and accountable nursing care

Medical Home model a mechanism to provide patients with a central primary care practice or provider who coordinates the patients' care across settings and providers

nurse-managed clinics nurse-run facilities that provide comprehensive primary care

professional practice model a schematic description of a theory, phenomenon, or system that depicts how nurses practice, collaborate, communicate, and develop professionally to provide the highest quality care for those served by the organization (American Nurses Credentialing Center [ANCC], 2019)

PROFESSIONAL PRACTICE MODELS

The **professional practice model** (PPM) is the driving force of nursing care (American Nurses Credentialing Center [ANCC], 2019, p. 158). The PPM of an organization illustrates the alignment and integration of nursing practice with the mission, vision, and values of the organization and the nursing department. It is the overarching conceptual framework for nurses, nursing care, and interprofessional patient care. It is usually presented as a schematic that describes how nurses practice, collaborate, and develop professionally to deliver care that meets the three aims of effectiveness, efficiency, and patient experience. At the center or forefront of such

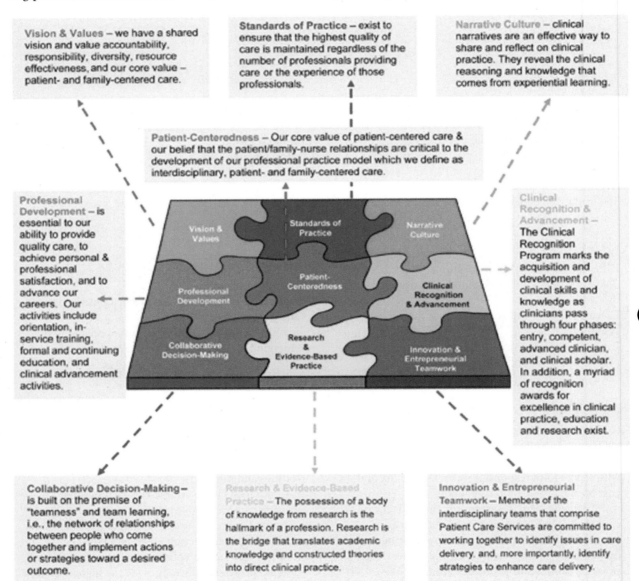

Vision & Values – we have a shared vision and value accountability, responsibility, diversity, resource effectiveness, and our core value – patient- and family-centered care.

Standards of Practice – exist to ensure that the highest quality of care is maintained regardless of the number of professionals providing care or the experience of those professionals.

Narrative Culture – clinical narratives are an effective way to share and reflect on clinical practice. They reveal the clinical reasoning and knowledge that comes from experiential learning.

Patient-Centeredness – Our core value of patient-centered care & our belief that the patient/family-nurse relationships are critical to the development of our professional practice model which we define as interdisciplinary, patient- and family-centered care.

Professional Development – is essential to our ability to provide quality care, to achieve personal & professional satisfaction, and to advance our careers. Our activities include orientation, in-service training, formal and continuing education, and clinical advancement activities.

Clinical Recognition & Advancement – The Clinical Recognition Program marks the acquisition and development of clinical skills and knowledge as clinicians pass through four phases: entry, competent, advanced clinician, and clinical scholar. In addition, a myriad of recognition awards for excellence in clinical practice, education and research exist.

Collaborative Decision-Making – is built on the premise of "teamness" and team learning, i.e., the network of relationships between people who come together and implement actions or strategies toward a desired outcome.

Research & Evidence-Based Practice – The possession of a body of knowledge from research is the hallmark of a profession. Research is the bridge that translates academic knowledge and constructed theories into direct clinical practice.

Innovation & Entrepreneurial Teamwork – Members of the interdisciplinary teams that comprise Patient Care Services are committed to working together to identify issues in care delivery, and, more importantly, identify strategies to enhance care delivery.

Fig. 11.1 The Massachusetts General Hospital professional practice model. (From Massachusetts General Hospital. (2014). Professional practice model. Retrieved July 31, 2019, from www.massgeneral.org/assets/MGH/pdf/nursing-patientcare/PPM-with-descriptions-091417.pdfhttps://www.massgeneral.org/assets/MGH/pdf/nursing-patientcare/PPM-with-descriptions-091417.pdf.)

models is the patient and family. Fig. 11.1 represents the PPM of Massachusetts General Patient Care Services.

This PPM represents the interconnected pieces of the "puzzle" that forms nursing practice at Massachusetts General Hospital. Nursing is delivered through the many pieces of the puzzle, and the expectation of how each nurse in the institution practices is defined in this model. This goes beyond the care delivery models described in Chapter 2. Those models, team nursing, functional nursing, and primary nursing, describe how the actual delivery of care is organized. The care delivery system is integrated within the PPM and promotes continuous, consistent, efficient, and accountable delivery of patient care. The care delivery system is adapted to meet evidence-based practice standards, national patient safety goals, affordable and value-based outcomes, and regulatory requirements (ANCC, 2019, p. 40) The PPM describes the environment in which the professional nurse practices. This professional nurse practice environment empowers nurses by providing them with opportunities for autonomy, accountability, and control over the care that they provide and the environment in which they deliver care (Zelauskas & Howes, 1992 as cited in American Nurses Credentialing Center ANCC, 2013). Shared governance, as discussed in Chapter 6 is the vehicle by which the decision making of the PPM occurs. In this model the patient remains at the center of all care decisions. The nursing vision and values, and the standards of practice, guide the activities of the professional nurse. The nurse is supported through professional development and clinical recognition and achievement. Practice is continually advanced and delivered through collaborative decision making, the narrative culture, research, evidence-based practice, and innovation and entrepreneurial teamwork.

The University of California, Los Angeles (UCLA) PPM (Fig. 11.2) is philosophically similar in many respects, but the schematic reflects the culture of the larger organization. The patient, family, and community are at the center of care. The overall mission of UCLA and the mission and values form the next circle of the model. This PPM is guided by the O'Rourke Model of the professional role, the Watson Theory of Human Caring, and the Swanson Five Caring Processes. Relationship-based care is the care delivery model. This schematic includes the theoretical models on which the PPM is based. The professional nurse as a decision maker is guided by the American Nurses Association (ANA) Code of Ethics,

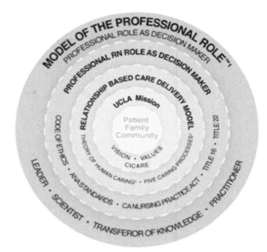

[1]O'Rourke Model of the Professional Role™   [2]Watson Theory of Human Caring
[3]Swanson Five Caring Processes

Fig. 11.2 The University of California Los Angeles professional practice model. (From University of California–Los Angeles (UCLA). (2014). *Professional Practice Model.* <https://www.uclahealth.org/nursing/professional-practice-model.>)

the ANA Standards, the State Nursing Practice Act, and State Titles. Last, the nurse has roles as leader, scientist, transferor of knowledge, and practitioner.

Both of the previously mentioned PPMs clearly describe the professional environment of nursing within the institution and the expectations of the nurse and the nursing department.

Knowledge of the PPM can be an important determinant in a nurse's decision to join a particular organization.

CARE DELIVERY SYSTEM

The care delivery system is integrated into the PPM. It is continually improved to adjust to national patient safety goals, value-based outcomes, regulatory requirements, and current best evidence. It describes the manner in which care is delivered, the context of care, and the expected outcomes of care. Nurses create care delivery systems that describe the nurses' accountability and shared authority for evidence-based practice, clinical decision making and outcomes, performance improvement initiatives, and staffing and scheduling processes (American Nurses Credentialing Center ANCC, 2013, p. 42).

Limitations of the more traditional definitions of care delivery (team, functional, primary care, etc.) have been documented, and many consider them inadequate for depicting the multiplicity of actual nursing work organization models in practice (O'Connor, Bennett, Crawford, & Korfiatis, 2006; Tiedman & Lookinland, 2004). The care delivery models described by Massachusetts General and UCLA reflect a taxonomy of nursing care organization models that incorporate a broader range of attributes than those found in the traditional care delivery models. Dubois et al. (2013) proposed that a nursing care delivery model should consist of the following five key dimensions:

1. Staffing intensity
2. Skill and nursing education mix
3. Professional scope of practice in six domains of practice (assessment and planning, teaching, communication, supervision, quality of care, and knowledge updating)
4. Nursing practice environment (nurse participation in hospital affairs, nursing foundations for quality, nurse manager leadership and support, resource adequacy and nurse–physician relations)
5. Unit-level capacity for innovation measured on five criteria (expanded RN roles, sharpened focus of care on the patient, attention to patient transitions, leveraging of technologies, and performance monitoring and feedback)

In a study comparing outcomes of such professional models and the more traditional functional models (Dubois et al., 2013), more positive patient outcomes were seen with the more innovative professional care delivery models. This supports the notion that patient safety results from more than just staffing models. The lowest rates of negative outcomes were seen in the professional models characterized by richer skill and education mix, higher staffing intensity, and a practice environment more supportive of professional practice and with greater investments in innovation. These associations are consistent with findings reported for Magnet hospitals, known for the excellence of their conditions for both nurses and patients.

Frameworks for the Delivery of Patient Care

In recognition of the unique characteristics of patients and their needs, each organization/unit/service/clinic develops a method of delivering care. Information provided in the development and improvement of the care delivery model should include the following:

- Populations served/patient characteristics
- Age, ethnic, cultural, and spiritual patient characteristics
- Scope and complexity of patients
- Admission characteristics
- Assessment/reassessment practices and standards
- Staffing ratios and staff mix
- Educational mix of the nursing staff
- Standards for assignment of patients
- Required competencies of the unit staff to meet patient needs
- The nursing philosophy, mission, vision, and values
- Interprofessionals who support care delivery
- Standards to ensure continuity of care
- Professional nursing standards that guide care delivery
- Use of evidence to drive innovation
- Performance improvement indicators to measure the effectiveness and efficiency of the care delivery system for the unit

It is imperative that the delivery of care is continually evaluated. Outcomes need to be evaluated throughout the shift as acuity changes and daily, weekly, monthly, quarterly, and annually.

The PPM and care delivery models are evaluated and revised based on new evidence and/or research and on outcome data such as the following:

- Accreditation standards and National Patient Safety Goals
- Patient satisfaction survey results
- National Database of Nursing Quality Indicators (NDNQI) nursing sensitive indicator outcomes
- Unit scorecards (quality and financial data)
- The NDNQI staff registered nurse (RN) satisfaction survey
- Centers for Medicare & Medicaid Services core measures
- Hospital Consumer Assessment of Healthcare Providers and Systems results
- Unit-based surveys

(Adapted from Jupiter Medical Center (2015). *Description of JMC Care Delivery System*. Jupiter, FL. Retrieved May 12, 2015, from www.jupitermed.com/care-delivery-system.)

EMERGING CARE DELIVERY MODELS

Many of these care delivery models can be adjusted to meet the needs of various populations, such as ambulatory centers, nurse-managed clinics, medical homes, and the wide variety of organizations that provide health care. But the role of nurses in emerging care delivery models will be a true test of the patient advocacy role of the professional nurse in the delivery of safe, efficient, and effective care. RNs are fundamental to the success of emerging patient-centered care delivery models.

The Patient Protection and Affordable Care Act of 2010 (PPACA) directs renewed attention and substantially more resources and incentives to promote those elements of care that are also the backbone of nursing practice. These essentials of nursing practice include patient-centered or "holistic" care, including family and community, care continuity, coordination and integration across settings and providers, chronic disease management, patient education, prevention and wellness care, and information management (American Nurses Association ANA Issue Brief, 2010, pp. 1–2).

In addition, PPACA recognizes the advance practice registered nurse (APRN) as a valuable provider of primary care services, and a potential leader in new integrated care systems. The Institute of Medicine defines primary care as "the provision of integrated, accessible health care services by clinicians who are accountable for addressing a large majority of personal health care needs, developing a sustained partnership with patients, and practicing in the context of family and community" (American Nurses Association ANA Issue Brief, 2010, pp. 1–2).

Three emerging care delivery models in particular, are addressed in PPACA. These are the Accountable Care Organization (ACO), the medical or health home, and the nurse-managed health center. Nurses and APRNs will play a major role in the planning, implementation, and success of these emerging care delivery models.

In an ACO a set of health care providers (including primary care physicians, nurses, specialists, and hospitals) work together collaboratively and accept collective accountability for the cost and quality of care delivered to a population of patients. Care is delivered across the transitions of care and includes primary care practices, hospitals, home health agencies, rehabilitation facilities, and other areas where health care is delivered.

The Patient-Centered Medical Home model was first proposed in 2007. It is, in essence, an enhanced primary care delivery model that strives to achieve better access, coordination of care, prevention, quality, and safety within the primary care practice, and to create a strong partnership between the patient and the primary care practitioner. ACOs are also based around a strong primary care core. However, ACOs are made up of many

TABLE 11.1	Four Surrogate Terms
Professional practice model	• Standards of practice • Professional development • Control over nursing practice • Increased job satisfaction • Accountability • Understanding of scope of practice • Shared vision/values • Practice changes • Evidence-based practice • Developing clinical expertise • Colleagueship • Foster professional identity
Care model	• Framework • Structure • Cost containment • Functional perspective • Response to downsizing and change in staffing
Care delivery model/system	• Structure • Framework • Cost containment • Functional perspective • Response to downsizing and change in staffing • Continuity of care • Guides daily work and nursing practice • Decentralization/flattening of levels • Systems model (involves many elements)
Shared governance model	• Mostly used at Magnet organizations • Participative management • Self-managed teams • Collaborative, interdisciplinary teams • Control over nursing practice • Increased job satisfaction • Autonomous nursing practice • Decentralized organizational models • Practice changes • Evidence-based practice • High patient satisfaction • Transformational leadership skills • Colleagueship

"medical homes," in other words, many primary care providers and/or practices that work together. Some have even dubbed ACOs the "medical neighborhood."

Nurse-Managed Health Clinics (NMHCs) (authorized under Title III of the Public Health Service Act) are health care delivery sites operated by APRNs. These clinics are often associated with a school, college, university, department of nursing, federally qualified health center, or independent nonprofit health care agency. Although managed by APRNs, NMHCs are staffed by an interdisciplinary team of health care providers that includes physicians, social workers, and public health nurses. NMHCs provide primary care, health promotion, and disease prevention to individuals with limited access to care, regardless of their ability to pay. Services available at these clinics include physical exams, cardiovascular checks, diabetes and osteoporosis screenings, smoking cessation programs, immunizations, and other prevention-focused services. These clinics provide care to vulnerable populations in America's rural, urban, and suburban communities. For many patients in medically underserved areas, NMHCs and nurse practitioners are the areas' only primary care providers. NMHCs serve as critical access points to keep patients out of the emergency room, saving the health care system millions of dollars annually.

One example of an emerging care delivery model is the Transitional Care Model (TCM) (Naylor, 2013). This nursing-developed model focuses on the care delivered through the varied transitions of care of those individuals with chronic illness.

Ten Essential Elements of Traditional Care Models

TCMs target older adults with two or more risk factors, including a history of recent hospitalizations, multiple chronic conditions, and poor self-health ratings.

1. The transitional care nurse (TCN), a master's-prepared nurse with advanced knowledge and skills in the care of this population, acts as the primary coordinator of care to ensure continuity throughout acute episodes of care.
2. In-hospital assessment, collaboration with team members to reduce adverse events and prevent functional decline, preparation and development of a streamlined, and evidenced-based plan of care.
3. Regular home visits by the TCN with ongoing telephone support (7 days per week) through an average of 2 months post-discharge.
4. Continuity of medical care between hospital and primary care providers facilitated by the TCN accompanying patients to first follow-up visit(s).
5. Comprehensive, holistic focus on each patient's goals and needs, including the reason for the primary hospitalization and other complicating or coexisting health problems and risks.
6. Active engagement of patients and family caregivers with a focus on meeting their goals.
7. Emphasis on patients' early identification and response to health care risks and symptoms to achieve longer-term positive outcomes and avoid adverse and untoward events that lead to readmissions.
8. Multidisciplinary approach that includes the patient, family caregivers, and health care providers as members of a team.
9. Physician-nurse collaboration across episodes of acute care.
10. Communication to, between, and among the patient, family caregivers and health care providers.

Outcomes of this model of care include the following:

- Reductions in preventable hospital readmissions for both primary and coexisting health conditions
- Improvements in health outcomes; short-term improvements in physical health, functional status, and quality of life were reported by patients who received TCM
- Enhancement of patient satisfaction
- Reductions in total health care costs; both total and average reimbursements per patient have been reduced in TCM 3

SUMMARY

Nurses are accountable for the delivery of safe, efficient, and effective patient/family care. The PPM and care delivery system and model serve as the vehicles for the delivery of such care. The decisions are based on a variety of information and current evidence and research. With the advent of the PPACA of 2010, nurses are at the forefront of the development and implementation of evidence-based models of care delivery to meet the needs of the population.

CLINICAL CORNER

Professional Practice Model Development

According to the American Nursing Credentialing Center, a **professional practice model** (PPM) is a schematic depiction of a theory, phenomenon, or system that depicts how nurses practice, collaborate, communicate, and develop professionally. It is the conceptual framework and philosophy of nursing at a specific organization. The creation of a schematic depiction of a theory or phenomenon of how nurses see themselves practicing nursing in an organization can be challenging. This challenge was accepted by the Professional Practice Council in collaboration with the Nurse Executive Council. One of the goals behind this challenge was that nurses at every level in the organization would participate in this endeavor. Making this model with frontline nurse involvement was essential for the enculturation. A task force was developed and a literature review begun. The PPM was to be grounded in theory, using a qualitative methodology to discover the embedded phenomenon that was in existence.

An invitation was sent out to all nurses in the organization requesting volunteers to participate in establishing a PPM for the organization. The response rate captured nurses at all levels in the organization. A focus group was created and the moderator and assistant moderator were assigned. Characteristics that the moderator needed to possess were the ability to exercise unobtrusive behavior, adequate knowledge of the PPM concept, and to identify as one of the participants. The assistant moderator would need to be able to handle the logistics, take careful notes, and use flip charts. In this case the Chair of the Professional Practice Council was selected for the moderator, and the Magnet Coordinator was selected for the assistant moderator. Data analysis was undertaken using the Colaizzi method by collecting and transcribing; extracting significant statements; collapsing into like categories; and clustering themes into categories, which reflected the elements of the PPM.

The first item on the agenda was education regarding the explanation of a PPM and its relationship to nursing theory as it pertains to the patient, nurse, environment, and health. Education about our Nursing Theorist, Jean Watson, was instrumental in capturing the true essence of the PPM and providing the groundwork for the philosophy of nursing in the organization. The organization's mission and vision statement were also presented during the education session. Identifying a nursing philosophy and depicting what is important to nursing within an organization is imperative and must be aligned with the organizational mission and vision. Giving examples of existing PPMs was the last step in the education part of the session.

Everyone then broke into different teams to brainstorm and describe how nursing practice could be depicted in a schematic model representing the organization and its vision, "pursuing excellence in health care." The statement pursuing excellence in nursing practice was the starting point for the development of the PPM. The elements that were important to the PPM such as practice, collaboration, communication, and professional development were recorded on flip charts. A fifth element, "caring," as in the Jean Watson Theory of Caring, was added to incorporate our nursing theory. Every element was a driving force for delivering high-quality health care with the nurse in the lead. Everyday nursing practice deals with communication, collaboration, professional development, and caring.

Nursing practice in our PPM encompasses many components including but not limited to patient-centered care, high-quality care, shared governance, evidence-based practice, and research in the delivery of care. When shared governance is strong and nurses have a voice, many changes based on evidence and research will occur. The philosophy of shared governance implies that nurses at every level play a role in the decisions that affect nursing, and it requires nurses to be accountable for their decisions (Porter-O'Grady, 1989, p. 350). These decisions should be based on evidence. Evidence-based practice is the "conscientious, explicit, and judicious use of the current best evidence in making decisions about the care of individuals" (Sackett, Rosenberg, Gray, Haynes, & Richardson, 1996, p. 71). It encompasses clinical and administrative practices that have been proven to consistently produce specific intended results. Research is vital to evidence-based practices. By definition, research is an organized study with methodical investigation into a subject to discover facts, to establish or revise a theory, or to develop a plan of action based on the facts discovered. It is the discovery of new knowledge. It is no longer the norm to say, we do it that way because we have always done it that way. Nurses are educated and knowledgeable and can apply evidence to their practice. When research is applied and evidence is presented, high-quality care will be delivered.

Another element in our PPM is collaboration, as evidenced by the statement in our model: "Nurses act as facilitators and advocates. We develop a partnership in care with our patients, their families, and with fellow

Continued

CLINICAL CORNER—Cont'd

Professional Practice Model Development

health care professionals." This is demonstrated through our care delivery model in which the nurse is considered to be the coordinator of care for patients as they navigate through a complex health care system. Our care delivery model needed to be updated to align with our PPM. This was done after the PPM was developed and disseminated. Our multidisciplinary rounds are nurse led and the collaboration between all disciplines is essential to providing high-quality care and establishing a strong discharge plan that will empower our patients and families to care for themselves at home. Our rounds include patient and family goals, projected length of stay, and any barriers that will hinder that length of stay. At present, our Nursing Informatics Council is working on a "rounding tool" that incorporates all aspects of our rounds including the disease-specific certification requirements of The Joint Commission. It is a proactive tool that will keep the patients' goals obtainable. This tool will be embedded in the electronic medical record.

Our communication element addresses our goal to promote the professional image of nursing through active engagement in patient education, quality initiatives, and innovation to promote continuity of care for patients and their families, including local and global outreach. There is a strong relationship between the communication and collaboration elements. The communication element has enhanced our nurses' ability to reach out to our communities, both local and global. Our Nursing Leadership meetings provide nurses with the opportunity to present their global and local outreach endeavors to other nurses within the organization. This forum also promotes nurses taking the lead in promoting the image of nursing and encourages nurses to give back to the community, at both the local and global level.

The promotion of professional development has blossomed within our organization and continues to grow since the implementation of our PPM. Certification is taken seriously, and we have celebrated Certification Day every year for the last 6 years. Our celebration includes having nurses within the organization set up booths to promote their professional organizations and has stirred up competition about which units have the largest increases in certified nurses for the past year. Every year follows a different theme, and money is raised to help buy appropriate tools to encourage nurses to join their organization and go for their certification. We are fortunate enough to have a certification champion who speaks to all nurses when they begin their orientation to the medical center.

This sends a strong message that certification means you are an expert in your specialty. It is also incorporated into our Clinical Ladder Program. In the past couple of years we have also partnered with area colleges to have the schools come to our campus to encourage nurses who have been nursing for years to return to school for their Bachelor of Science in Nursing degree. An educational assistant program has also been implemented to streamline the reimbursement process and provide counseling for those returning to school.

The caring element is what connects all the components. As our model states: "Our Professional Practice Model is based on Jean Watson's Theory of Caring, which is a convergence of the art, theory, and science of nursing." According to Gallup polls, nurses are historically the most trusted profession, having always looked after the patients and families entrusted to their care. There is now an awareness of the importance of caring for each other. We are now working hard to encourage nurses to care for themselves. Our Nurses' Day celebrations encompass caring modalities, such as providing the nurses with reiki and massages. We have also established a Caritas Committee, which has educated all of the practice, peer, and unit-based councils about the importance of the Jean Watson Theory of Caring. All the council meetings begin with an inspirational reading and deep breathing and relaxation techniques before starting the meeting. The effect has been contagious. In the last year we have offered reiki certification classes to staff at all levels and are in the process of instituting a policy to offer reiki to our patients. The Caritas Committee has also been instrumental in obtaining a Care Channel for our patients to help them heal in a healing environment.

The nurses at our organization are constantly improving the care they render to patients and their families at our medical center, and our PPM has empowered our nurses to be at the forefront of change. This change includes, but is not limited to, creating a healing environment, creating a healthy work environment, and establishing practices based on evidence and research.

References

Porter-O'Grady, T. (1989). Shared governance: reality or sham? *American Journal of Nursing, 89*(3), 350–351.

Sackett, D. L., Rosenberg, W. M. C., Gray, J. A. M., Haynes, R. B., & Richardson, W. S. (1996). Evidence based medicine: what it is and what it isn't. *BMJ, 312*(71), 71–72.

Catherine Herrmann, BSN, RN, CCRN
Hackensack UMC

EVIDENCED-BASED PRACTICE

(From Chamberlin, B., Bersick, E., Cole, D., Craig, J., Commins, K., Duffy, M., Hascup, V., Kaufman, M., McClure, D., & Skeahan, L. (2013). Practice models: a concept analysis. *Nursing Management, 44*(10), 16–18.)

The members of the Research Committee of the Organization of Nurse Executives of NJ (now Organization of Nurse Leaders of NJ) discussed the need to clarify the meaning of a professional practice model in nursing. Confusion regarding this term and its essential elements exists. Terms such as *patient care delivery model, professional care model, professional practice model, contemporary care delivery model,* and *integrated delivery system* are common in the nursing community. These terms are often used interchangeably or have overlapping elements. The members of this committee completed a literature review, with a goal to establish clarification of professional practice models and to propose a definition. They concluded that the term *professional practice model* can be used to describe "any practice model that relies on the professionalism of the care delivery term to improve patient outcomes."

As the science of nursing continues to build its knowledge base, professional frameworks and models of care are used to guide practice. Practice models, as a blend of professional behaviors and clinical leadership, are a foundation that allows for mutual goal setting and facilitates the prioritization of patient care by the interdisciplinary team. When a clear model guides practice, nurses can articulate the effect of their care. Use of such structures helps foster autonomous decision making; professional identity, job satisfaction, high quality, consistent nursing care; improved patient and nurse outcomes; and interdisciplinary communication.

A practice model reflects nursing values that exemplify the culture of the organization. The dominant attributes shared among models include nursing autonomy, empowerment, and cost-effective care. The primary goal of a nurse practice model is to support the relationship between the nurse and the patient. Nurses' participation in decision making improves the quality of care, enhances patient and family satisfaction, and contributes to overall nursing satisfaction. These attributes are also associated with increased nursing engagement and retention. For nurses, the positive outcomes are improved practice and communication, shared governance, autonomy, empowerment, engagement, powerful work teams, and increased job satisfaction.

Practice models may be found in any area where nurses are providing care. The professional practice model is the overarching term for guiding care delivery. It is the total system in which nurses provide care. It is made up of the care delivery model (structure and processes), teamwork (relationships), and values that facilitate nurses' contributions to both patient outcomes and the environment. Each element in the model strengthens the other components, and requires the integrated system to function effectively and efficiently in today's practice environment.

▮ NCLEX® EXAMINATION QUESTIONS

1. Which of the following is a collaboration among primary care clinicians, a hospital, specialists, and other health professionals who accept joint responsibility for the quality and cost of care provided to patients?
   A. Medical home model
   B. Accountable Care Organization (ACO)
   C. Professional practice model
   D. Care delivery system
2. Which of the following is a schematic description of a theory, phenomenon, or system that depicts how nurses practice, collaborate, communicate, and develop professionally to provide the highest quality for those by the organization (American Nurses Credentialing Center (ANCC, 2019)?

   A. Medical home
   B. ACOs
   C. Professional practice model
   D. Care delivery system
3. The professional nurse practice environment empowers nurses by providing them with opportunities for:
   A. Autonomy, accountability, and control over the care that they provide and the environment in which they deliver care
   B. Access, accountability, and control over the care that they provide and the environment in which they deliver care

C. Autonomy, accountability, and administration over the care that they provide and the environment in which they deliver care

D. Accuracy, accountability, and control over the care that they provide and the environment in which they deliver care

4. The professional nurse as a decision maker is guided by:
   A. The American Nurses Association Code of Ethics
   B. The ANA Standards of the State Nursing Practice Act
   C. State titles
   D. All of the above

5. Who is the fundamental health care provider to meet the success of emerging patient-centered care delivery models?
   A. Registered nurse
   B. Physician
   C. Physician's assistant
   D. Nurse practitioner

6. The professional practice model and care delivery models are evaluated and revised based on new evidence and/or research and on outcome data such as the following:
   A. Accreditation standards and National Patient Safety Goals
   B. Patient satisfaction survey results
   C. National Database of Nursing Quality Indicators (NDNQI) nursing sensitive indicator outcomes
   D. All of the above

7. The Patient Protection and Affordable Care Act of 2010 (PPACA) directs renewed attention and substantially more resources and incentives to promote those elements of care that are also the backbone of nursing practice. These essentials of nursing practice **do not** include:
   A. Patient-centered or "holistic" care, including family and community
   B. Care continuity, such as coordination and integration across settings and providers
   C. Chronic disease management, such as patient education, prevention, and wellness care
   D. Patient's ability to pay for services, use of referral system

8. Three emerging care delivery models are:
   A. The ACO, the inpatient care, and the nurse-managed health center
   B. The ACO, the medical or health home, and the nurse-managed health center
   C. The ACO, the medical or health home, and the nurse-managed health center
   D. The ACO, the inpatient rehabilitation, and the nurse-managed health center

9. There are ten essential elements of traditional care models. Which of the following is not included as an essential element?
   A. In-hospital assessment
   B. Home visits
   C. Continuity of care
   D. Use of telehealth system

10. Transitional Care Model target:
   A. Older adults with two or more risk factors
   B. Middle-age adults with one risk factor
   C. Childbirth at home
   D. Teenagers with type 2 diabetes mellitus

Answers: 1. B   2. C   3. A   4. D   5. A   6. D
7. D   8. B   9. D   10. A

BIBILOGRAPHY

Accountable Care Facts. www.accountablecarefacts.org/topten/what-is-the-difference-between-a-medical-home-and-an-aco-1.

American Association of Critical-Care Nurses [AACN] Policy Brief. (2013). *Nurse-managed health clinics: Increasing access to primary care and educating the healthcare workforce.* Retrieved July 31, 2019, from www.aacn.nche.edu/government-affairs/FY13NMHCs.pdf.

American Nurses Association [ANA] Issue Brief. (2010) *New care delivery models in health system reform: Opportunities for nurses and their patient.* Retrieved July 31, 2021, from www.nursingworld.org/MainMenu Categories/Policy-Advocacy/Positions-and-Resolutions/Issue-Briefs/Care-Delivery-Models.pdf.

American Nurses Credentialing Center [ANCC]. (2013). *2014 Magnet application manual.* Silver Spring, MD: ANCC.

American Nurses Credentialing Center. (2019). *2019 Magnet Application Manual.* Silver Spring, MD: ANCC.

Brannon, R. L. (1994). *Intensifying care: The hospital industry, professionalization, and the reorganization of the nursing labor process.* Amityville, NY: Baywood Publishing Company.

Chamberlain, B, Bersick, E, Cole, D, Craig, J, Cummins, K, &, Duffy, M, et al. (2013). Practice models: A concept analysis. Nursing Management,. *Nursing Management*, doi:10.1097/01.NUMA.0000434465.90084.eb

Dubois, C., D'Amour, D., Tchouaket, E., Clarke, S., Rivard, M., & Blais, R. (2013). Associations of patient safety outcomes with models of nursing care organization at unit level in hospitals. *International Journal Quality Health Care, 25*(2), 110–117.

Gardner, K. (1991). A summary of findings of a five-year comparison study of primary and team nursing. *Nursing Research, 40*(2), 113–117.

Jupiter Medical Center. (2015). *Description of JMC care delivery system.* Retrieved July 31, 2019, from www.jupitermed.com/care-delivery-system.

Kimball, B., Joynt, J., & Cherner, D. (2007). The quest for new innovative care delivery models. *Journal of Nursing Administration, 37*(9), 392–398.

Lake, E. T. (2002). Development of the practice environment scale of the Nursing Work Index. *Research in Nursing & Health, 25*(3), 176–188.

Massachusetts General Hospital. (2014). Professional practice model. Retrieved July 31, 2019, from www.massgeneral.org/assets/MGH/pdf/nursing-patientcare/PPM-with-descriptions-091417.pdf.

Naylor, M. (2013). *Transitional Care Model.* Retrieved July 31, 2019, from www.nursing.upenn.edu/media/transitional-care/Documents/Information%20on%20the%20Model.pdf.

O'Connor, B., Bennett, M., Crawford, S., & Korfiatis, V. (2006). The trials and tribulations of team nursing. *Collegian, 13*(3), 11–17.

O'Connor, S. E. (1994). A re-organization that improves patient care: An evaluation of team nursing in acute clinical setting. *Professional Nurse, 9*, 808–811.

Sjetne, I. S., Helgeland, J., & Stavem, K. (2010). Classifying nursing organization in wards in Norwegian hospitals: Self-identification versus observation. *BMC Nursing, 9*(3). doi:10.1186/1472-6955-9-3.

Tiedman, M., & Lookinland, S. (2004). Traditional models of care delivery: What have we learned? *Journal of Nursing Administration, 34*(6), 291–297.

University of California–Los Angeles (UCLA). (2014). *Professional Practice Model.* www.uclahealth.org/nursing/professional-practice-model.

Yoder-Wise, P. S. (2011). *Leading and managing in nursing* (4th ed.). St. Louis: Mosby.

UNCITED REFERENCES

(Brannon, 1994; D'Amour et al., 2012; Gardner, 1991; Kimball, Joynt, & Cherner, 2007; Lake, 2002; O'Connor, 1994; Sjetne, Helgeland, & Stavem, 2010; Yoder-Wise, 2011; Accountable Care Facts; American Association of Critical-Care Nurses AACN Policy Brief, 2013; Jupiter Medical, 2015; Massachusetts General, 2014; University of California–Los Angeles UCLA, 2014)

Staffing and Scheduling

OBJECTIVES

- Discuss the information required for the determination of staffing needs.
- Review the different types of assignment systems.
- Identify the difference between centralized and decentralized staffing.

- Differentiate between the various types of staffing patterns.
- Discuss activities used by the nurse manager to support fluctuating staffing needs.

KEY TERMS

average length of stay (ALOS)

block scheduling using the same schedule repeatedly

centralized scheduling scheduling done in one location

decentralized scheduling scheduling done in local areas

full-time equivalent (FTE) full-time equivalent; equal to the equivalent of a full-time employee

nursing care hours per patient day total paid hours for nursing personnel for a specific time period divided by the number of patient days in the same period

patient acuity measure of nursing workload that is generated for each patient

permanent shifts personnel working the same hours repeatedly

rotating work shifts alternating work hours among days, evening, and nights

self-scheduling staff coordinating their own work schedules

staffing pattern plan that articulates how many and what kind of staff are needed by shift and day to staff a unit or department

staffing ratios number of nursing staff per patient

staffing schedules work schedules for personnel

variable staffing determining the number and mix of staff based on patient needs

variance reports noting differences in budgeted or planned staffing and costs

STAFFING

One of the most time-consuming concerns of most nurse managers is the staffing of the unit. Staffing requires having enough staff to deliver care and that the staff present are qualified to deliver that care. Hospital nurse staffing has an important relationship to patient safety and quality of care. The available evidence indicates that there is a statistically and clinically significant association between registered nurse (RN) staffing and the adjusted odds ratio of hospital-related mortality, failure to rescue, and other patient outcomes (Kane, Shamliyan, Mueller, Duval, & Wilt, 2007). Staffing schedules are also a major concern of nurses as they enter a health care environment. Issues with schedules are often cited as a major job dissatisfier by nurses leaving the workplace (Halm, Peterson, & Kandelis, 2005).

There have been multiple studies in recent literature supporting the importance of safe staffing and its relation to patient safety (Aiken, Clarke, Sloan, Sochalski, & Silber, 2002; Hugonnet, Chevrolet, & Pittet, 2007; Marine, Meehan, Lyons, & Curley, 2013; Stone, Mooney-Kane, & Larson, 2007; Weissman, Rothschild, & Bendavid, 2007). Higher numbers of hours of nursing care provided by RNs and a greater number of hours of care by RNs per day are associated with better care for hospitalized patients ((American Nurses Association 2019); Choi et al., 2013; Park, Blegen, Spetz, Chapman, & DeGroot, 2015).

Health care staffing is a complicated issue requiring knowledge of patient acuity, nursing productivity, nursing competence, organization finance, and health care regulations.

The Joint Commission

The Joint Commission (TJC) and other accrediting agencies survey hospitals on the quality of care provided. They do not mandate staffing levels, but they do assess an organization's ability to provide the right number of competent staff to meet the needs of patients served by the hospital (The Joint Commission TJC, 2019).

The American Nurses Association *Principles for Nurse Staffing*

In 2012, the ANA published *Principles for Nurse Staffing* (2nd ed.), which emphasizes the importance of the nursing work environment in providing safe patient care (Box 12.1). Appropriate nurse staffing is the match of RN expertise with the needs of the recipient of nursing care services in the context of the practice setting and situation. The provision of appropriate nurse staffing is necessary to reach safe quality outcomes; it is achieved by dynamic, multifaceted decision-making processes that must take into account a wide range of variables (American Nurses Association ANA, 2012). The ANA *Principles for Nurse Staffing* are organized into five sets according to the following topics (note the relationship with the data required for care delivery decisions [Chapter 2]):

- The characteristics and considerations of the health care consumer
- The characteristics and considerations of the RNs and others
- Interprofessional team members and staff
- The context of the entire organization in which the nursing services are delivered
- The overall practice environment that influences the delivery of care
- The evaluation of staffing plans

After the first edition of *Principles for Nurse Staffing* in 1999, the ANA advocated a work environment that supports nurses in providing the best possible patient care by budgeting enough positions, administrative support, good nurse–physician relations, career advancement options, work flexibility, and personal choice in scheduling (ANA, American Nurses Association ANA, 2012). This advocacy continues today.

State departments of health have staffing regulations for health care institutions; these regulations are often broad. Additionally, California has mandatory staffing

BOX 12.1   The American Nurses Association *Principles for Nurse Staffing*

Core components of nurse staffing.
- Appropriate nurse staffing is critical to the delivery of quality, cost-effective health care.
- All settings should have well-developed staffing guidelines with measurable nurse sensitive outcomes specific to that setting and health care consumer population that are used as evidence to guide daily staffing.
- Registered nurses are full partners working with other health care professionals in collaborative, interdisciplinary partnerships.
- Registered nurses, including direct care nurses, must have a substantive and active role in staffing decisions to ensure the necessary time with patients to meet care needs and overall nursing responsibilities.
- Staffing needs must be determined based on an analysis of health care consumer status (e.g., degree of stability, intensity, and acuity) and the environment in which the care is provided. Other considerations to be included are professional characteristics, skill set and mix of the staff, and previous staffing patterns that have been shown to improve outcomes.
- Appropriate nurse staffing should be based on allocating the appropriate number of competent practitioners to a care situation; pursuing quality of care indices; meeting consumer-centered and organizational outcomes; meeting federal and state laws and regulations; and attending to a safe, quality work environment.
- Cost effectiveness is an important consideration in delivery of safe, quality care.
- Reimbursement structure should not influence nurse staffing patterns or the level of care provided.

Principles Related to the Health Care Consumer
Staffing decisions should be based on the number and needs of the individual health care consumers, families, and population served. These include the following:
- Age and functional ability
- Communication skills
- Cultural and linguistic diversities
- Severity, intensity, acuity, complexity, and stability of condition
- Existence and severity of multimorbid conditions
- Scheduled procedure(s)
- Ability to meet health care requisites
- Availability of social supports
- Transitional care, within or beyond the health care setting
- Continuity of care
- Complexity of care needs
- Environmental turbulence (i.e., rapid admissions, turnovers, and/or discharges)

- Other specific needs identified by the health care consumer, the family, and the registered nurse

The following elements are to be considered when making the determination:
- Governance within the setting (i.e., shared governance)
- Involvement in quality measurement activities
- Quality of the work environment of the nurses
- Development of comprehensive plans of care
- Practice environment
- Architectural geography of the unit and institution
- Evaluation of practice outcomes that include both quality and safety
- Available technology
- Evolving evidence

Principles Related to Registered Nurses and Other Staff
The following nurse characteristics should be taken into account when determining staffing:
- Licensure
- Experience with the population being served
- Level of experience (i.e., novice to expert)
- Competency with technology and clinical interventions
- Professional certification
- Educational preparation
- Language capabilities

Principles Related to Organization and Workplace Culture
These include at a minimum:
- Effective and efficient support services (e.g., transport, clerical, housekeeping, and laboratory)
- Timely coordination, supervision, and delegation as needed to maximize safety
- Access to timely, accurate, relevant information provided by communication technology that links clinical, administrative, and outcome data
- Sufficient orientation and preparation, including nurse preceptors and nurse experts to ensure registered nurse competency
- Preparation and ongoing training for competency in technology or other tools
- Sufficient time for patient documentation
- Necessary time to collaborate with and supervise other staff
- Necessary time to accommodate increased documentation demands created by integration of technology, electronic records, surveillance systems, and regulatory requirements
- Support in ethical decision making

Continued

> ## BOX 12.1 The American Nurses Association *Principles for Nurse Staffing*—Cont'd
>
> - Resources and pathways for care coordination and health care consumer/client and/or family education
> - Adequate time for coordination and supervision of nursing assistive personnel by registered nurses
> - Processes to facilitate transitions during work redesign, mergers, and other major changes in work life
> - Supporting the registered nurse's professional responsibility to maintain continuing education and engagement in lifelong learning
>
> ### Principles Related to the Practice Environment
> Staffing is a structure and process that affects the safety of patients, as well as others in the environment and nurses themselves. Institutions employing a culture of safety must recognize appropriate nurse staffing as integral to achieving goals for patient safety and quality.
>
> Registered nurses have a professional obligation to report unsafe conditions or inappropriate staffing that adversely impacts safe, quality care and the right to do so without reprisal.
>
> Registered nurses should be provided a professional nursing practice environment in which they have control over nursing practice and autonomy in their workplace.
>
> Appropriate preparation, resources, and information should be provided for those involved at all levels of decision making. Opportunities must be provided for individuals to be involved in decision making related to nursing practice.
>
> Routine mandatory overtime is an unacceptable solution to achieve appropriate nurse staffing. Policies on length of shifts, management of meal and rest periods, and overtime should be in place to ensure the health and stamina of nurses and prevent fatigue-related errors.
>
> ### Principles Related to Staffing Evaluation
> Organizations should evaluate staffing plans based on factors including but not limited to the following:
> - Outcomes, especially as measured by nurse-sensitive indicators
> - Time needed for direct and indirect patient care
> - Work-related staff illness and injury rates
> - Turnover/vacancy rates
> - Overtime rates
> - Rate of use of supplemental staffing
> - Flexibility of human resource policies and benefit packages
> - Evidence of compliance with applicable federal, state, and local regulations
> - Levels of health care consumer satisfaction and nurse satisfaction

(From American Nurses Association [ANA]. (2012). *Principles for nurse staffing* (2nd ed.). Silver Spring, MD: American Nurses Association.)

guidelines. These guidelines have provoked court challenges and much discussion and review in other states. On October 10, 1999, California became the first state in the country to require mandatory, safe licensed nurse-to-patient ratios in all units in acute-care facilities. The legislation (AB 394) requires that additional nurses be added to a minimum ratio in accordance with a patient classification system based on the severity of the patient's condition. As mandated by state law, the California Department of Health Services requires acute-care hospitals to maintain minimum nurse-to-patient staffing ratios. Required ratios vary by unit from 1:1 in operating rooms to 1:6 in psychiatric units (Agency for Healthcare Research and Quality [AHRQ], 2014). Thirteen other states address nurse staffing in hospitals with official Department of Health regulations (CT, IL, MA, MN, NV, NJ, NY, OH, OR, RI, TX, VT, and WA). Seven states require hospitals to have staffing committees responsible for plans and staffing policy (CT, IL, NV, OH, OR, TX, and WA). Lawmakers in the District of Columbia, New York, Texas, Florida, New Jersey, Iowa, and Minnesota are also considering legislation. Some states are attempting to introduce mandated staffing ratios in long-term care facilities.

PROCESS OF STAFFING

A staffing plan addresses the requirements of the unit or organization over a defined period of time. Daily staffing plans outline what is necessary to meet the needs of the patients over a 24-hour period. An annual staffing plan is created to determine the budgetary needs of an organization. "Daily staffing" refers to filling in open shifts on the current work schedule.

"Scheduling" refers to making work assignments for the next work period. It is done from 4 to 8 weeks in advance depending on the institution (Fig. 12.1).

Process of Daily Staffing

The process of daily staffing begins with an assessment of the current staffing situation. The assessment includes

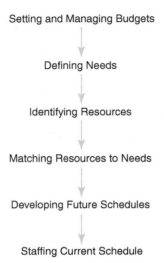

Setting and Managing Budgets

↓

Defining Needs

↓

Identifying Resources

↓

Matching Resources to Needs

↓

Developing Future Schedules

↓

Staffing Current Schedule

Fig. 12.1 Nurse scheduling and staffing. (From California Health Care Foundation. [2005]. *Adopting online nurse scheduling and staffing systems.* Oakland, CA: California Health Care Foundation. Used with permission.)

the qualifications and competence of the staff needed and available to meet the needs of the current patients (ANA, American Nurses Association ANA, 2012). The next step is to formulate a plan to meet future needs. The staffing process culminates in a schedule (organized plan) of personnel to provide patient care services. Scheduling variables are defined as (adapted from (Jones, 2007) p. 280):

1. The number of patients, complexity of patients' conditions, and nursing care required
2. The physical environment in which nursing care is to be provided
3. The nursing staff members' competency levels, qualifications, skill range, knowledge or ability, and experience levels
4. The level of supervision required
5. Availability of nursing staff members for the assignment of responsibilities
6. Availability of staff needed for participation in shared governance activities

The Staffing Plan

The staffing plan consists of four different elements that must be addressed:

1. The health care setting
2. The care delivery model
3. Patient acuity
4. Nursing staff

These are then incorporated into the next step in the process—the scheduling and staffing system. A staffing plan can also be referred to as the "staffing matrix."

Staffing and Scheduling Systems

There are various types of staffing systems in place in health care. The four major types are as follows:

1. **Centralized scheduling:** Decision making occurs in a "centralized" location for the entire institution.
2. **Decentralized scheduling:** Decision making occurs with the nurse manager on the unit.
3. **Mixed scheduling:** Blends aspects of items 1 and 2. Individual units may manage staffing, but if they cannot fill open shifts, they might forward their needs to a centralized office.
4. **Self-scheduling:** Individual staff members schedule themselves. The nurse manager then works with staff members to fill empty slots.

Many organizations are moving toward computer-assisted staffing.

Centralized Scheduling

There are two major advantages of centralized scheduling: fairness to employees through consistent, objective, and impartial application of policies and opportunities for cost containment through better use of resources (Marquis & Huston, 2017).

Decentralized Scheduling

When managers are given authority and assume responsibility, they can staff their own units through decentralized scheduling.

Scheduling staff, which is very time consuming, takes managers away from other duties or forces them to do the scheduling while off duty. Decentralized scheduling may use resources less effectively and consequently make cost containment more difficult (Marquis & Huston, 2017).

Mixed Scheduling

An individual may manage staffing but with the option of consulting a centralized office to help fill open shifts.

Self-Scheduling

Staff nurses coordinate the scheduling. This saves the manager considerable scheduling time. It also increases staff members' ability to negotiate with each other and

TABLE 12.1   Pros and Cons of Centralized and Decentralized Scheduling

Scheduling Method	Pros	Cons
Centralized	Fairness Cost containment	Lack of individualized treatment
Decentralized	Managers have authority Staff get personalized attention Staffing is easier Staffing is less complicated	Schedule used to punish and reward Time consuming for managers Cost containment is more difficult

BOX 12.2   Types of Pattern Scheduling

- Alternating or rotating work shifts: Work schedule is based on a predefined pattern, such as alternate weekends off, or rotating from days to evenings every 3 weeks. Sometimes, however, the rotating of shifts may only occur as needed, such as when the night nurse is off.
- Permanent shifts: Individuals are hired to work specific shifts, such as nights only.
- Block, or cyclical, scheduling: This type of scheduling system uses the same schedule repeatedly. It may be similar to alternating or rotating shifts but may also include a pattern of days on and days off (4 on, 2 off). It is often used as part of another type of scheduling pattern (see below).

  8-hour shift, 5-day work week: This method uses the traditional 5-day, 40-hour work week. This does not mean that weekends are not covered; the nurse works 5 days a week with 2 days off, and the nurse may work alternating weekends.

  10-hour day, 4-day work week: This method requires careful block scheduling to cover all shifts.

  12-hour shifts: 3 days on and 4 days off. Some studies demonstrate that this method allows for better use of nursing personnel, increased continuity of care, and improved job satisfaction and morale (Garrett, 2008).

  Baylor plan—weekend alternative: Baylor University Medical Center in Dallas, Texas, started a 2-day alternative plan. Nurses have the option to work two 12-hour days on the weekends and be paid for 36 hours for day shifts, or 40 hours for night shifts, or five 8-hour shifts Monday through Friday. This plan requires a larger nursing staff, filled weekend positions, and reduced turnover. Some hospitals have implemented the Baylor plan, indicating that the extra pay on weekends compensated for vacations, holidays, and sick time (Toomey, 2008, p. 393).

- Variable staffing: This type of staffing is dependent on the patient acuity and needs of the unit. If acuity is higher than budgeted, extra staff may be called in on overtime, or additional staff, such as agency or float staff, may be used.

has been associated with perceptions of increased nursing autonomy and satisfaction.

Table 12.1 provides pros and cons of centralized and decentralized scheduling.

Health care organizations must have a system in place to track available personnel. To match personnel with staffing needs, the organization must be able to determine an individual's skills, competencies, license, certifications, and so on. Most scheduling is done in advance, and therefore future scheduling is used. Institutions use one or more of the following four types of future scheduling in their planning:

1. Pattern scheduling: Staff commit to work a set number of shift types in a given timeframe. At the end of the time period, the pattern repeats (such as 3 weeks of day shift followed by 1 week of night shift, repeated every 4 weeks). Pattern scheduling can also include permanent shifts, block shifts, and rotating shifts (Box 12.2).
2. Preference scheduling: Staff define their preferences for shift type, days of the week, and unit. Defined rules can override preferences.
3. Rules scheduling: This is based on an organization's scheduling policies. Because it does not take pattern or preference into account, it is rarely used alone.
4. Self-scheduling: Scheduling needs are defined, and then staff sign up for available shifts on a rotating, first-come, first-served basis.

Table 12.2 provides pros and cons of scheduling types.

Table 12.3 lists advantages and disadvantages of the types of pattern scheduling.

FULL-TIME EQUIVALENT

No matter what the shift, the needs of the patient, unit, and organization must be accommodated. There is no end to the creative ways that staffing can be accomplished, but the basic number that is used in staffing is the

TABLE 12.2   Pros and Cons of Scheduling Types

Scheduling Type	Pros	Cons
Rules-based	Incorporates regulatory issues (hours of work, time off overtime, staffing ratios)	Does not take preferences into account Does not take staffing patterns into account Scheduling can be erratic
Pattern	Predictable schedules	Little flexibility Impairs recruitment
Preference	Considers staff needs	Preferences may not match rules
Self	Enables more creativity in covering shifts Increased staff satisfaction Saves time for nurse managers	Less organization and manager control of staffing

(From California Health Care Foundation. (2005). *Adopting online nurse scheduling and staffing systems* (p. 13). Oakland, CA: California Health Care Foundation. Used with permission).

TABLE 12.3   Advantages and Disadvantages of Types of Pattern Scheduling

Type	Advantages	Disadvantages
Rotating work shifts	Can rotate teams	Rotates among shifts Increases stress Affects health Affects quality of work Disrupts development of work groups High turnover
Permanent shifts	Can participate in social activities Job satisfaction	Most people want day shifts New graduates predominantly staff evenings and nights
	Commitment to the organization	Difficulty of evaluating evening and night staff
	Few health problems	Nurses may not appreciate the workload or problems of other shifts
	Less tardiness Less absenteeism Less turnover	Rigidity
Block, or cyclical, scheduling	Same schedule repeatedly Nurses not so exhausted Sick time reduced Personnel know schedule in advance Personnel can schedule social events Decreased time spent on scheduling Staff treated fairly Helps establish stable work groups Decreases floating Promotes team spirit Promotes continuity of care	
Variable staffing	Use census to determine number and mix of staff Little need to call in unscheduled staff Efficient	

(From Tomey, A. M. (2008). *Guide to nursing management and leadership* (8th ed.). St. Louis: Mosby).

TABLE 12.4   FTE Calculation for Varying Levels of Work Commitment
1.0 FTE = 40 hours per week or five 8-hour shifts per week
0.8 FTE = 32 hour per week or four 8-hour shifts per week
0.6 FTE = 24 hours per week or three 8-hour shifts per week
0.4 FTE = 16 hours per week or two 8-hour shifts per week
0.2 FTE = 8 hours per week or one 8-hour shift per week

(From Kelly-Heidenthal, P. (2003). *Nursing leadership and management* (p. 240). Clifton Park, NY: Thomson Delmar Learning).

full-time equivalent (FTE). An FTE is a measure of the work commitment of a full-time employee. A full-time employee works to qualify for full-time employment. In institutions with a 40-hour full-time work week, this works out to 2080 hours of work time per year (40 hours per week for 52 weeks a year equals 2080 hours of work time). In organizations with a 37.5-hour work week, this would be (37.5 × 52 weeks) 1950 hours of work time per year. Most institutions use a 40-hour work week for the definition of an FTE (Table 12.4).

Therefore, if the nurse manager needed to cover 40 hours of work per week, it could be done by one full-time employee or two half-time employees, and so on. For budget purposes, it would be important to know the state rules and regulations covering benefits. When does an employee receive benefits (health care, vacation time, etc.)? Staff benefits are a costly expense to health care institutions. Benefits are presently estimated as up to 53% beyond actual pay in some institutions.

Another variable in the staffing decision will be the amount of productive versus nonproductive hours. Not all of the 2080 hours of the FTE are productive. Benefit time, such as vacation, sick time, and education time are considered nonproductive time. To determine the amount of productive time of an employee, you would subtract the hours of benefit time from the FTE of 2080 hours. So if an employee had:

5 sick days (5 days × 8 hours/day) = 40 hours
20 vacation days (20 × 8 hours/day) = 160 hours
Holidays (5 days × 8 hours/day) = 40 hours
Education time (3 days × 8 hours/day) = 24 hours

Then this all adds up to 264 hours of nonproductive time, thus 2080 hours per year minus 264 hours = 1816 hours of productive time. When calculating the number of FTEs needed to staff the unit, you would count only the number of productive hours available.

To determine staffing needs, the nurse manager needs to know the number of FTE employees and the amount of nursing hours per patient day. Nursing care hours per patient day are the number of hours worked by nursing staff that have direct patient-care responsibilities. To calculate nursing care hours per patient day, use only productive hours.

Calculation of nursing care hours per patient day (Bernat, 2003):

20 patients on the unit
5 staff on each of three shifts = 15 staff
15 staff each working 8 productive hours = 120 hours ÷ 24 hours
120 nursing care hours ÷ 20 patients = 6.0 nursing care hours per patient

The Nursing Care Hours Per Patient Day (NCH/PPD) as a workload measurement tool may be too restrictive because it does not represent the "churn" of the unit, the reality of the patient unit where patient population and staffing fluctuates within shifts.

DEVELOPMENT OF A STAFFING PATTERN

One cannot assume that the number of nursing care hours is a permanent number. This number will change based on patient acuity. Patient acuity data are used to predict the amount of nursing care required by a group of patients. The higher the acuity level, the more nursing care is needed by the patient. There are several types of patient acuity measurement tools. The critical indicator PCS uses broad indicators such as IV fluid/medications, positioning, diet, and so on to summarize patient care activities. The summative task type uses the frequency of occurrence of specific activities, treatments, and procedures for each patient. Once adopted hours of patient care must be assigned for each patient classification. With patient acuity systems organizations can adjust staffing to documented need rather than perceived need.

To develop a staffing pattern using nursing hours per patient day (NHPPD) and patient acuity, you will need to determine the NCH/PPD needed for each shift depending on the acuity level of the patients on the unit during the shift.

What is important to realize is that any approach to predicting staffing needs and actualities must be flexible and based on expert nursing judgment that takes into consideration patient complexity and staff ability. Many health facilities are utilizing "flex-up" and "flex-down" staffing across all shifts to meet patient needs.

There are other options that health care facilities use to effectively and efficiently flex-up staffing when required.

Part-Time Staff

Part-time staff are used to decrease staffing shortages in an institution.

Part-time employment has the following benefits for nurses. It can:
- Broaden horizons beyond home
- Increase income
- Provide ego satisfaction
- Help maintain nursing skills
- Continue education

Benefits for the institution include:
- Maintain a flexible work pool
- Decrease benefit costs

Another option is for two nurses to share one full-time position. The disadvantages to an institution of position sharing are that educational and administrative expenses are higher proportionately for part-time than for full-time help because it costs as much to orient a part-time nurse as it does a full-time nurse, thereby costing more per hours worked. Also, maintaining continuity of care is complicated if two or more part-time people fill budgeted full-time positions. The disadvantages for the nurses are that there are not full-time benefits, such as vacation and sick time.

External Temporary Agencies

Usually as a last resort, an institution may use temporary agency nurses. The staffing agency is a business that has a registry of nurses who have highly flexible schedules. Matching of nurses' credentials with the position is sometimes daunting. Replacement staff from agency pools are usually an expensive means of maintaining staffing. Most hospitals prefer to minimize the use of agency nurses because of the extra cost to the institution. The extra costs arise from the mandated orientations, evaluation of competencies, and the agency fee.

BOX 12.3   Options Used for Sick Calls

- Use a float, per diem, or agency nurse.
- Ask a nurse to work for the sick person and cancel a shift for that person later in the week.
- Ask a part-time person to work an extra shift, substituting one type of classification for another, such as a licensed practical nurse (LPN) for an RN.
- Ask one staff member to work a few hours of overtime and another to come in a few hours early.
- Do without a substitute.
- Manager covers the shift.

Travel Nurses

"Travelers" are per diem nurses working for a business that places them in contracted hospitals. Unlike agency nurses, travelers usually sign longer-term contracts with hospitals (3–6 months or longer).

There are many options used by health care institutions to deal with staffing and daily absences because of sick calls (Box 12.3).

Overtime

In a staffing emergency, institutions may ask nurses to work overtime. Overtime pay is usually at a higher rate than regular pay, and many nurses depend on the extra money provided by overtime. There are a number of issues with overtime that need concern the nurse and nurse manager.

- Length of time the nurse will be working. In a normal shift, the nurse will have already worked up to 12 hours and an additional shift could have them working a full 24 hours! This can be ameliorated by only allowing 4 hours of overtime in such a situation.
- The nurse manager must be careful to evaluate the exhaustion level of the staff.
- There are documented instances of increased errors when the staff members are exhausted (Garrett, 2008).
- With regard to budget, overtime may increase the dollars spent on care provided. This budget variance will need to be documented.
- State labor law and union guidelines will need to be reviewed. These may define the number of hours required between shifts.

Mandatory overtime is never a solution to staffing concerns.

Automated Staffing Systems

Many health care institutions are moving toward the use of computerized staffing and scheduling systems. These systems greatly enhance the manager's ability to properly schedule staff. They also free up much of the time that the manager spends on the creation of the schedule. Integrated online scheduling and staffing products are available for purchase under license.

Evaluation of Staffing Measures

As discussed in the ANA *Principles for Nurse Staffing* (2012), the evaluation of the effectiveness of nurse staffing is of utmost importance. As a nurse manager, you will be evaluated in areas of patient outcomes and budget performance. The ever-evolving management of daily staffing with the patient outcomes and budget requirements is a daunting challenge for nurse administrators. The patient outcomes that are reviewed on a daily/weekly/monthly/quarterly basis are also related to nurse staffing. They include the following:

- Accreditation Standards and National Patient Safety Goals
- Patient Satisfaction survey results
- National Database of Nursing Quality Indicators (NDNQI) nursing sensitive indicator outcomes
- Unit scorecards
- The NDNQI Staff RN Satisfaction Survey
- Centers for Medicare and Medicaid Services (CMS) core measures
- Hospital Consumer Assessment of Healthcare Providers and Systems (HCAHPS) results
- Unit-based surveys

They also relate to the organizational budget performance and expected productivity. Typical unit productivity report indicators include:

Variance reports for areas of alteration (positive or negative!) must be shared with the key stakeholders. Performance is an ever-changing and evolving science.

BOX 12.4   Typical Unit Activities Productivity Report Indicators

- Volume statistic: number of units of service for the reporting period
- Capacity statistic: number of beds or blocks of time available for providing services
- Percentage of occupancy: number of occupied beds for the reporting period
- Average daily census (ADC): average number of patients cared for per day for the reporting period
- Average length of stay (ALOS): average number of days that a patient remained in an occupied bed

Formulas for Calculating Volume Statistics
Assume that a 20-bed medical-surgical unit *(capacity statistic)* accrued 566 patient days in June *(volume statistic)*. Ninety-eight of these patients were discharged during the month.

Average Daily Census (ADC) on this unit is 18.9
Formula: patient days for a given time period divided by the number of days in the time period
a. 30 days in June
b. 566 patient days/30 days = ADC of 18.9

Percentage of Occupancy for June is 95%
Formula: daily patient census (rounded) divided by the number of beds in the unit
19 patients in a 20-bed unit
19 patients/20 beds = 95% occupancy

Average Length of Stay for June is 5.8
Formula: number of patient days divided by the number of discharges
566 patient days/98 patient discharges = 5.8 (rounded)

SUMMARY

Staffing and scheduling represents one of the most challenging of the nurse manager's responsibilities. It requires an accurate sense of the day-to-day workings of the unit as well as a keen awareness of the staff's abilities and personalities. It also requires evaluation of the care delivered and the flexibility to create staffing levels that best meet patient needs.

CLINICAL CORNER

Staffing Innovation
Josephine Bodino, DNP, MPA, RN, NEA-BC, HN-BC, The Valley Hospital, Ridgewood, NJ

Health care organizations are embarking on strategic initiatives to become a high-reliability organization (HRO). HROs have systems in place to make them consistent and to avoid errors. One of the five tenets of an HRO is "sensitivity to operations," or having leaders who are in touch with work that is being done and the effect of that work on day-to-day operations. Observations could lead to new operational initiatives (Gamble, 2013).

Part of this sensitivity is to ensure that patient needs are met through appropriate labor management and the use of well-developed staffing models. Adequate staffing is critical to our ability to provide safe, reliable, high-quality care to our patients and their families. On any given day, some units experience staffing challenges while there are other units with a low census, which results in canceling staff.

There are challenges to staffing, and according to the Bureau of Labor Statistics (2013), nurse job openings are expected to be 1.05 million in 2022 due to growth and replacements. A Klynveld, Peat, Marwick, and Goerdeler (KPMG) survey (as cited in American Association of Colleges of Nursing [AACN], 2014) indicated that there is a turnover rate of 14% for RNs annually. The contributing factors to turnover are as follows: restrictions to nursing program enrollments, retiring workforce, demographic change with an aging population, and increased stress levels (AACN, 2014). Health care organizations are experiencing difficulty in recruitment, especially in specialized areas such as labor and delivery and the operating room.

Managing the current workforce in specific departments is an ongoing challenge due to fluctuations in patient flow, the daily staffing complement, and workload volume. Nurse leaders are charged with ensuring that the right caregivers providing the proper care at the right time and in the right setting meet the needs of acutely ill patients. Nurse leaders have a heavy responsibility for managing their full-time equivalents (FTEs) and positions.

To address staffing issues and workplace factors, some hospitals have a structure in place called nurse workplace environment and staffing councils (Caruso et al., 2019) or a healthy work environment and staffing committee. Some hospitals use shared governance structures with their councils/committees to empower nurses, giving nurses the ability to make decisions about their practice environment and job satisfaction (Allen-Gilliam et al., 2016). The council/committee addresses how to better meet organizational staffing needs and engages employees by asking them to come up with

new ideas and innovative processes. Having a staffing council or committee provides an avenue for nurses to share ideas, improve the work environment, and impact patient care (Kroning et al., 2019).

The Valley Hospital in Ridgewood, New Jersey, experienced high volume and staffing challenges. The dilemma of nurses being dissatisfied with floating to other areas was addressed at the Healthy Work Environment Staffing Committee (HWESC).

The committee decided to conduct a survey to gain feedback about floating. A literature review was undertaken to investigate queries about comfort level with floating to other units. The survey was developed and adopted questions from a "A Descriptive Study of Resources Needed During Floating Among Nurses in a Tertiary Pediatric Facility" (Hoffman & von Sadovszky, 2016).

A new question was asked during the survey: The committee wanted to know if nurses would float and be a resource to a unit experiencing high census and activity, including being a resource on a group in a different division. The question was, "If given a task list and not a full patient assignment, would you help a critically short unit outside your division?" (Some examples of crossing divisions include medical-surgical to critical care, emergency department [ED] to medical-surgical to ED, women's and children's services to medical-surgical.)

The committee reviewed the survey results, and the majority of respondents stated that instead of being canceled they would be willing to help other units with specific tasks, including groups in a different division. During the discussion of staffing and floating, the HWESC meeting also reviewed the cancelation hours of nurses. An idea was formulated by the HWESC not to cancel nurses and instead develop a program by which Valley could assist nursing units that are critically short across the division. Adequate staffing is critical to Valley's ability to provide safe, reliable, high-quality care to patients and their families when nursing units experience high census and activity and staffing gaps.

Through the shared governance model, the HWESC voted, and a decision was made to use a new innovative approach wherein nurses can help other nurses across divisions. The program is called the Helping Hands Program, the goal of which is to help critically short-staffed units. The HWESC developed a general task list to assist with tasks that nurses could do across divisions. The RN task list included patient education, dressing changes, rounding, emotional support, transporting, and medication administration.

Continued

CLINICAL CORNER—cont'd

The staff on the units receiving help are so appreciative when a Helping Hands nurse arrives. Many of the staff providing the support feel they have been a great asset to the staff of the unit to which they are sent. This new program has been instrumental in assisting Valley to provide a safer environment for patients. The Helping Hands Program received some great feedback:

- "Critical Care float nurse was phenomenal in helping us on a busy day in Peds." –Pediatrics staff
- "Staff in ED truly appreciated all your work! You jumped in and helped with medication reconciliation on many patients." –ED CSS to Med-Surg nurse
- "Nurse helped with tasks. Walked patient to the bathroom, helped with IV insertions, transport." –Mother/Baby and Labor & Delivery staff

Of course, it has not been entirely smooth sailing. Understandably, some staff members are uncomfortable going to a division where they have no experience, and there have been requests made for Helping Hands staff to perform tasks that are not always appropriate. There was a request to discontinue the program, but ethically does it feel right to cancel nurses if there are critically short units that require help?

The Helping Hands Program continues to be refined with task lists/processes and constant oversight over the program in real time. Helping Hands resource nurses receive a face-to-face check-in by the clinical shift supervisors, nurse managers, and hospital operations supervisor. Feedback is vital to ensure the success of the program. This new innovative approach to staffing is shared with all of the nursing leaders in the organization. Health care organizations have to look at new strategies to address staffing gaps, and this new innovative practice has made an impact on the nursing environment.

References

Allen-Gilliam, J., Kring, D., Graham, R., Freeman, K., Swain, S., Faircloth, G., & Jenkinson, B. (2016). The Impact of Shared Governance Over Time in a Small Community Hospital. *Journal of Nursing Administration, 46*(5), 257–264.

American Association of Colleges of Nursing. (2014). Nursing shortage. Retrieved from http://www.aacn.nche.edu/media-relations/fact-sheets/nursing-shortage.

Bureau of Labor Statistics. (2013). Table 8. Occupations with the largest projected number of job openings due to growth and replacement needs, 2012 and projected 2022. Retrieved February 8, 2015, from http://www.bls.gov/news.release/ecopro.t08.htm.

Caruso, J., Smith, R., Steingall, P., Cholewka, S., & Borenstein, K. (2019). Call to Action: Implementing Nurse Workplace Environment and Staffing Councils in New Jersey Hospitals. *Nurse Leader, 17*(4), 299–302.

Gamble, M. (2013 April, 29). *5 Traits of High Reliability Organizations: How to Hardwire Each in Your Organization*. Becker's Hospital Review. Retrieved September 29, 2019 from https://www.beckershospitalreview.com/hospital-management-administration/5-traits-of-high-reliability-organizations-how-to-hardwire-each-in-your-organization.html.

Hoffman, A. and von Sadovszky, V. A Descriptive Study of Resources Needed During Floating Among Nurses in a Tertiary Pediatric Facility. (2016). Sigma Theta Tau International. Indianapolis, Indiana.

Kroning, M., Yezzo, P., Leah, M., & Foran, A. (2019). TEAM CONCEPTS. The idea board: A best practice initiative. *Nursing Management, 50*(6), 12–14.

EVIDENCE-BASED PRACTICE

In 2004, California became the first state to implement minimum nurse-to-patient staffing requirements in acute-care hospitals. The U.S. federal government (through 42 codes of federal regulation) requires that hospitals certified to participate in Medicare have adequate staffing. However, only 14 states currently address nurse staffing in laws. Regulations required states to maintain appropriate nurse staffing in hospitals that participate in Medicare. The current law is ambiguous in that the federal government lets each state enact specific laws about nurse staffing related to patient safety. The 11 states studied in this review have established current laws on nurse staffing, and New Mexico, North Carolina, the District of Columbia, and Maine are in the process of enacting nursing laws. participate in Medicare (see). The current law is ambiguous in that the federal government lets each state enact specific laws about nurse staffing related to patient safety. The 11 states studied in this review have established current laws on nurse staffing, and New Mexico, North Carolina, the District of Columbia, and Maine are in the process of enacting nursing laws.

EVIDENCE-BASED PRACTICE—cont'd

Law	Definition	Main Characteristics
42 Code of Federal Regulations (42CFR 482.23(b))	Requires Medicare-certified hospitals to maintain all levels of adequate direct-care staff.	11 states have staffing laws. CA is the only state that stipulates minimum nurse-to-patient ratios; MA has laws specific to ICUs requiring 1:1 or 1:2 ratios, depending on patient stability.

California: California is the only state that enacted a law about minimum staffing ratios of nurses. In the Nurse Staffing Standards for Patient Safety and Quality Care Act of 2013 (H.R., 1907), California Nurse-to-Patient Ratio law A.B.394 1999-2000 Reg. Sess., the state proposed a plan for each unit to have an appropriate ratio of nurses to the number of patients and limited mandatory overtime.

New York: The Safe Staffing for Quality Care Act, S3691A-2013, provided an appropriate nurse-to-patient ratio for every unit, requiring facilities to announce nurse staffing information to the public. The New York law suggested the hours per resident day for nursing homes as 0.75 hours per RN day, 1.3 to LPNs per day, and 2.8 to CNAs per resident day. In the Safe Staffing for Hospital Care Act Bill S1634-2013 (pending), the legislature not only presented minimum nurse staffing but also suggested that more than 50% of nursing staff must provide direct care to patients, except for administrative workers and education personnel.

Massachusetts: In Massachusetts, on the basis of Bill H. 4228, every intensive care unit has to arrange a nurse-to-patient ratio of 1:1 or 1:2, depending on patient's severity of need.

Connecticut: On the basis of Public Act 08-79, An Act Concerning Hospital Staffing, Connecticut law requires that every hospital organize a staffing committee. Each facility must make regulations that specify use of temporary nurses, and the law suggests a minimum nursing skill-mix ratio.

Illinois: On the basis of Public Act 095-0401, Illinois law requires that every hospital organize a staffing committee that includes a majority of members who are direct-care nurses. Also, the hospital must administrate general matters about nurse staffing such as records, representativeness, and quality management.

Nevada: On the basis of the Patient Protection and Safe Staffing Bill (SB 362), Nevada law requires that every hospital organize a staffing committee and establish standards for high-quality patient care. If hospitals do not develop a staffing plan, Nevada law suggests they will be investigated and incur penalties and fines.

Oregon: On the basis of the Nurse Practice Act (Oregon Revised Statutes, Chapter 678.010–678.445), Oregon law requires that every hospital make a hospital nurse-staffing plan that includes direct-care nurses.

Rhode Island: On the basis of Rhode Island Law §23-17.17-8, hospitals in Rhode Island must submit a nurse-staffing plan to present the average nursing-skill mix for each unit and each shift.

Texas: On the basis of the Health and Safety Code Chapter 257, Nurse Staffing, Texas law requires that each medical center organizes a committee on nurse staffing of which 60% must be nurses who provide direct care to patients for more than 50% of their duty hours. The committee has to develop the nurse-staffing guidelines, efficient operation of nurse staffing, and an evaluation plan.

Vermont: On the basis of VT Statute Title 18 §1854, medical centers in Vermont must provide public notice of information on nurse staffing.

Washington: On the basis of RCW §70.41.420, Washington law requires that each medical center organize a staffing committee, 50% of whom must be nurses who provide direct care to patients. The committee must develop plans about an appropriate number of nurses for each unit and shift and provide public notice of information about nurse staffing.

A common feature of nursing law in the United States is a minimum nurse-staffing plan that must include direct-care nurses, with exceptions for administrative staff and assistive personnel. Each state has to organize a staffing committee and must establish a staffing plan suited for each hospital and unit. Nursing law in Illinois, Oregon, Washington, and Texas mandates inclusion of at least 50% to 60% direct-care nurses on committees. Some states, such as Vermont, mandate public notification of information about nurse staffing to ensure the public's right to know.

(From Shin, J., Koh, J., Kim, H., Lee, H., & Song, S. (2018). Current status of nursing law in the United States and implications. *Health Systems and Policy Research, 5*(1):67. doi:10.21767/2254-9137.100086.)

NCLEX® EXAMINATION QUESTIONS

1. One advantage of centralized scheduling is:
   A. Better use of resources
   B. Lack of cost containment
   C. Decrease use of resources
   D. Increase in cost

2. What is the average number of patients cared for per day for the reporting period called?
   A. Nursing hours per patient
   B. The average daily census
   C. The average length of stay
   D. Direct care hours

3. Which of the following requires knowledge of patient acuity, nursing productivity, nursing competence, organization finance, and health care regulations?
   A. Self-scheduling
   B. Health care staffing
   C. Health care scheduling
   D. Staff mix

4. What is the type of scheduling that blends aspects of centralized and decentralized scheduling whereby individual units may mange staffing?
   A. Self
   B. Centralized
   C. Mixed
   D. Decentralized

5. One of the most time-consuming concerns of nurse managers is the staffing of the unit. Staffing requires having enough staff to deliver care, and that the staff present are qualified to deliver that care. What must the nurse manager keep in mind?
   A. Use of unlicensed personnel saves the health care facility money.
   B. Better patient care and less errors are made when a unit is staffed by RNs.
   C. When a nurse calls out sick, ask present staff to work overtime.
   D. The use of travel nurses is better for cost containment.

6. The Joint Commission (TJC) and other accrediting agencies survey hospitals on the quality of care provided, but they:

   A. Do not mandate staffing levels
   B. Do assess an organization's ability to provide the right number of competent staff to meet the needs of patients served by the hospital
   C. Do not assess safe quality outcomes
   D. Do require mandatory, safe licensed nurse-to-patient ratios in all units in acute-care facilities at the state level

7. The staffing plan consists of four different elements that must be addressed. They are:
   A. The care delivery model, patient acuity, nursing staff, and staff experience
   B. The health care setting, care delivery model, patient acuity, and nursing staff
   C. The health care setting, patient acuity, nursing staff, and shift
   D. The number of patients, care delivery model, patient acuity, and nursing staff

8. As a new nurse you will need to ask how your unit's schedule is done. What type of scheduling is using the same schedule repeatedly?
   A. Block scheduling
   B. Rotation scheduling
   C. Permanent shifts
   D. Self-scheduling

9. As mandated by state law, which state requires acute-care hospitals to maintain minimum nurse-to-patient staffing ratios?
   A. New Jersey Department of Health Services
   B. New York Department of Health Services
   C. California Depaw rtment of Health Services
   D. Oregon Department of Health Services

10. What type of scheduling allows an individual to manage staffing, but with the option of consulting a centralized office to help fill open shifts?
    A. Self-scheduling
    B. Mixed scheduling
    C. Block scheduling
    D. Decentralized scheduling

REFERENCES

Agency for Healthcare Research and Quality [AHRQ]. (2004). *Hospital nurse staffing and quality of care: research in action,* (Issue 14. March 2004). Agency for Healthcare Research and Quality: Rockville, MD. http://www.ahrq.gov/research/findings/factsheets/services/nursestaffing/index.html.

Agency for Healthcare Research and Quality [AHRQ]. (2014). State-mandated nurse staffing levels alleviate workloads, leading to lower patient mortality and higher nurse satisfaction. http://www.innovations.ahrq.gov/content.aspx?id=3708.

Aiken, L., Clarke, S., Sloan, D., Sochalski, J., & Silber, J. (2002). Hospital nurse staffing and patient mortality, nurse burnout, and job dissatisfaction. *Journal of the American Medical Association, 288*(16), 1987–1993.

American Nurses Association. (2019). *Safe Staffing Literature Review.* Retrieved October 31, 2019 from https://www.nursingworld.org/~4a2a14/globalassets/practiceandpolicy/wor-environment/nurse-staffing/safe-staffing-literature-review.pdf.

American Nurses Association [ANA]. (2004). *Scope and standards for nurse administrators* (2nd ed.). Silver Spring, MD: ANA.

American Nurses Association [ANA]. (2012). *Principles for nurse staffing.* Silver Spring, MD: ANA.

Bernat, A. (2003). Effective staffing. In Kelly-Heidentha., P, (Ed.), *Nursing leadership and management* (pp. 238–265). Clifton Park, NY: Thomson Delmar Learning.

California Health Care Foundation. (2005). *Adopting online nurse scheduling and staffing systems.* Oakland, CA: CHCF.

Choi, J., & Boyle, D. (2013). RN Workgroup Job Satisfaction and Patient falls in Acute Care Hospital Units. *Journal of Nursing Administration, 43*(11), 586–591.

Garrett, C. (2008) The effect of nurse staffing patterns on medical errors and nurse burnout. AORN Journal (87) 1191–1192. 1194, 1196–1200, 1202–1204.

Halm, M., Peterson, M., & Kandelis, M. (2005). Hospital nurse staffing and patient mortality, emotional exhaustion, and job dissatisfaction. *Clinical Nurse Specialist, 19*(5), 241–251.

Heidenthal, K. (2003). *Nursing leadership & management.* Clifton Park, NY: Thomson/Delmar Learning.

Hugonnet, S., Chevrolet, J., & Pittet, D. (2007). The effect of workload on infection risk in critically ill patients. *Critical Care Medicine, 35*(1), 76–81.

Jones, P. (2007). *Nursing leadership and management: Theories, processes and practice.* Philadelphia, PA: F.A. Davis.

Kane, R. L., Shamliyan, T. A., Mueller, C., Duval, S., & Wilt, T. J. (2007). The association of registered nurse staffing levels and patient outcomes. *Systematic Review and Meta-analysis Medical Care, 45*(12), 1195–1204.

Marine, K., Meehan, P., Lyons, A., & Curley, M. (2013). Inequity of patient assignments: fact or fiction. *Critical Care Nurse, 33*(2), 74–77.

Marquis, B.L., & Huston, C.J. (2017). *Leadership roles and management functions in nursing: Theory and application* (9 ed.), Philadelphia: Lippincott Williams and Wilkins.

Needleman, J., Buerhaus, P., Stewart, M., Zelevinsky, K., & Mattke, S. (2006). Nurse staffing in hospitals: Is there a business case for quality? *Health Affairs, 25*(1), 204–211.

Needleman, J., Buerhaus, P., Mattke, S., Stewart, M., & Zelevinsky, K. (2002). Nurse staffing levels and the quality of care in hospitals. *New England Journal of Medicine, 346,* 1715–1722.

Park, S., Blegen, M., Spetz, J., Chapman, S., & DeGroot, H. (2015). Comparison of Nurse Staffing Measurments in Staffing-Outcomes Research. *Medical Care, 53*(1), 1–8. doi:10.1097/MLR0b01e318277eb50.

Siebert, S. & Chiusano, J. (2015). Understanding the charge nurse's role in staffing. American Nurse Today, 10(9), 9–10.

Stone, P., Mooney-Kane, C., & Larson, E. (2007). Nurse working conditions and patient safety outcomes. *Medical Care, 45*(6), 571–578.

The Joint Commission [TJC]. (2019). *Comprehensive accreditation manual for hospitals.* Oakbrook Terrace, IL: Author.

Toomey, A.M. (2008). *Guide to nursing management and leadership.* St Louis, MO: Mosby.

Weissman, J., Rothschild, J., & Bendavid, E. (2007). Hospital workload and adverse events. *Medical Care, 45*(5), 448–455.

Yoder-Wise. P. (2011). *Leading and managing in nursing* (5th ed.). St Louis: Elsevier.

Delegation of Nursing Tasks

OBJECTIVES

- Define delegation.
- Identify the five rights of delegation.
- Review the circumstances where delegation is appropriate.
- Identify tasks appropriate for delegation.
- Discuss the role of unlicensed personnel in the delivery of health care.
- Identify the role of the nurse in the delegation of health care.
- Review the legal ramifications of delegation of care.

KEY TERMS

accountability acknowledgment and assumption of responsibility for actions, decisions, and policies within the scope of the role or employment position and encompassing the obligation to report, explain, and be answerable for resulting consequences

assignment delegation of work to a selected group of patient care givers. The downward or lateral transfer of the responsibility of an activity from one individual to another while retaining accountability for the outcome

authority refers to an individual's ability to complete duties within a specific role. The authority derives from nurse practice acts and organizational policies and job descriptions

delegation transferring the authority to perform a selected nursing task in a selected situation to a competent individual

direct patient care activities activities such as hygienic care, feeding patients, taking vital signs, and so on that are performed on the patient indirect patient care activities routine activities of the patient unit that deal with the day-to-day functioning of the unit, such as restocking supplies

supervision active process of directing, guiding, and influencing the outcome of an individual's performance of an activity

unlicensed assistive personnel (UAP)/ noncredentialed assistive personnel individuals who are not licensed by the state but are trained to assist nurses by performing patient care tasks as allowed by the organization. There are many job titles for such employees, such as nursing assistant (NA), patient care associate (PCA), and UAP

DELEGATION

Delegation is defined as the "transfer of responsibility for the performance of an activity from one individual to another while retaining accountability for the outcome; for example, the nurse, in delegating an activity to an unlicensed individual, transfers the responsibility for the performance of the activity, but retains professional accountability for the overall care" (American Nurses Association [ANA], 1992, ANA (2019)). It is the entrusting of a selected nursing task to an individual who is qualified, competent, has the authority, and is able to perform such a task.

The following principles provide guidance and inform the registered nurse's (RN's) decision making about delegation:

- The nursing profession determines the scope and standards of nursing practice.
- The RN takes responsibility and accountability for the provision of nursing practice.
- The RN directs care and determines the appropriate use of resources when providing care.
- The RN may delegate tasks or elements of care, but he or she does not delegate the nursing process itself.
- The RN considers facility/agency policies and procedures and the knowledge and skills, training, diversity awareness, and experience of any individual to whom the RN may delegate elements of care.
- The decision to delegate is based on the RN's judgment concerning the care complexity of the patient, the availability and competence of the individual accepting the delegation, and the type and intensity of supervision required.
- The RN acknowledges that delegation involves the relational concept of mutual respect.
- Nurse leaders are accountable for establishing systems to assess, monitor, verify, and communicate ongoing competence requirements in areas related to delegation.
- The organization/agency is accountable to provide sufficient resources to enable appropriate delegation.

- The organization/agency is accountable for ensuring that the RN has access to documented competency information for staff to whom the RN is delegating tasks.
- Organizational/agency policies on delegation are developed with the active participation of RNs (American Nurses Association [ANA] and National Council of State Boards of Nursing [NCSBN], 2008).

The majority of health care institutions have care delivery systems that include various levels of caregivers. The acuity of patients within hospitals has increased during the last 10 years, and many hospitals have moved from total patient care, primary care, and other care delivery systems that require an all–RN staff. To meet the needs of the higher-acuity patients, nurses must delegate aspects of care to non-RN team members. Delegation changes as the health care environment changes. Since the advent of the nursing shortage, unlicensed assistive personnel (UAP) have been used to help fill the workforce gaps. The role of these assistive personnel is set by the institution that employs them and defines their practice. They may be called **noncredentialed assistive personnel**, and UAP. Individuals hired into these jobs are trained and evaluated by the facility. They may use a variety of titles, such as nursing assistant (NA), patient care associate (PCA), attendants, nursing technician, unit technician, and others (Marquis & Huston, 2017). They cannot practice nursing, and they must be directed, supervised, and evaluated by an RN, who is ultimately responsible for all patient care (see Box 13.1 for the nurse's responsibility in delegation). One form of licensed personnel, the licensed practical nurse (LPN), is used by many facilities. The LPN works under the direction and supervision of the RN. Licensed personnel work according to the state board regulations (see Chapter 11), but the job descriptions will vary from institution to institution. Various patient care roles are listed in Table 13.1.

There are two types of nursing activities that may be delegated, direct and indirect. **Direct patient care activities** include assisting with feeding, grooming, hygienic care, taking vital signs, ambulation, electrocardiogram

BOX 13.1 Nurse's Responsibility in Delegation

1. Before delegating a nursing task, the nurse shall determine the nursing care needs of the patient. The nurse shall retain responsibility and accountability for the nursing care of the patient, including nursing assessment, planning, evaluation, and nursing documentation.
2. Before the delegation of the nursing task to unlicensed assistive personnel, the nurse shall determine that the unlicensed person has been trained in the task and deemed to be competent.

Criteria for Delegation

1. The delegated nursing task shall be a task that a reasonable and prudent nurse would find within the scope of sound nursing judgment and practice to delegate.
2. The delegated nursing task shall be a task that can be competently and safely performed by the unlicensed personnel without compromising the patient's safety.
3. The nursing task shall not require the unlicensed personnel to exercise independent nursing judgment or intervention.
4. The nurse shall be responsible for ensuring that the delegated task is performed in a competent manner by the unlicensed personnel.

Supervision

1. The nurse shall provide supervision of the delegated nursing task.
2. The degree of supervision required shall be determined by the nurse after an evaluation of the following factors:
   a. Stability and acuity of the patient's condition
   b. Training and competency of the unlicensed personnel
   c. Complexity of the nursing task being delegated
   d. Proximity and availability of the nurse to the unlicensed personnel when the nursing task is being performed

(Adapted from *State of Kentucky. Delegation of nursing tasks.* (1999). KRS 311A.170, 314.011, 201 KAR 20:400.).

TABLE 13.1 Roles of Patient Team Members

Patient Care Team Members and Their Roles

Registered Nurses (RNs)
- Determine the scope of nursing practice
- Are responsible and accountable for the provision of nursing services
- Supervise and determine the appropriate use of any unlicensed assistive personnel involved in patient care
- Define and supervise the education, training, and use of any unlicensed assistive personnel

Licensed Vocational Nurse/Licensed Practical Nurse (LVN/LPN)
- Complete a 1-year to 18-month educational program
- Provide basic patient care that includes, but is not limited to taking vital signs, changing dressings, performing phlebotomy, and assisting with activities of daily living under the supervision of the RN

Unlicensed Assistive Personnel (UAP)
- Work under the direct supervision of a RN to implement the delegated aspects of nursing care
- Assist the RN in providing patient care
- Enable the RN to provide nursing care for the patient
- May include but are not limited to the following titles:
- Patient care assistant
  - Nurse's aide
  - Technician
  - Multiskilled worker
  - Practice partner
  - Nursing assistant
  - Nurse extender
  - Orderly
  - Support personnel
  - Practice partner

(From American Association of Critical-Care Nurses. (2004). Retrieved July 1, 2019, from http://www.aacn.org/wd/practice/docs/aacndelegationhandbook.pdf.)

THE FIVE RIGHTS OF DELEGATION

The NCSBN (1997) has defined the Five Rights of Delegation as:
1. Right task
2. Right circumstance
3. Right person
4. Right direction/communication
5. Right supervision

To assist you in reviewing these five rights, Box 13.2 will help you to determine whether you are following

tracing, and measuring blood sugar levels. **Indirect patient care activities** are those routinely done to support the functioning of the patient care unit. Such activities include the restocking of supplies, the transport of patients, and clerical activities.

BOX 13.2   The Five Rights of Delegation

Right Task
- Has the nursing department established policies and standards consistent with the nurse practice act of the state and professional nursing standards?
- Are you aware of the specific polices and standards of your institution?
- Do you know to whom you can delegate what?
- Can this task be delegated to any staff, or only to certain staff?

Right Circumstance
- Are the setting and resources conducive to safe care?
- Do the job description and competency of the caregiver match the patient requirements?
- Do staff members understand how to do the task safely?
- Do staff members have the appropriate resources and equipment to carry out the task safely?
- Do staff members have the appropriate supervision to carry out the task safely?

Right Person
- Is the right person delegating the task, and is the right person being delegated to?
- Is the patient condition appropriate for the level of delegation?
- Do hospital policy and the nurse practice act of the state allow the delegation of this activity?
- Can you verify the knowledge and competency of the staff member to whom you are delegating a specific task?

Right Direction/Communication
- Have you clearly communicated the task with directions, limits, and expected outcomes?
- Are times for feedback specified in the assignment?
- Does the staff member understand what is to be done?
- Can the staff member ask questions as needed?

Right Supervision
- Will you be able to appropriately monitor and evaluate patient response to the delegated task?
- Will you be able to give feedback to the staff member if needed?

these rights in your delegation (National Council of State Boards of Nursing NCSBN, 2016). The Delegation Model described by the National Council of State Boards of Nursing NCSBN, 2016, is as follows:

New figure…….. (National Council of State Boards of Nursing NCSBN, 2016). National Guidelines for Nursing Delegation. *Journal of Nursing Regulation 7*(1), 6.

Right Task

State boards of nursing regulate nursing practice within each state. It is important for you to know the nurse practice act of the state in which you are practicing and to be aware of the delegation regulation within your state. In addition, most hospitals have policies that very carefully describe what nursing tasks can be delegated to whom; there are differing standards of delegation depending on the type of health care facility in which you practice. Many long-term care facilities assign LPNs as charge nurses, with RNs supervising that care. In ambulatory care settings, medical assistants play a major role in the delivery of care. Just because your institution uses patient care technicians to measure all vital signs and blood sugar levels and to make blood draws, it does not mean that all facilities can or do use such personnel. It is vital to know your institution's standard on delegation and the specific job descriptions and competencies of each level of personnel with whom you will be working. A sample hospital policy on delegation is shown in Fig. 13.1. The scope of practice will vary from state to state, so this will vary across the country.

Generally, appropriate tasks for consideration in delegation decision making include those
- that frequently recur in the daily care of a client or group of clients,
- that do not require the UAP to exercise nursing judgment,
- that do not require complex and/or multidimensional application of the nursing process,
- for which the results are predictable and the potential risk is minimal, and
- that use a standard and unchanging procedure.

(The Five Rights of Delegation, see https://www.ncsbn.org/search.htm?q=The+Five+Rights+of+Delegation)

Right Circumstance

The right circumstance refers to the workplace. The circumstance is the context in which the delegation takes place. As stated earlier, a LPN will be performing different tasks under different circumstances. In a long-term facility, it is not unusual to have a LPN as the "charge nurse" with a RN covering multiple units for supervision. However, it would be unusual to have a LPN assigned as a "charge nurse" in an acute care facility with a high acuity of patients. There may be differences in extreme circumstances such as disasters, but in such a situation, the right communication/direction needs to occur.

THE VALLEY HOSPITAL
Ridgewood, New Jersey

PATIENT CARE SERVICES (PCS) POLICY AND PROCEDURE

SUBJECT: Delegation – Nursing Tasks

POLICY:
1. In delegating selected nursing tasks to licensed practice nurses and other health care team members, the registered professional nurse shall be responsible for exercising that degree of judgment and knowledge reasonably expected to assure that a proper delegation has been made.
2. A registered professional nurse may not delegate the performance of a nursing task to persons who have not been adequately prepared by verifiable training and education and have not demonstrated the adequacy of their knowledge, skill and competency to perform the task being delegated.
3. A RN may not delegate non-PCA tasks to staff employed as PCA II or PCA I who are RNs from a foreign country or those enrolled in nursing school. In order to function/perform tasks that are approved under the scope of practice of a RN, staff must be licensed as a RN in New Jersey.
4. No task may be delegated which is within the scope of nursing practice and requires:
   a. The substantial knowledge and skill derived from completion of a nursing education program and the specialized skill, judgment and knowledge of a registered nurse; and
   b. An understanding of nursing principles necessary to recognize and manage complications which may result in harm to the health and safety of the patient.

WHO CAN PERFORM: RN

RESPONSIBILITY:
It is the responsibility of nursing leadership or management member, as appropriate to implement, maintain, evaluate, review and revise this policy.

APPROVED: Nurse Practice Education Council, January 10, 2003.

Beverly S. Karas-Irwin, RN
Chairperson, Nurse Practice Education Council

Linda C. Lewis, RN
Vice President, Paient Care Services

Fig. 13.1 Sample hospital policy on delegation. (With permission from Valley Hospital.).

Right Person

The requirement of the right person means that you must know the competency level, job description, individual level of skill, and standard of education of the individual to whom you are delegating. Job descriptions will give you a broad view of what an individual is expected to do, but you must know the individual's capabilities, experience, attitude, and skills. A novice nurse will not have the competency that a nurse with 10 years of experience, a professional certification, and a clinical ladder position will have. It is also necessary to have knowledge of the individual strengths and weaknesses of each team member. A team member who just lost her mother to breast cancer may not be the best person to delegate to perform tasks for a patient with breast cancer.

The Right Direction/Communication

The right direction/communication is required of nurses as they delegate tasks to staff members. It is not enough to assign a task to staff members; they must know what is expected of them. "You will take Ms. Smith's temperature every hour starting at 8 a.m., and report the temperature back to me immediately." If you tell the staff member to take the temperature every hour, he or she may not know when to start and may report a sudden increase in temperature to you because the staff member has not been trained to determine when an independent nursing action is needed. Your directions must follow the 4 Cs: be clear, concise, correct, and complete. A clear communication is one that is understood by the listener. If you say, "Can you get Mrs. Jones?" What are you asking? For that patient to be transported back to the unit from a test? For the staff member to assume full care for Mrs. Jones? Or to answer Mrs. Jones's bell? Tell the staff member exactly what you want done. A concise communication is one in which the right amount of communication has been given. If you are asking a PCA to take a patient's temperature, he or she does not need to know the physiologic response to an increased temperature. It confuses the communication and wastes time. Tell the associate what they need to know. A correct communication is one that is accurate. You may have two patients named Edward Norton on your unit. It is not enough to tell the LPN to give Mr. Norton his pain medication. Which Mr. Norton are you referring to? Last, a complete communication leaves no questions on the part of the delegate. Do not assume that just because you asked a PCA to take a patient's temperature that he or she will know to report it to you.

Communication is a two-way activity, and it is important to create an environment in which staff members feel free to say that they are not comfortable doing a task, for instance, because they have not done it for a long time.

Right Supervision

The nurse remains accountable for the total care delivered to the patients on the unit. The right supervision includes "the provision of guidance, direction, oversight, evaluation, and follow-up by the licensed nurse for accomplishment of a nursing task delegated to nursing assistive personnel" (National Council of State Boards of Nursing NCSBN, 2016). Although you will not directly perform the tasks delegated, you will be responsible for determining patient progress and outcomes of the care delivered and evaluating and improving staff performance. This requires you to be able to communicate effectively to support team performance.

ACCEPTANCE OF DELEGATED ASSIGNMENT

In accepting a delegated assignment, the following decision-making algorithm is appropriate (State of New Jersey, 1999):

- Is the act consistent with your defined scope of practice?
- Is the activity authorized by a valid order and in accordance with established institutional/agency or provider protocols, policies, and procedures?
- Is the act supported by research data from nursing literature/or research from a health-related field? Has a national nursing organization issued a position statement on this practice?
- Do you possess the knowledge and clinical competence to perform the act safely?
- Is the act to be performed within acceptable "standards of care" that would be provided under similar circumstances by reasonable, prudent nurses with similar education and clinical skills?
- Are you prepared to assume accountability for the provision of safe care?
- This model will assist you if you have a question about nursing practice or the delegation of work to you.

DELEGATION FACTORS

To recap, what to delegate will depend on a number of factors (adapted from Heidenthal & Marthaler, 2005):

- Your state's nurse practice act (authority)
- Hospital policies and procedures
- Job descriptions
- Staff competencies
- Clinical situation
- Professional standards
- Patient needs

What activities can usually be delegated? The following is a list of potential activities that may be delegated.

Direct Patient Care Activities

Vital signs
- Take and record blood pressure, respirations, temperature, and pulse rate
- Obtain daily weight
- Apply leads and connect to cardiac monitor

Intake and output
- Measure and record intake and output
- Collect specimens

Activities of daily living
- Perform total or partial bed bath
- Perform perineal care
- Shave
- Wash hair
- Perform mouth care
- Change linen and assist with making occupied bed

Nutrition
- Feed patient
- Calculate and record calorie count

Skin care
- Perform back care
- Prepare skin for procedure
- Perform skin prep for operative procedure

Activity and mobility
- Assist in ambulating patient
- Perform passive and active range of motion
- Position
- Turn and reposition patient
- Assist with transfers

Respiratory support
- Set up oxygen
- Assist patient with using an incentive spirometer
- Assist patient with coughing and deep breathing exercises

Procedures
- Set up patient room (suction canisters, cables for continuous cardiac monitoring, tubing for chest tubes)
- Orient patient to room environment
- Obtain necessary supplies for sterile procedure
- Perform postmortem care

Indirect Patient Care Activities

Cleaning
- Clean equipment in use and stored equipment
- Clean environment, including countertops and desktops
- Clean and defrost food refrigerators
- Clean patient care area after transfer or discharge
- Clean patient care area after procedures are completed
- Empty waste baskets in patient rooms and unit
- Empty linen hampers
- Remove meal trays
- Clean supply carts
- Clean and restock procedure rooms
- Make unoccupied beds

Errands
- Deliver meal trays
- Obtain and deliver supplies
- Obtain and deliver equipment
- Obtain and deliver blood products
- Check laboratory specimens for appropriate labeling
- Deliver specimens to clinical laboratory

Clerical tasks
- Place pages
- Place and answer phone calls
- Assemble, disassemble, and maintain patient charts
- Transcribe physician and nursing patient care orders
- Schedule diagnostic tests and procedures
- Order necessary office supplies and forms
- Sort and deliver mail
- Keep unit log books up-to-date with patient admissions, transfers, and discharges
- Maintain awareness of nursing bed assignments

Stocking and maintenance
- Stock patient bedside supplies
- Stock unit supplies
- Stock utility rooms
- Stock treatment, examination, and procedure rooms
- Stock nourishments and kitchen supplies
- Check electrical equipment for inspections due dates
- Stock linen carts

Activities That May Not Be Delegated

Nursing activities that may not be delegated include the following:

- Performing an initial patient assessment and subsequent assessments or nursing interventions that require specialized nursing knowledge, judgment, and/or skill
- Formulating a nursing diagnosis
- Identifying nursing care goals and developing the nursing plan of care in conjunction with the patient and/or family
- Updating the patient's plan of care
- Providing patient education to patient and/or family.
- Evaluating a patient's progress, or lack thereof, toward achieving desired goals and outcomes
- Discussing patient issues with physician.
- Communicating with physicians or implementing orders from physician
- Documenting the patient's assessment or response to therapeutic interventions in the patient's plan of care.
- Administering medications
- Providing direct nursing care
- (Adapted from American Association of Critical-Care Nurses AACN, 2004.)

OBSTACLES TO DELEGATION

There are obstacles to delegation. Nurses who have worked with primary care models for much of their professional life may have difficulty in giving up aspects of nursing care. It is important to keep in mind that "effective teams focus on integrative work processes while working toward a common goal" (Anthony, Standing, & Hertz, 2000).

Barriers to delegation can arise not only on the part of the delegator, the RN, but also on the part of the delegatee, the UAP, and the situation/environment. Characteristics that create barriers in the delegator include the following:

- Preference for operating by oneself
- Demand that everyone know all the details
- "I can do it better myself" fallacy
- Lack of experience in the job or in delegating
- Insecurity
- Fear of being disliked
- Refusal to allow mistakes
- Lack of confidence in subordinates
- Perfectionism, leading to excess control

- Lack of organizational skill in balancing workloads
- Failure to delegate authority commensurate with responsibility
- Uncertainty over tasks and inability to explain
- Disinclination to develop subordinates
- Failure to establish effective controls and to follow-up

Characteristics that create barriers in the delegate include the following:

- Lack of experience
- Lack of competence
- Avoidance of responsibility
- Overdependence
- Disorganization
- Overload of work
- Immersion in trivia

Characteristics that create barriers related to the situation/environment include the following:

- One-person-show policy
- No toleration of mistakes
- Criticality of decisions
- Urgency, leaving no time to explain (crisis management)
- Understaffing

(Adapted from AACN, 2004.)

LEVELS OF CLINICAL EXPERIENCE

The use of effective delegation has been related to levels of clinical experience (Benner & Benner, 1984, cited in Carroll, 2006) including:

- The novice nurse has limited experience with tasks and needs rules to guide actions.
- The advanced beginner has enough experience to recognize patterns in work but continues to need help in setting priorities; relies on rules and protocols.
- The competent nurse has been practicing 2 to 3 years, can prioritize and cope with various contingencies, and requires assistance working through various situations not yet experienced.
- The proficient nurse has enough experience to see the "big picture" rather than a series of individual accidents/actions, decision making is more efficient and accurate, and is able to prioritize and plan even more challenging patient care.
- The expert no longer relies on rules to understand a situation or to act appropriately, focuses quickly on viable solutions and is able to lead a team efficiently, and can organize others' work and supervise them effectively.

It is important to know the nurses with whom you are working on any given day so that you can also use their level of expertise in the planning of your delegation. The following guidelines may help RNs delegate more effectively:
- Be aware of your internal barriers to delegation.
- Never delegate a task you would not do yourself.
- Delegate to the most appropriate person, carefully considering these factors:
  - Patient acuity
  - The activity to be performed
  - The support person's job description
  - Competencies of the individual who will complete the task
- Communicate clearly. How one communicates a task can determine how successfully it will be completed. Ineffective communication is the most commonly cited reason delegated activities are not completed as expected. (American Association of Critical-Care Nurses AACN, 2004)

Koloroutis, Felgen, Person, and Wessel (2007) described three scenarios that can be used as a means of determining the most appropriate method of delegation to become part of the staffing assignments of a unit: unit based, pairing, and partnering.

Unit-Based Scenarios

In the unit-based scenario, assistive personnel, such as the ward secretary and NA, serve the unit. The NA works off a task list usually found in the job description and has minimal direction from or interaction with the RNs. An example of the unit-based scenario is assigning a NA to take all the vital signs or bathe all the patients. Another nurse may ask the NA to help with picking up medications from the pharmacy, while another nurse may ask the NA to assist with feeding a patient.

Pairing

In a pairing scenario, one RN works with a LPN and/or a NA for the shift. However, the RN and LPN and/or assistant are not intentionally scheduled to work the same shift each day. Delegation usually increases with pairing. In this scenario, the RN and the LPN or NA are able to discuss how care is to be prioritized and how it is to be done and identify expected individualized outcomes for the shift.

Partnering

In partnering, one RN and one LPN and/or NA are consistently scheduled to work together, making a commitment to maintain healthy interpersonal relationships, trust each other, and advance each other's knowledge.

PRIORITY SETTING

Proper delegation also requires priority setting. One of the most difficult challenges facing both the nurse and the nurse manager is the prioritization of care delivered to the patients on a unit. The priorities change rapidly and the nurse manager should be aware of the unit needs at all times. To manage your priorities and to control the activity of the workplace around you, Carrick, Carrick, & Yurkow, 2007 suggested the three I's:
1. Identify your priorities
2. Interact differently with others
3. Initiate action

To identify your priorities, list your entire job-related responsibilities on a piece of paper. Then classify the top priorities, and create a "to-do" list that you can work from during the day. Remember, this list will change as the day progresses, but keep updating it and rank your priorities as they change. This list serves as a reference for the actions of the day.

To interact differently with others, Carrick, Carrick, & Yurkow, 2007 recommended the following four tactics to maintain control over your time, energy, and priorities:
1. *Identifya time when you can handle an issue:* You cannot refuse a task or patient request, but you will be able to say when you will be available to do the task. Reassuring a person that you will complete the task and giving a timeline helps control requests and interruptions that compete for your time.
2. *Ask questions before taking on an assignment:* Before you take on any assignment, you need to understand the scope, the intended outcome, and the deadlines.
3. *Ask for help when you need it:* Quickly do a reality check of your time, prioritize alternatives, and then meet with the person who can help you make the right decision or complete the assignment. When asking for help, be realistic about the expectation of the other person, and be open to alternative decision making.
4. *Use delegation to manage your responsibilities:* You cannot do it all! When delegating, be sure to explain the scope, expectations, roles, responsibilities, and authority for the task. Always be available as a resource.

To initiate action, you need to set realistic goals. To set realistic goals, be SMART: the goals need to be specific, measurable, attainable, relevant, and time bound.

As a nurse manager, you have a responsibility to control time, set appropriate priorities, and act on the priorities. In setting priorities, you will always need to keep in mind the following question: Of all of the important things that I need to do right now, which is the most important for the patient(s)? Is it urgent? Or just important?

SUMMARY

Delegation is one of the most challenging activities of the new manager. There is more nursing care needed than nurses to provide that care. In addition, not all care needed for a patient requires a professional nurse. Nurses must work within an interdisciplinary team and with individuals of varying capabilities and talents.

Delegation skills are developed by the new nurse over time. It involves an awareness of the total patient care needs for the patients assigned and a thorough knowledge of the capabilities and competencies of staff members. Delegation is a process that results in safe and efficient patient care if it is used appropriately. It is a critical step in the delivery of nursing care.

In summary, the Four Delegation Steps identified by the NCSBN of Nursing and the ANA will serve as a guideline for effective delegation: Step One, Assessment and Planning; Step Two, Communication; Step Three, Surveillance and Supervision; and Step Four, Evaluation and Feedback (https://www.ncsbn.org/Delegation_joint_statement_NCSBN-ANA.pdf, pp. 7–9).

CLINICAL CORNER

When nurses share their stories about how they learned, (or if) they had formal education specific to nursing delegation, a wide range of emotions are expressed. Experiences vary in degree and sentiment. Often, reactions tend to run the gamut – some are explosive: "It was trial by fire!" most are questionable: "I don't remember learning about that!" And all were learning experiences on what not to do or what to do in the future. Often, the responses are reflective of how the nurse was "formed." Educational background, years of experience, and formal vs. extemporaneous education figure into the equation.

Delegation is an essential, core nursing skill, to be sure. However, in the era of Covid-19, the ability to delegate, assign, and supervise was stretched to the limit and beyond. Stories "from the front" wrench the gut and reveal a very different learned experience. While the world catapulted into an altered universe, healthcare agencies and all members of the frontline navigated in every direction and in uncharted waters. Remembering the early days of the pandemic, one recalls severe staffing shortages, workplace hardships, moral dilemmas, and well documented stresses daily *(Impact of Covid-19 pandemic on the nursing profession in …2020)*. Despite these enormous challenges, nurses also experienced accelerated growth, resilience, a heightened sense of teamwork and collaboration with various members of the healthcare team, and an ability to create and innovate *(Fauteux, N. 2021)*.

Clinical staff are directly impacted by these experiences. It can make or break a positive orientation/on-boarding process, develop or degrade teamwork and collaboration, and it can even be a factor when or if a newly hired nurse or other hospital worker decides to re-think their decision on whether to stay or leave the institution – or to leave the field altogether. Again, the pandemic was a strong "push factor" that influenced a nurse's decision to leave both job and profession *(Africa & Trepanier, 2021)*.

Therefore, it is critical for faculty and staff development specialists to create solid curriculum to implement a variety of learning modalities aside from the dry (and sometimes tedious) lecture, by mixing it up with simulations, discussions, anecdotes, role-playing, and the like. The goal of the education of nurses in the art of delegation is to develop skilled, professional clinical leaders who are excellent communicators, efficient and conscientious, and who achieve positive patient care experiences and outcomes.

Delegation keeps costs down, builds effective and solid teams across healthcare disciplines, and involves education, collaboration and creativity. It relies on an enormous team effort and mandates clear, coordinated communication skills. It is an expected nursing competency – and if/when a nurse becomes proficient in delegation, it allows her/him to make sound judgments about patients and coordinate optimal patient care *(National guidelines for Nursing Delegation, 2019, April 29)*.

CLINICAL CORNER—cont'd

Reflecting on my past early experiences as a new nurse 'delegator,' I decided to ask RN to BSN students the following questions:

What do you remember about the subject of delegation? Were you taught this subject in nursing school? Did you have a degree of mastery or comfort with this skill? Would you share your nursing delegation initiation story with me? I share with you these stories, and of course, mine.

Personal reflection #1 Kimberly

"I went to nursing school at a community college. I graduated in 1997 with an Associate's degree in Nursing. We were not taught how to delegate in school at all! When I started on the floor, we had a 4-6 week orientation. During that orientation, my preceptors showed me how to assign certain tasks to the tech. They were the ones who instructed me on what could and could not be assigned to the techs, and what had to be done by me as the nurse. They also made it clear that whatever I assigned to the tech, I was still ultimately responsible. Then one day I came in to work to find out that I was in charge. My delegation education at this level was baptism by fire. I was put in charge with no training, and part of the responsibility was to complete the assignment for the floor, as well as assign admissions as they came up. Oh, and if you screw it up, everyone will be miserable for the shift!"

Reflection #2 - Deborah

"When I attended Nursing School 32 years ago, we were never formally taught nursing or peer delegation. We learned how to delegate from our nursing instructors. My nursing clinical rotations consisted of eight hours of direct patient care followed by post evaluations. Upon graduation, we knew how to function on the floor.

Today, as a preceptor for new RNs in Labor & Delivery, I think that the new graduates are not well prepared in the role of delegation. Prioritization skills are lacking and they are more focused on "tasks" rather than the bigger picture – or the 'whole picture.' ….I lead by example and support them in every way to make them feel comfortable and not to feel intimidated. I am currently orienting a PCA and utilize the same techniques as mentioned above."

Reflection #3 Michelle

"Let me share with you my operating room experience today… I needed to turn our room around quickly, but of course, safely. We had the same surgeon following himself; therefore, I needed to manage my time wisely. I helped the surgical tech open all of the instrumentation, so she would not feel as if I put it all on her. Really, I should be seeing the patient, going over their history, obtaining the meds needed for the case and putting some of the information in the computer. But because I was a tech at one time, I know how it feels to be left on your own and open up an entire room by yourself.

Meanwhile, after helping her, I went to see my patient. It took me about 15 minutes to do that; she had a long history. When I brought my patient to the room, the tech was gone and did not communicate to me where she was going. There should always be two people in a room with a patient in case of a code, etc. She felt it was unfair that she did not get a break and I did. I said you could have said something, I would of given you more time for lunch to make up for a break...Communication is key.

And, safety is first! She was not being responsible by leaving the room and not letting me know where she was. I work hard and do lead by example."

Reflection #4 - Donna

"As a new RN working nights on an orthopedic unit, I remember feeling that I had to do it all. I was afraid to ask for help from the nursing assistants because I felt intimidated by their veteran status and I was not at all confident in my new role. I didn't have a good sense of what the big picture was, how it impacted my patients, my team, and my ability to be a better nurse. I remember many times leaving late from work because I couldn't complete all my work in a timely manner. Charting was always put off until the bitter end – and when it came time to remember what needed to be charted – that became another brutal memory game."

Delegation Experience #5 Kathleen

"As a relatively new RN, I was partnered with an LPN for an assignment of 10 patients.

I was told I needed to hang all IV meds, since they needed to be mixed and that is not in the scope of an LPN.

Looking back now, I was unclear of the Scope of LPN Practice and the job description for what I could expect from her.

These were all my patients and my responsibility. The situations were difficult as I was unclear what I could delegate to the LPN; she was happy to keep busy with her patients and reminded me she could not administer certain meds.

I found myself unprepared to delegate; not even sure what that looked or sounded like -and therefore, cared for the full patient load myself (at least this was my perception). Delegating to this LPN also seemed difficult to me as she was an older nurse there much longer than me.

Delegation to unlicensed care providers such as a nursing assistant (NA)and unit clerk was also something I struggled with. In this case, I had been a nursing assistant in another hospital before becoming a nurse. I

CLINICAL CORNER—cont'd

think this helped me know 'what nursing assistants do'. However, the NAs were very experienced, and again, they were older than me. As a new and inexperienced nurse, this was a barrier for me. The NAs did not always like a young, new nurse telling them what to do. That is not to say that I didn't have any good experiences with NAs. I had many excellent experiences with NAs, and I learned so much from them!

A valuable lesson my nurse manager taught me early on was to communicate with the person you are delegating to within the framework of the patient. Instead of asking the NA, " Could you please do me a favor and take Mr. Smith to the bathroom," you need to say, " Our patient Mr. Smith needs to use the bathroom. Will you assist him as I am beginning a dressing change for our patient Mrs. Johnson." She taught me that this language is more respectful and builds the staff as a team with the care of the patient in the center. The care I am requesting is to meet the patient's need, not purely my need. One other lesson learned is to be well aware of job descriptions and scope of practice for those with licenses."

Common themes come to the surface. Often, the RN with the delegation dilemma is a new RN, with limited (if any experience). A certain baseline level of discomfort exists and causes anxiety. Initially, the nurse views delegation as a "to do" list of tasks that need to be completed during a certain prescribed time. Most of the delegation decisions are based on job description: Patient Care Associate, RN, other ancillary help. Rarely, does a new delegator use their nursing judgment and take into consideration each person's strengths and weaknesses, who is suited to the various subtitles, etc. Delegation is a process. The nurse assesses if, when or where assistance is needed. She/he then selects the appropriate person. The assistance is carried out under that "umbrella" supervision, and lastly, the delegation process is evaluated, and feedback is shared. The nurse prioritizes the patient's needs, considers his or her condition, differentiates between nursing versus non-nursing tasks, and selects tasks to be delegated. The nurse then chooses the appropriate member of the team to assume the task. Nurses need to know the skill level of each team member to match the assignment appropriately (Curtis and Nicholl 2004).

Donna Grotheer RN, MSN

References

Africa, L., & Trepanier, S. (2021). The role of the nurse leader in reversing the new graduate nurse intent to leave. *Nurse leader, 19*(3), 239–245 https://doi.org/10.1016.j/m/2021.02013

ANA, NCSBN. (2019, April 29). *National Guidelines for Nursing Delegation.* Retrieved October 30, 2021 from https://www.ncsbn.org/NGND-PosPaper_06.pdf

Curtis E. Nicholl H. Delegation: a key function of nursing. Nurs Manag (Harrow) 2004 Jul;11(4):26–31.doi: 10.7748.nm200407.11.4.26.c1985.PMID: 15296057

Impact of covid-19 pandemic on the nursing profession in… (n.d.). Retrieved October 30, 2021, from https://nursing.jnj.com/2020-quantitative-research-summary.

EVIDENCE-BASED PRACTICE

(From Magnussin, C., Allan, H., Horton, K., Evans, K., & Ball, E. (2017). An analysis of delegation styles among newly qualified nurses. *Nursing Standard, 31*(25), 46–53.)

Delegation is one skill new nurses often have challenges with. The aim of this research project was to explore how novice nurses learn to organize, delegate, and supervise care in hospital units when working with patient care assistants and other licensed personnel. This was part of a larger research project across the United Kingdom to explore how novice nurses recontextualize the knowledge they gained in the nursing education programs for use in clinical practice.

Method ethnographic case studies were conducted at three large acute care hospitals. Data collection methods included participant observations and semistructured interviews with novice nurses, unit managers, and patient care assistants. A thematic analysis was used to examine the data collected.

Five styles of how the novice nurses delegates care to the patient care assistant were identified:
- The "do it all" nurse, who completes most of the work themselves.
- The "justifier," who over explains the reasons for decisions and is sometimes defensive.
- The "buddy," who wants to be everyone's friend and avoids assuming authority.
- The "role model" who hopes that others will copy his or her best practice but has no way of ensuring how.
- The "inspector," who is acutely aware of his or her responsibility and constantly checks the work of others.

This study validates the importance of delegation content and competency development in novice nurse residency programs.

NCLEX® EXAMINATION QUESTIONS

1. Acknowledgment and assumption of responsibility for actions, decisions, and policies within the scope of the role or employment position and encompassing the obligation to report, explain, and be answerable for resulting consequences is referred to as:
   A. Accountability
   B. Autonomy
   C. Authority
   D. Assessment

2. The Five Rights of Delegation are:
   A. Right direction, right circumstance, right person, communication
   B. Right task, right circumstance, right person, right direction, communication
   C. Right task, right circumstance, right person, right direction, communication
   D. Right task, right circumstance, right person, right discussion

3. The person accountable for establishing systems to assess, monitor, verify, and communicate ongoing competence requirements in areas related to delegation is:
   A. Nurse manager
   B. Nurse leader, vice president of nursing
   C. Nursing supervisor
   D. All of the above

4. Who works under the direction and supervision of the registered nurse?
   A. Licensed practical nurse
   B. Unlicensed personnel
   C. Patient care technicians
   D. All of the above

5. You have just received report on a patient with an acute myocardial infarction, and are delegating patient case load to a patient care technician (PCT). Which of the following can be delegated to the PCT?
   A. Dietary teaching
   B. Physical care
   C. Admission assessment
   D. Asking the patient what pain level he or she is experiencing

6. You just received report from the night shift nurse. You must assign both direct patient care and indirect patient care to staff members. An example of a direct patient care task is:
   A. Restocking shelves and patient rooms
   B. Performing an electrocardiogram

   C. Asking patient what they are requesting when their light is on, then informing the RN
   D. Transporting patients

7. Which of the following are delegation factors?
   A. State nurse practice act, hospital policies and procedures, job descriptions, patient needs, staff competencies, professional standards, clinical situation
   B. State nurse practice act, hospital policies and procedures, job descriptions, patient needs, staff competencies, professional standards
   C. State nurse practice act, hospital policies and procedures, job descriptions, patient needs, staff competencies, professional standards
   D. State nurse practice act, hospital policies and procedures, job descriptions, patient needs, staff competencies, professional standards

8. Appropriate tasks for consideration in delegation decision making include those that frequently recur in the daily care of a client or group of clients. These include:
   A. Tasks that do not use a standard and unchanging procedure.
   B. Tasks related to medication delivery.
   C. Tasks that do not require the unlicensed assistive personnel to exercise nursing judgment and do not require complex and/or multidimensional application of the nursing process.
   D. Tasks that require nursing process assessment.

9. At the end of a shift, a new RN tells the charge nurse that she has not documented her medications. You should:
   A. Ask her why she was unable to chart medications
   B. Tell the nurse manager about the situation
   C. Tell her you will pay her overtime for proper documentation completion
   D. Ask her if she would like the charge nurse to complete the documentation

10. When delegating:
    A. You will directly perform, together with the nursing assistant, the tasks delegated
    B. You will not be responsible for determining patient progress
    C. You will need excellent communication skills very clear

Answers: 1. A   2. B   3. D   4. D   5. B   6. B   7. A   8. C   9. A   10. C

REFERENCES

American Nurses Association [ANA]. (2019). *Decision tree for delegation by registered nurses.* Retrieved July 1, 2019 from www.nursingworld.org/MainMenuCategories/ThePracticeofProfessionalNursing/NursingStandards/ANAPrinciples/PrinciplesofDelegation.pdf.aspx p. 12.

American Nurses Association [ANA]. (1992). *Position statement: Registered nurse education relating to the utilization of unlicensed assistive personnel.* http://ana.org/readroom/position/uap/uaprned.htm. Accessed July 1, 2019.

American Association of Critical-Care Nurses [AACN] (2004). *AACN delegation handbook* (2nd ed.). Aliso Viejo, CA: AACN.

American Nurses Association [ANA] and National Council of State Boards of Nursing [NCSBN] (2008). Joint statement of delegation. ANA, NCSBN. https://www.ncsbn.org/index.htm. (Accessed 1 July 2019).

Anthony, M. K., Standing, T., & Hertz, J. E. (2000). Factors influencing outcomes after delegation to unlicensed assistive personnel. *Journal of Nursing Administration, 30*(10), 474–481.

Benner, P., & Benner, R. (1984). *From novice to expert: Excellence and power in clinical nursing practice.* Menlo Park, CA: Addison-Wesley Publishing.

Carrick, L., Carrick, L., & Yurkow, J. (2007). A nurse leader's guide to managing priorities. *American Nurse Today,* 40–41.

Carroll, P. (2006). *Nursing leadership and management: A practical guide.* Clifton Park, NY: Thomson Delmar Learning.

Heidenthal, P., & Marthaler, M. (2005). *Delegation of nursing care.* Clifton Park, NY: Thomson Delmar Learning.

Koloroutis, M., Felgen, J., Person, C., & Wessel, S. (2007). *Field guide: Relationship-based care visions, strategies, tools and exemplars for transforming practice.* Minneapolis, MN: Creative Health Care Management, Inc.

Marquis, B.L., & Huston, C.J. (2017). *Leadership roles and management functions in nursing* (9th ed.). Philadelphia, PA: Lippincott Williams and Wilkins.

National Council of State Boards of Nursing. (1997). *The five rights of delegation.* Chicago, IL: NCSBN.

National Council of State Boards of Nursing [NCSBN]. (2016). National guidelines for nursing delegation. *Journal of Nursing Delegation, 7*(1), 4–12.

State of Kentucky. (1999) Delegation of nursing tasks. KRS 311A.170, 314.011, 201 KAR 20:400 www.lrc.state.ky.us/kar/201/020/400.htm.

State of New Jersey. (1999). New Jersey State Board of Nursing fact sheet: Decision making model for delegations of selected nursing tasks. *New Jersey Administrative Code, 13*(3), 7–36. .state.nj.us/lps/ca/nursing/ago1.htm. (Accessed 1 July 2019).

Providing Competent Staff

OUTLINE

OBJECTIVES

- Discuss hospital-wide and unit-based new employee orientation.
- Analyze the role of preceptor in nurse orientation.
- Compare and contrast the roles of the nurse, preceptor, and human resources in orientation.
- Analyze the progression of nursing clinical competence.
- Review the annual mandatory competencies for patient care staff.
- Compare and contrast the roles of manager and staff in performance appraisal.
- Identify the steps and progression of the staff registered nurse in the clinical ladder program.
- Discuss activities used by the nurse manager to support promotion of staff members.

KEY TERMS

competencies areas in which employees are judged to be qualified to perform

mandatories mandatory education educational sessions and competencies that are required by accrediting agencies

orientation process in which initial job training and information are provided to staff

peer review the process by which practicing registered nurses systematically assess, monitor, and make judgments about the quality of nursing care provided by peers as measured against professional standards of practice

performance appraisal process in an organization by which employees are routinely evaluated according to performance standards

preceptors experienced individuals who assist new employees in acquiring the necessary knowledge and skills to function effectively in a new environment

BENNER FIVE STAGES

When new nurses enter the workforce, it is important to realize that this is just the beginning of their professional journey. As discussed in Chapter 10, Benner (1984) posited that the nurse moves through five stages of clinical competence: novice, advanced beginner, competent, proficient, and expert. As you read this content, think of your own areas of experience in nursing. Decide where you think you fit.

Remember that you progress in professional competence as you work. Self-assessment of your current level of performance is an important function in nursing. Much of your progression will also greatly depend on the work environment. The organization provides the environment for the clinical progression of all staff, both for organizational needs and for the personal development of the nurse. Such professional work environments are evidenced in the various health care organizations that have achieved Magnet status (American Nurses Credentialing Center [ANCC], 2019).

The first experience of a novice nurse in the continuing progression toward competency occurs in the health care agency as a new employee.

STAFF COMPETENCY

The Joint Commission (2019) stated that a hospital must provide the right number of competent staff to meet the needs of the patients. Competent staff members are qualified and able to perform the work according to professional standards. To meet the goal of providing adequate competent staff, the hospital must carry out the following processes and activities:

- Orienting, training, and educating staff
- Ongoing in-service and other education and training to increase staff knowledge of specific work-related issues
- Assessing, maintaining, and improving staff competence
- Ongoing, periodic competence assessment evaluating staff members' continuing abilities to perform throughout their association with the organization
- Transitioning staff to new roles

NEW EMPLOYEE ORIENTATION

Orientation is a process in which initial job training and information are provided to staff. Staff orientation promotes safe and effective job performance. Some elements of orientation need to occur before staff begin to provide care, treatment, and services. Other elements of orientation can occur when staff are providing care, treatment, and services (The Joint Commission, 2019). Employees, regardless of level of competence, are required to attend orientation. Basic-to-new employee orientation is education on organization-specific functions, policies, and expectations, such as mission, vision, values, stakeholder expectations, performance improvement, basic skill evaluation, and mandatory policy review. Traditional hospital orientations can range from 3 weeks to 6 months depending on the organization and responsibilities of the nurse. The newer residency programs are ranging from 6 weeks to 1 year.

For new graduates the orientation is often expanded to allow for mentoring to the new role. The time-frame for new nurse socialization to the role, or the process of developing clinical judgment in practice, has been suggested to be as follows (Ferguson et al., 2007):

- Orientation (0 to 20 days)
- Learning practice norms (orientation 4 to 6 months)
- Developing confidence (6 to 12 months)
- Consolidating relationships (12 to 18 months)
- Seeking challenges (18 to 24 months)

This does not mean that the formal orientation is 2 years, but that the length of time for a new nurse to become fully socialized to the profession and organization takes that amount of time. Once an employee accepts a new position, the orientation process is outlined. The length of orientation varies from hospital to hospital and for different groups of employees. Some hospitals differentiate between experienced staff and novice staff. Before this, a new employee will also have to complete a health physical and meet all of the medical criteria for employment, such as hepatitis B immunization and immunity status, tuberculosis testing, and so forth. Some institutions require criminal background checks and drug screens.

Mandatory Content

The first part of orientation is usually organization specific and includes a hospital-wide orientation that may include speakers, such as the human resources representative, the infection control coordinator, the safety officer, the employee health coordinator, and the process improvement coordinator. This organization-specific orientation usually includes those educational topics that are considered mandatory by the accreditation

> **BOX 14.1   New Employee Orientation: Mandatory Content**
>
> - Mission and governance
> - Organizational strategic plan and objectives
> - Customer contact requirements
> - Code of conduct
> - Fire safety
> - Service excellence
> - Age-specific patient content
> - Infection control
> - Process improvement
> - Corporate compliance
> - Health Insurance Portability and Accountability Act (HIPAA)
> - Benefits

agencies. These mandatory topics are usually reviewed on an annual basis in most health care institutions. This mandatory review allows for the determination of employee competency in knowledge in the content areas shown in Box 14.1.

Unit-Based Content

Next, there is unit-based or nursing-based orientation. Unit-based orientations are designed by the unit educator and nurse manager to orient the new nurse to the unit, its policies, patient needs, procedures, and protocols. For example, a nurse in a cardiac unit will receive education on electrocardiogram interpretation, cardiac drugs, cardiac arrest protocols, and so forth. A nurse in the labor room will receive education on fetal monitoring, neonatal resuscitation, and so forth. Patient care assignments will be made to match the learning of orientation. A description of the progression of new nurse orientation is shown in Fig. 14.1.

PRECEPTOR MODEL

There are numerous models of nursing orientation, but most use **preceptors** to work with and evaluate the new employee during the orientation phase. New nurses are traditionally oriented to the professional role by "experienced" registered nurses (RNs) who are knowledgeable in the "ways of nursing" in the organization. Such preceptors are also used when experienced nurses move into new roles, such as a staff nurse moving to a nurse manager role, or a new advanced practice nurse (APN)

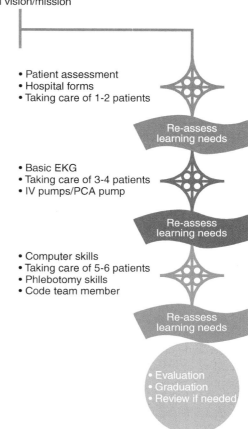

Fig. **14.1** A sample training roadmap. (Adapted from Lee, V., & Harris, T. [2007]. Mentoring new nursing graduates. www.minoritynurse.com/features/other/080207d.html.)

entering a first-time APN role. A preceptor can be defined as an experienced staff member who possesses excellent clinical skills and facilitates learning through caring, respect, compassion, understanding, nurturing, role modeling, and the excellent use of interpersonal communication (Speers et al., 2004). There are varied methods of choosing preceptors and pairing them with orientees and transitioning staff. In hospitals with clinical ladders, experienced nurses are required to serve as preceptors as part of their normal responsibilities. In other institutions, preceptors are chosen based on their competencies, although in other institutions, nurses are chosen based on availability. This last method often results in multiple preceptors for one orientee, depending on who is available. This can result in frustration for the orientee, who may be receiving multiple messages from multiple preceptors (Hardy & Smith, 2001). Research demonstrates that proper pairing is key to the success of the preceptor program (Hardy & Smith, 2001; Horton et al., 2012). Proper pairing occurs with preceptors who are selected into the role based on competencies in both clinical nursing and the ability to facilitate learning (Speers et al., 2004; Bower et al., 2012).

This model can be used to assist new employees and to reward experienced staff nurses. It provides a means for orienting and socializing the new nurse and providing a mechanism to recognize exceptionally competent staff nurses (Sullivan & Decker, 2013). Box 14.2 lists various functions of the preceptor.

There are also rewards for the preceptor in assisting the orientation of new nurses. The experienced nurses often feel more enthusiasm and more involved with the new staff, whereas the orientees express a sense of belonging to the unit (Hardy & Smith, 2001). Many preceptors use their precepting activities to support their progression up the institution's clinical ladder (Chapter 10). New graduate nurses require time to move from the role of student to expert clinician. Acting as a preceptor is an essential part of that transition (Neuman et al., 2004; Bower et al., 2012).

Other roles involved in this orientation are discussed in Box 14.2.

BOX 14.2   Preceptor Functions

- Assist new nurse to acquire knowledge and skills
- Tailor program specifically to needs
- Orient to unit
- Socialize within group
- Orient to unit functions
- Teach unfamiliar procedures
- Assist in development of skills
- Act as resource person
- Familiarize with policies and procedures
- Act as counselor
- Act as role model
- Act as time management coach
- Delegate tasks
- Assist with priority setting
- Mentor to shared governance

RESIDENCY PROGRAMS

The Institute of Medicine report, *The Future of Nursing* (2006), called for the development of nurse residency programs to assist in the transition process of the new graduate, both at the new RN and advanced practice registered nurse levels. Although nurse residency programs vary in length and pay, they are usually 12-month programs designed to support baccalaureate nursing graduates as they transition into their first professional nursing role. The programs consist of a series of work and learning experiences that emphasize and develop the clinical and leadership skills necessary for the novice nurse to become a successful part of the interdisciplinary health care team. Before the development of such residency programs, new nurses often reported a lack of confidence, difficulty with work relationships, frustrations relating to the work environment, lack of time and guidance for developing organizational and priority-setting abilities, and overall high levels of stress. These factors likely contributed to the high turnover rate among new nurses, estimated at between 35% and 60% within the first year (Casey et al., 2004; Halfer & Grad, 2006). Evaluation of 12 1-year postbaccalaureate nurse residency programs found improved communication and organization skills, and higher perceived levels of support and reduced stress. The 12-month turnover rate among the first and second group of residents to graduate from the program was significantly lower (12% and 9%, respectively) than the average rate of 35% to 60% reported in the literature for hospitals without such a program (Krugman et al., 2006; Williams et al., 2007; Goode et al., 2009). Such 12-month residencies are highly competitive.

CONTINUED EMPLOYEE DEVELOPMENT

Accrediting agencies require that staff competence to perform job responsibilities must be assessed, demonstrated, and maintained by the human resources department in conjunction with the education department and the nurse manager (The Joint Commission, 2019). Competency in the required organizational and unit "mandatories" must be annually evaluated. Simulation is playing a large role in the assessment of required unit competencies for many nurses. The current licensure of the individual must be maintained on record. Some states require contact hours for professional license renewal. Many health care organizations provide these contact hours through their internal education or through employee benefits, which include educational advancement.

As the employee moves from novice to expert, the organization supports the individual in achieving the required competencies and additional learning required for growth. The basis for the assessment of the individual's needs and abilities is determined through the performance appraisal, peer review processes, and the educational needs assessment. These processes allow for the evaluation of the employee against stated standards. They also allow the employee to set annual goals for future development. The aggregation of these individual learning goals then becomes part of the annual education and human resources plan of the organization.

PEER REVIEW

Peer review in nursing is the process by which practicing RNs systematically access, monitor, and make judgments about the quality of nursing care provided by peers as measured against professional standards of practice. It is different from the standard performance appraisal in that it forms part of an annual performance appraisal process by which professional nurses judge the performance of professional peers. The peer review process stimulates professionalism through consistent accountability and promotes the self-regulation of nursing practice (ANCC, 2019). Such peer review is also a major component of recertifications of APNs in many states.

The six principles of peer review are as follows:
1. A peer is someone of the same rank.
2. Peer review is practice focused.
3. Feedback is timely, routine, and a continuous expectation.
4. Peer review fosters a continuous learning culture of patient safety and best practice.
5. Feedback is not anonymous.
6. Feedback incorporates the nurse's developmental stage.

Peer Review Principles
1. A peer is someone of the same rank.
   - Peer review implies that nursing care delivered by a group of nurses or an individual nurse is evaluated by individuals of the same rank or standing, according to established standards of practice.

- Peer reviewers are nurse colleagues with clinical competence similar to that of the nurse seeking peer review.
- Steps in the peer review process are the same for all nurses and all settings.
- The key difference lies in identifying the purpose, peer group, and appropriate professionally defined standards on which to base the review.

2. Peer review is practice focused.
   - Standards of nursing practice provide a means for measuring the quality of nursing care a client receives.
   - Peer review in nursing is a process by which practicing RNs systematically access, monitor, and make judgments about the quality of nursing care provided by peers, as measured against professional standards of practice.
   - Peer review activities are focused on practice decisions of professional nurses to determine the appropriateness and timeliness of those decisions.

3. Feedback is timely, routine, and a continuous expectation.
   - This should occur in every health care facility in which nurses practice, and for each nurse it is a continuous expectation.
   - Individual practice and provision for peer review should be an ongoing process.
   - An organized program makes peer review timely and objective.

4. Peer review fosters a continuous learning culture of patient safety and best practice.
   - The goals of every agency providing nursing care should include peer review as a culture of patient safety and best practice. It is one means of maintaining standards of nursing practice and upgrading nursing care.
   - With respect to the individual, participation in the peer review process stimulates professional growth; clinical knowledge and skills are updated.
   - The purpose of peer review is to determine strengths and weaknesses of nursing care, taking into consideration local and institutional resources and constraints; to provide evidence for use as the basis of recommendations for new or altered policies and procedures to improve nursing care; and to identify areas where practice patterns indicate more knowledge is needed.

- Nurse reviewers need, or must strive to develop, a judicial temperament and the capacity and willingness to make critical decisions on the basis of evidence.
5. Feedback is not anonymous.
   - Feedback to the nurse under review is most effective when both verbal and written communication are combined.
6. Feedback incorporates the nurse's developmental stage.
   - Individuals, institutions, and the nursing profession benefit from an effective developmental stage.
   - Peer review program. With respect to the individual, participation in the peer review process stimulates professional growth; clinical knowledge and skills are updated.

(Adapted from Haag-Heitman & George, 2011b).

Peer review forms the basis of nursing accountability for current practice and the continual improvement of practice. Many institutions include peer review as the first step in the performance appraisal process. Roles involved in orientation are shown in Box 14.3.

PERFORMANCE APPRAISAL PROCESS

Performance appraisal originally began as a method to justify salary increases for employees. Today the performance appraisal is still used to determine rewards and to further assist the employee in setting performance goals for the year. Staff career progression begins with goal setting at the annual performance appraisal process.

Guidelines for Overall Performance Rating

Formal performance evaluations occur on an annual basis for most employees. These are most often done at a

---

BOX 14.3 Roles Involved in Orientation

Role of Nurse Manager
- Provide leadership in the culture of the nursing unit
- Provide supportive evaluation feedback to new nurses and experienced nurses
- Demonstrate valuing of mentoring activities
- Provide workloads that are reasonable and safe (with monitoring)
- Provide full-time employment on a single nursing unit
- Provide educational experiences
- Provide collaborative team experiences when possible

Nurse Managers' Retention Strategies
- Assist new nurses to manage stress
- Increase levels of responsibility slowly
- Maintain a level of challenge through provision of additional responsibilities
- Acknowledge continuing education needs
- Provide encouragement and support in nurses' transition
- Maintain an appropriate staff mix wherein nurses can practice safely

Human Resources Role
- Provide adequate orientation programs
- Provide ongoing support to address higher levels of learning

- Approve leaves of absence or educational study
- Support educational opportunities
- Coordinate new nurse employment on single units
- Initiate formal evaluative processes for performance appraisal
- Support a learning organization approach
- Provide resources and learning opportunities
- Acknowledge the contributions of mentors

Creative Engagement and Retention Strategies
- Support and encourage certification programs
- Facilitate service for education agreements
- Support clinical leadership
- Invest in the employee
- Provide extended learning experiences to enhance practice
- Provide adequate staff for safe patient care
- Provide oversight of new nurses by experienced nurses
- Encourage institutional commitment to mentorship
- Support "respectful workplace" initiatives

(From Ferguson, L., Day, R., Anderson, C., & Rohatinsky, N. (2007). The process for mentoring new nurses into professional practice. Conference presentation at the National Healthcare Leadership Conference, 2007. www.healthcareleadershipconference.ca/assets/PDFs/Presentation%20PDFs/June%2012/Pier%209/The%20Process%20of%20Mentoring%20New%20Nurses%20into%20Professional%20Practice.pdf.)

predetermined time, based on the human resources policies of the institution. The formal evaluation is part of the employee record and is usually a competency-based assessment of the performance of the employee during the past year. In many institutions, the competencies are related to the overall mission, vision, and goals of the organization. The evaluation forms the basis for the retention/promotion of the individual and the compensation adjustment. It also provides information that assists in the development of the employee's goals and objectives for the upcoming evaluation period. Box 14.4 provides guidelines for performance rating.

The nurse and the nurse manager should know the bases on which the individual is being rated. If you are

---

BOX 14.4   Guidelines for Overall Performance Rating

University of Michigan Health System
Important Points
- There should be no surprises at evaluation time that influence an employee's overall rating.
- Overall principle is preponderance
- Applicable to level of nurse
- Developmental tool to initiate discussion in regard to level movement
- Any rating other than "meets behavioral expectations" requires rationale

Scale	Guidelines
Behavioral expectations not met/NA	• This category is used when employees have consistently not met their job expectations over the course of the last year • It would be expected that you would have already documented and counseled the employee on the issues that led to this overall rating

Approaching behavioral expectations	• This category can be used for two purposes: to indicate performance issues that need attention and to indicate performance for a new hire or someone at a new level who has not been in the position long enough to fully evaluate their performance
	• For staff that are new to University of Michigan Hospitals and Health Centers or their roles:
	  • Employment or transfer of less than 4 months (or any timeframe that is appropriate for you to evaluate performance)
	  • Still mastering new skills and responsibilities
	  • You expect the employee will be able to meet expectations next year
	• For staff whose performance is less than meeting expectations:
	  • Inconsistent demonstration of framework behaviors for applicable level
	  • Need to demonstrate growth and improvement to meet behaviors
	  • Specific action plan should be developed to improve performance that includes measurable goals and expected outcomes

Meets behavioral expectations	• This category is used when the employee is meeting behavioral expectations, is effective, and provides value for the organization • Work is thorough and accurate; is accountable for own outcomes • Contributes to the goals of the organization and the unit • Exhibits professional demeanor • Demonstrates commitment to meeting level expectations

Exceeds behavioral expectations	• This category is used when the employee regularly meets expectations plus:
	  • Demonstrates excellence and exceeds expectations consistently; goes above and beyond
	  • Continuously increases the quality and/or quantity of contribution
	  • Demonstrates self-awareness related to performance

the nurse being evaluated, ask for a copy of the tool being used. If the evaluation is based on the job description, make sure that both the nurse and manager have a copy. Most nursing departments develop department-wide or unit-specific goals, and all nurses, regardless of their position, are expected to contribute to these goals. Other organizations expect nurses to accomplish individual goals. It is important to know how you are evaluating or being evaluated. Behaviors appropriate during the evaluation process are listed in Box 14.5.

As a nurse being evaluated:

- Know what you are being rated on
- Acknowledge the peer review results
- Before the review, carefully think about the period since your last review
- Review the previous year's goals
- Keep track of your performance and accomplishments along the way
- Use examples to illustrate how you met the standard
- Remain positive; acknowledge errors and show how you learned from them
- Receive criticism well
- Clarify expectations
- Accept praise

There are three main phases of the performance appraisal process:

1. Planning for the appraisal interview
2. Participating in the appraisal interview
3. Using evaluation results from both the peer review and performance appraisal

Planning for the Appraisal Interview

Preparing for the evaluation is important. In preparing, one should always list strengths and weaknesses, accomplishment of last year's goals, and future goals.

The nurse manager must also be prepared with proper documentation for this interview with specific examples of performance. There must be a correlation between the evaluation and the job description and goals of the institution.

Participating in the Appraisal Interview

This is the time for discussion specific to the employee only. The first topic of discussion is the individual's accomplishments and successes. This begins the interview on a positive note. The process should be carried out in a professional and sequential manner. If the employee is being recommended for improvement in certain areas, these specific areas must be addressed at the interview and the employee be granted a certain amount of time to improve on the lacking skills or performance. If disciplinary action is warranted because of inferior performance, the nurse manager should have the means to correct the performance, such as counseling or reeducation, readily available to the employee.

BOX 14.5   List of Recommended Supervisor and Staff Nurse Behaviors for Performance Appraisal

Manager Behaviors	Staff Nurse Behaviors
Records routinely schedule observations of the nurse's performance relative to position, professional standards, and job description competencies in a variety of situations	Uses position and professional standard expectations daily
Validates interpretation of nurse's performance	Documents specific patient outcomes that reflect planned nursing interventions
Offers counsel and support as required, citing position and professional standard expectations	Asks for clarification of expectations when there is doubt, citing position responsibilities and professional standards
Plans a date and time collaboratively with the nurse	Summarizes accomplishments during the evaluation period
Communicates to nurse what will be needed for evaluation meeting	Prepares a list of activities that advance career to the next level
Confirms the interview in writing	Collaborates with the supervisor relative to date, time, and expected preparation for the evaluation interview
Reviews nurse's past evaluation record	
Completes the written evaluation	

(Modified from Grohar-Murray, M. E., DiCroce, H. R., & Langan, J. (2011). *Leadership and management in nursing* (5th ed.). Upper Saddle River, NJ: Prentice Hall.)

Using Evaluation Results

Health care organizations have in place a method for goal attainment and outcome management. This plan may include items such as whether employee goals were met and, if not, what the plan is to assist the employee in meeting these goals in a timely manner. There may be a process improvement plan in place for evaluation of this process. Also, the employee is asked to set goals for the upcoming year along with outcome measures. These goals and outcome measures will form a portion of the next performance appraisal. The responsibilities of the supervisor and the staff nurses during the performance appraisal are listed in Box 14.6.

A sample evaluation process for a beginning nurse and a peer evaluation process is shown in Box 14.7.

The goals of the individual employees must match the goals of the unit, the department, and the institution as a whole. As the goals of all employees are set and the organizations set the strategic challenges and objectives for the next year, education and human resources plans are developed. Ongoing education, is mandated by The Joint Commission (2014) and includes in-services, training, and other activities that should, at a minimum:

- Occur when job responsibilities or duties change
- Increase knowledge of work-related issues
- Be appropriate to the needs of the population(s) served and comply with law and regulation
- Emphasize specific job-related aspects of safety and infection prevention and control
- Incorporate methods of team training, when appropriate
- Inform when and how to report adverse and sentinel events
- Be offered in response to learning needs identified through performance improvement findings and other data analysis (i.e., data from staff surveys, performance evaluations, or other needs assessments)
- Result in documented outcomes
- Be documented

Health care organizations develop myriad educational programs to further support the professional growth of employees and the mission of the organization.

As nurses progress from novice to expert, many health care facilities have a system that allows for promotion of nurses along clinical ladders. Education and benefits for progression in clinical competence form the basis for such ladders.

BOX 14.6   Supervisor and Staff Nurse Responsibilities

Supervisor Responsibilities	Staff Nurse Responsibilities
Conducts the interview	Shares documented evidence of significant professional outcomes
States judgments about the nurse's performance	
Provides justification for salary	Clarifies performance
Encourages new goals	States future goals
Agrees on future goals	States actions to meet goals

(Modified from Grohar-Murray, M. E., DiCroce, H. R., & Langan, J. (2011). *Leadership and management in nursing* (5th ed.). Upper Saddle River, NJ: Prentice Hall.)

BOX 14.7   University of Michigan Health System

Performance Evaluation Process: Self-Evaluation With Peer Input

1. The nurse will select a minimum of three peers to perform a peer review:
   - Those selected must be educated in the peer review process.
   - At least one peer must be an RN.
   - Each nurse will be asked to evaluate the person on one or two different Framework domains, so that all five Framework domains are reviewed overall by peers. The Clinical Skills and Knowledge domain must be completed by an RN whenever possible.
2. The nurse will submit the names of their chosen peers to the manager that will be completing their performance evaluation. The nurse distributes one or two domains of the peer feedback tool to selected peers.
3. The reviewers will use the current Development Framework Peer Input tool for their appraisal. They will complete their peer tool, sign it, and return it to the nurse within 7 days.

Continued

BOX 14.7   **University of Michigan Health System—cont'd**

- Peers should circle the appropriate behavioral level. Peer reviewers would be encouraged to support their views with concrete examples on the right side of the page.
- Each peer will comment on one or two different Framework domains.
4. The Peer Review forms are returned to the nurse, who shall review the content and summarize the information on the performance review form. The nurse will complete the level appropriate self-evaluation portion of the staff.
5. Performance Planning and Evaluation form, with consideration of the input provided by the peer evaluation.
6. The nurse will submit their completed Staff Performance Planning and Evaluation form and their Peer Review forms to the manager. If materials are not submitted within 2 weeks of the established due date, then the managers may proceed with completing the evaluation process.

- The manager will review the Peer Review form, peer summary, and self-evaluation and then complete the manager section of the evaluation form.
- The manager will use peer and self-evaluations and his or her own knowledge of employee performance in determining ratings on the Performance Planning and Evaluation form.
- Rationale for rating other than "meets expectations" must be provided in the evaluation summary section after each domain.
- The manager will arrange an appointment with the nurse for the performance review.
7. The Peer Review forms will be returned to the nurse after the performance evaluation process, and a copy of the completed Performance Plan/Evaluation will be given to the nurse.
8. Completed evaluations are given to the administrative assistant for processing.

(From University of Michigan Health System. *Performance evaluation process—Self-evaluation with peer input.* Used with permission.)

SUMMARY

Health care organizations are responsible for the level of competency of all employees. Competency assessment starts with the initial orientation for all employees and continues throughout the term of employment. Nurses progress on a continuum of competency from novice to expert during their careers according to the work of Benner (1984). This continuum forms the basis for many career development opportunities available to the nurse. These opportunities are related to job function during the peer review and performance appraisal process.

CLINICAL CORNER

Nursing Peer Feedback: Engage in Your Practice

"There is only one corner of the universe you can be certain of improving, and that is your own self."
Aldous Leonard Huxley
Peer review is often connected with providing feedback to an author and editor after assessing submitted scholarly work. Peer experts in the same field ensure scholarly standards are met prior to publication. The process of peer input into a nurse's practice is not standardized across nursing. The process of peer input has been reported in the literature as nurse peer feedback/review to enhance professionalism (Goble, 2017; Pinero et al., 2019; Ryiz-Semmel et al., 2019), case-based nursing incident peer review (Thielen, 2014; Garner, 2015; Cortez, 2017; Herrington & Hand, 2019), face-to-face or clinical observation nursing peer feedback/review (Karas-Irwin

& Hoffmann, 2014; LeClair-Smith et al., 2016; Mangold et al., 2018; Murphy, 2018), and most recently nurse peer-to-peer accountability (Lockett et al., 2015). Regardless of the process, the individual nurse receives constructive feedback and suggestions for professional development or improvement in practice.

Frequently when we hear "peer feedback," these two words often invoke fear in our hearts. Many express that they "feel uncomfortable" giving and receiving peer feedback, but they are okay with receiving feedback from a direct nurse supervisor who does not share the same role-specific competencies and spends less time working side by side with the nurse. You need to ask yourself, even if you might feel uncomfortable receiving feedback from a peer, do you think your peers are not assessing and evaluating your practice? Do you think your peers have not formed opinions on the skills you excel at and the skills that you might need some mentoring in? Might your peer not have some suggestions for your professional development that could assist you to grow in your role or advance? These are important questions to contemplate, and peer feedback is a tool to assist you on your journey through your professional nursing career.

The American Nurses Association (ANA, 1988) deems that primary accountability for quality nursing care resides with the individual nurse. The nursing peer feedback process recognizes that, in a self-regulating professional practice model, the clinical accountability for care rests solely with the clinical practicing nurse (Haag-Heitman & George, 2011b, p. 6). Peer feedback is a mechanism to maintain nursing standards. Each nurse is responsible for interpreting and implementing the standards of nursing practice in their specialty.

The ANA's (2010) *Nursing's Social Policy Statement: The Essence of the Profession* discussed the need for all practicing nurses at any level to participate in peer feedback to regulate their own practice. The Institute of Medicine (2010) recognized that nursing plays a vital role in the frontlines of health care and nurses should be considered full partners in redesigning health care. Peer feedback is one element to assist nurses in taking responsibility for their professional growth and redesigning the work environment. More recently the ANA's (2015a) *Code of Ethics for Nurses with Interpretive Statements* discussed the nurse's responsibility to safeguard patients, nurses, and colleagues. A component of the safeguards is a peer feedback process. Quality of practice and professional practice evaluation standards in the ANA's (2015b) *Nursing Scope and Standards of Practice* calls for nurses to seek and engage in feedback from peers and others regarding their practice and role performance. Additionally, a periodic self-appraisal and peer feedback for assurance of accountability, competence, and autonomy must be demonstrated in all levels of nursing in order to achieve and maintain Magnet designation (American Nurse Credentialing Center, 2017). Nurses are stewards for patient safety and have a professional and societal responsibility to maintain competence and participate in improvement activities.

What is Nursing Peer Feedback?

The ANA (1988, p. 3) defined nursing peer review as "an organized effort whereby practicing professionals review the quality and appropriateness of services ordered or performed by their professional peers. Peer review in nursing is the process by which practicing registered nurses systematically assess, monitor, and make judgments about the quality of nursing care provided by peers as measured against professional standards of practice."

Current-day peer feedback guiding principles include feedback from someone of the same rank, education, practice focus, and level of licensure; timely, routine, and continuous feedback; a continuous learning culture of best practice; feedback that is not anonymous; and feedback that incorporates the developmental stage of the nurse (Haag-Heitman & George, 2011a).

Nursing peer feedback is often confused with peer and annual evaluations. The annual evaluation is a supervisory function and focuses on the nurse's goal alignment with the organization. In addition to the annual evaluation, organizations often have nurses give "peer" feedback about the nurse being evaluated to the nurse's direct supervisor. The direct supervisor summarizes the feedback and delivers this anonymous feedback to the nurse at the time of the annual evaluation. This peer evaluation method described violates current-day nursing peer feedback principles. The annual evaluation is retrospective and does not allow for real-time practice assessments of the nurses' practice. A direct supervisor is not a peer of the nurse and the feedback is delivered anonymously. Nursing peer feedback needs to focus on role-specific competencies, professional development, and outcomes. Peer feedback should be independent of the annual evaluation, should not be blinded from the nurse, and should be delivered by a peer of the same rank (George & Haag-Heitman, 2012). Instead of delivering blinded peer feedback at the time of the annual evaluation, the nurse's direct supervisor needs to create a supportive environment for giving and receiving peer feedback and carve out protected time to complete peer feedback (George & Haag-Heitman, 2015). This support will foster a continuous learning culture.

Think of peer feedback as an opportunity to own your nursing practice and develop a plan on how you want to grow as a professional. We tend to not reflect on our practice as often as we should. Things you need to ask yourself:

- Professionally, where do I want to practice 5 years from now? Do I want to stay in the same specialty? Am I interested in transitioning to a new specialty?
- What formal education or professional development will I need to achieve my professional goal(s)?
- Am I knowledgeable about the external forces affecting health care and nursing?

Continued

CLINICAL CORNER—Cont'd

- How can I be a nurse advocate in my organization, community, and at the state and federal level? What skills do I need to be a nurse advocate?
- Do I have the skills needed for an outpatient setting or managing population health?
- Am I nationally board certified? How will I get there?
- Who is a role model for me? What nurse can I work with to improve? What mentoring do I need?

Take the time to reflect on these questions and evaluate your professional practice. Peer feedback can help you grow and develop. It also strengthens a nurse's commitment to a culture of excellence and enriches relationships with colleagues.

Benefits of Nursing Peer Feedback

The benefits of peer feedback are an integration of improved communication, professional autonomy, and accountability. In 2016 the American Association of Critical-Care Nurses (AACN) reaffirmed their original *Six Standards of a Healthy Work Environment*. Skilled communication is one of the six standards. Skilled communication is a critical element in a healthy work environment and the lack of communication can be costly to an organization (Ulrich et al., 2019). Blinded peer feedback violates the principle of skilled communication. Blinded feedback does not provide for clarification of the comment(s) or constructive pointers for behavior change to enhance growth. Through ongoing peer feedback of equal rank, the peer feedback process provides the nurse with an increased awareness of professional conduct, enhances interprofessional collaboration, and allows the nurse time to reflect on his or her practice. This allows nurses to develop each other and improve nurse-to-nurse interactions. Taking full ownership of one's practice engages and inspires others.

Implications

Nurses have an obligation to themselves, each other, and the profession to actively participate in nursing peer feedback. Nurses are the only health care professional at the frontline of patient care delivery around the clock and are required to be knowledgeable about chronic disease, medication management, evidenced-based practice, ethical decision making, evaluating trended data, and the use of complex technology, just to name a few. Nurses working to ensure a healthy work environment cannot be overlooked. Healthy work environments are essential to ensure patient safety, enhance nurse's career and job satisfaction, and maintain an organization's financial viability (Ulrich et al., 2019).

The ANA and Magnet Recognition Program calls for nurses to engage in peer feedback. Typically, the attention of peer feedback has been a clinical focus to improve systems of care to reduce occurrences of negative events. This type of peer feedback is essential for nurses to deliver quality care. But just as the role of the clinical nurse has expanded, so has all specialty roles in nursing. A robust peer feedback process must be in place for all roles and settings in which nurses practice. If the nurse is involved in direct care, an advanced practice registered nurse, nursing management, or a nurse executive peer feedback is needed to assist the nurse to gain insight, draw from each other's expertise, create more cohesive teams, improve the culture, professional socialization, and organizational growth.

Conclusion

Peer feedback is an essential element that defines all professional disciplines and is not optional for a practicing professional. Until all nurses embrace the principles of peer feedback and implement a continual structure for peer feedback, nursing will not achieve significant and sustainable changes in quality and safety outcomes for patient, families, and society (George & Haag-Heitman, 2011).

Challenge yourself to think about peer feedback in a different light and move away from a state of uneasiness that peer feedback often creates. Strive to be a lifelong learner. Let this clinical corner be the spark that will catapult you to make a vital contribution, or lead a team in your organization, to develop or redefine your peer feedback process to align with contemporary principles. Feedback is a gift. Be open to hearing your strengths. Let your peers help you to develop your potential and provide insight for you to continue to grow and improve. Your peer is the most suited to give you this feedback because your peer is working in the same specialty and role. We often see ourselves with one lens, and receiving feedback from a peer can open our eyes to opportunities for development. How does an individual nurse grow in his or her practice and in the profession without honest, direct peer feedback on his or her performance? The true value of peer feedback is to assist us in improving ourselves in the wonderful professional that we have chosen—nursing.

"We all need people who will give us feedback. That's how we improve."

Bill Gates

Beverly S. Karas-Irwin, DNP, RN,
NP-C, HNB-BC, NEA-BC
New York-Presbyterian

CLINICAL CORNER—Cont'd

References

American Association of Critical-Care Nurses. (2016). *AACN Standards for establishing and sustaining healthy work environments: A journey to excellence* (2nd ed.). Aliso Viejo, CA: Author.

American Nurses Association. (1988). *Peer review guidelines.* Kansas City, MO: Author.

American Nurses Association. (2010). *Nursing's social policy statement: The essence of the profession* (3rd ed.). Silver Spring, MD: Author.

American Nurses Association. (2015a). *Code of ethics for nurses with interpretive statements.* Washington, D. C: American Nurses Publishing.

American Nurses Association. (2015b). *Nursing scope and standards of practice* (3rd ed.). Silver Spring, MD: Author.

American Nurses Credentialing Center. (2017). *2019 Magnet® Application Manual.* Silver Spring, MD: Author.

Cortez, W. (2017). Peer feedback drives improved injury rates. *Nursing Management, 48*(10), 16–19. https://doi.org/10.1097/01.NUMA.0000524820.33911.87.

Garner, J. K. (2015). Implementation of a Nursing Peer-Review Program in the Hospital Setting. *Clinical Nurse Specialist: The Journal for Advanced Nursing Practice, 29*(5), 271–275. https://doi.org/10.1097/NUR.0000000000000149.

George, V., & Haag-Heitman, B. (2011). Nursing peer review: the manager's role. *Journal of Nursing Management, 19,* 254–259.

George, V., & Haag-Heitman, B. (2012). Differentiating Peer Review and the Annual Performance Review. *Nurse Leader, 10*(1), 26–28.

George, V., & Haag-Heitman, B. (2015). Essential Components of a Model Supporting Safety and Quality. *Journal of Nursing Administration, 45*(7/8), 398–403. https://doi.org/10.1097/NNA.0000000000000221.

Goble, P. H. (2017). The power of peer review: a pathway to professionalism. *Nursing Management, 48*(2), 9–12. https://doi.org/10.1097/01.NUMA.0000511927.05764.77.

Haag-Heitman, B., & George, V. (2011a). Nursing peer review: principles and practice. *American Nurse Today, 6*(9), 48.

Haag-Heitman, B., & George, V. (2011b). *Nursing Peer Review: Strategies for Successful Implementation.* Burlington, MA: Jones & Bartlett.

Herrington, C. R., & Hand, M. W. (2019). Impact of Nurse Peer Review on a Culture of Safety. *Journal of Nursing Care Quality, 34*(2), 158–162. https://doi.org/10.1097/NCQ.0000000000000361.

Institute of Medicine. (2010). *The future of nursing: Leading change, advancing health.* Retrieved from http://nationalacademies.org/hmd/~/media/Files/Report%20Files/2010/The-Future-of-Nursing/Future%20of%20Nursing%202010%20Recommendations.pdf on August 18, 2019.

Karas-Irwin, B. S., & Hoffmann, R. L. (2014). Facing the facts: in-person peer review. *Nursing Management, 45*(11), 14–17. https://doi.org/10.1097/01.NUMA.0000455736.01991.b2.

LeClair-Smith, C., Branum, B., Bryant, L., Cornell, B., Martinez, H., Nash, E., & Phillips, L. (2016). Peer-to-Peer Feedback. *Journal of Nursing Administration, 46*(6), 321–328. https://doi.org/10.1097/NNA.0000000000000352.

Lockett, J. J., Barkley, L., Stichler, J., Palomo, J., Kik, B., Walker, C., & O'Byrne, N. (2015). Defining peer-to-peer accountability from the nurse's perspective. *Journal of Nursing Administration, 45*(11), 557–562. https://doi.org/10.1097/NNA.0000000000000263.

Mangold, K., Tyler, B., Velez, L., & Clark, C. (2018). Peer-Review Competency Assessment Engages Staff and Influences Patient Outcomes. *Journal of Continuing Education in Nursing, 49*(3), 119–126. https://doi.org/10.3928/00220124–20180219-06.

Murphy, J. (2018). Comprehensive nursing peer review: our voice, our practice, our growth. *Nursing Management, 49*(8), 49–53. https://doi.org/10.1097/01.NUMA.0000542301.90248.30.

Pinero, M., Bieler, J., Smithingell, R., Andre-Jones, C., Hughes, A., & Fischer-Cartlidge, E. (2019). Integrating Peer Review into Nursing Practice. *AJN American Journal of Nursing, 119*(2), 54–59. https://doi.org/10.1097/01.NAJ.0000553206.67083.65.

Ryiz-Semmel, J., France, M., Bradshaw, R., Khan, M., Mulholland, B., Meucci, J., & McGrath, J. (2019). Design and Implementation of a Face-to-Face Peer Feedback Program for Ambulatory Nursing. *Journal of Nursing Administration, 49*(3), 143–149. https://doi.org/10.1097/NNA.0000000000000728.

Thielen, J. (2014). Failure to Rescue as the Conceptual Basis for Nursing Clinical Peer Review. *Journal of Nursing Care Quality, 29*(2), 155–163. https://doi.org/10.1097/NCQ.0b013e3182a8df96.

Ulrich, B., Barden, C., Cassidy, L., & Varn-Davis, N. (2019). Critical care nurse work environments 2018: Findings and implications. *Critical Care Nurse, 39*(2), 67–84.

EVIDENCE-BASED PRACTICE

(From Eckerson, C. (2018). The impact of nurse residency programs in the United States on improving retention and satisfaction of new nurse hires: an evidence based literature review. *Nurse Education Today, 71*(2018), 84–90.)

Transitioning from student nurse to practicing nurse has been identified as a stressful and challenging time for new nurses. The challenging evolution has been shown to be a contributing factor for high turnover rates among new nurses during their first year (Olsen-Sitki et al., 2012). Research studying the effect of hospital work environments on retention of new nurses found that new nurses experience less anxiety and stress in environments that foster a safe learning environment and effective communication and support (Cochran, 2017).

In an effort to evaluate the effect of Nurse Residency Programs the following PSCOT (population, strategy, comparison, outcomes, and time) was developed: In newly hired BSN graduates, how would the use of a 1-year residency program compared with a traditional orientation affect turnover rates and reported satisfaction of the new nurse hires over a 1-year period? Twelve articles met the inclusion criteria for the review.

Review of the evidence analyzed in this review yielded two important findings. Based on the literature review there is a strong correlation between the uses of an NRP and increased retention of new nurses in their first year of hire (Fiedler et al., 2014; Edwards et al., 2015; Chappy & Van Camp, 2017; Cline et al., 2017). The improved retention rates were also shown to have positive financial implications, saving some facilities up to $15,228,000 (Trepanier et al., 2012). Through the use of the NRP, it can be assumed based on the literature that more nurses will remain in their role within the first year of hire, which will also have positive financial outcomes for the facility.

Furthermore, newly graduated nurses may be more prone to apply to a hospital offering an NRP because of the positive outcomes presented by NRPs.

There is moderate evidence to support an increase in satisfaction with the use of an NRP. Although literature showed a decrease in satisfaction in new nurse hires after 6 months of employment, satisfaction rates stabilized and were still considered to be high based on the McCloskey Mueller Satisfaction Scale (Goode et al., 2013; Fiedler et al., 2014).

These findings reinforce the need for health care institutions to develop NRPs in place of traditional orientations for new nurse hires. Increased retention and satisfaction of new nurse hires have proven outcomes of NRPs positively affecting nurse turnover rates and finances in health care institutions.

References

Chappy, S., & Van Camp, J. (2017). The effectiveness of nurse residency programs on retention: a systematic review. *AORN J, 106*(2), 128–143.

Cline, D., La, Frentz, & Fellman, B. (2017). Longitudinal outcomes of an institutionally developed nurse residency program. *Journal of Nursing Administration, 47*(7), 384–390.

Edwards, D., Hawker, C., Carrier, J., & Rees, C. (2015). A systematic review of the effectiveness of strategies and interventions to improve the transition from student to newly qualified nurse. *International Journal of Nursing Studies, 52*(2015), 1254–1268.

Fiedler, R., Read, E., Lane, K., Hicks, F., & Jegier, B. (2014). Long term outcomes of a post baccalaureate residency program. *Journal of Nursing Administration, 44*(7), 73–79.

Goode, C., Lynn, M., & McElroy, D. (2013). Lessons learned from 10 years of research on a postbaccalaureate nurse residency program. *Journal of Nursing Administration, 44*(7), 417–422.

Trepanier, S., Early, S., Ulrich, B., & Cherry, B. (2012). New graduate nurse residency program: a cost benefit analysis based on turnover and contract labor usage. *Nursing Economics, 30*(4), 207–2014.

NCLEX® EXAMINATION QUESTIONS

1. Benner (1984) posited that the nurse moves through five stages of clinical competence: novice, advanced beginner, competent, proficient, and expert. Once you have graduated and begun your new job it is important to know that you are considered what level of nurse?
   A. Novice
   B. Expert
   C. Advanced beginner
   D. Competent

2. Your nurse manager has been in her nursing profession in the same position for 8 years. She is an MSN, and is board certified through the American Nurses Credentialing Center (ANCC). According to Benner, which of the following would this nurse leader be in?
   A. Novice
   B. Expert
   C. Advanced beginner
   D. Competent

3. Throughout nursing school your nursing professors have taught you that in the nursing profession there is lifelong learning. An example of this is:
   A. Attending conferences in your field of expertise
   B. Keeping your annual competencies up-to-date
   C. Reading nursing journals
   D. All of the above

4. When you are hired it is key that you see the competence evaluation so that you are aware of the facilities' expectations of you as an RN. You will sit with your nurse manager when you have your evaluation at 6 months, for example. What will not be on this evaluation?
   A. How much overtime you worked
   B. Tardiness
   C. History of incident reports
   D. Input from peers

5. The Joint Commission (2019) stated that a hospital must provide the right number of competent staff to meet the needs of the patients. Competent staff members are qualified and able to perform the work according to professional standards. Which of the following is not included in the assessment of competent staff members?
   A. Orienting, training, and educating staff.
   B. Ongoing in-service and other education and training to increase staff knowledge of specific work-related issues.
   C. Assessing, maintaining, and improving staff competence.
   D. Nurses age and number of years as an RN

6. Which of the following is an advantage for the nurse to act as preceptor to new nurses?
   A. It supports the progression in the institution's clinical ladder
   B. Higher pay per hour is awarded to precept
   C. Enhanced job promotion prospects
   D. The preceptor decides if the new nurse should stay on or be let go

7. Newly hired RNs will be required to have a health physical and meet all of the medical criteria for employment. Some of the medical requirements are:
   A. Hepatitis B immunizations and titer
   B. Two-step TB test
   C. Drug screening
   D. All of the above

8. The Joint Commission (2014) states that a hospital must provide the right number of competent staff to meet the needs of the patients. Which of the following is not a criterion that must be present to meet the goal of providing adequate competent staff?
   A. Orienting, training, and educating staff
   B. The hospital provides ongoing in-service and other education and training
   C. Assessing, maintaining, and improving staff competence
   D. Providing full monetary compensation for conferences and nurse certifications

9. According to the Institute of Medicine's report, *The Future of Nursing* (2006), there was a call for the development of _____ programs to assist in the transition process of the new graduate:
   A. Residency
   B. Preceptor
   C. Clinical ladder
   D. Peer review

10. The part of the orientation process that includes speakers from human resources, infection control, hospital safety and security, and process improvement, is called:
    A. Hospital-wide orientation
    B. Unit-specific orientation
    C. Staff competencies
    D. Nursing orientation

Answers: 1. A   2. B   3. ?   4. A   5. D   6. A   7. D   8. D   9. A   10. A

BIBLIOGRAPHY

Alexander, C. S., Weisman, C. S., & Chase, G. A. (1982). Determinants of staff nurses' perceptions of autonomy within different clinical outcomes. *Nursing Research, 31*, 48–52.

American Nurses Association. (1988). *Peer review guidelines.* Kansas City, MO: Author.

American Nurses Association. (2010). *Nursing's social policy statement: The essence of the profession.* Silver Spring, MD: ANA.

American Nurses Credentialing Center. (2018). *2019 Magnet application manual.* Silver Spring, MD: ANCC.

Barden, C. (Ed.), (2005). *AACN standards for establishing and sustaining healthy work environments.* Aliso Viejo, CA: AACN.

Combes, J. (2009). Peer perspective deepens. *Hospital Health Network, 83*(9), 56.

George, V., & Haag-Heitman, B. (2011). Nursing peer review: the manager's role. *Journal of Nursing Management, 19*, 254–259.

George, V., & Haag-Heitman, B. (2012). Differentiating peer review and the annual performance review. *Nurse Leader, 10*(1), 26–28.

Graham, G. (2009). Introducing the new principles-based peer review standards. *Journal of Accountancy, 207*(5), 39–43.

Haag-Heitman, B., & George, V. (2011a). Nursing peer review: principles and practice. *American Nurse Today, 6*(9), 48.

Haag-Heitman, B., & George, V. (2011b). *Nursing peer review: Strategies for successful implementation.* Burlington, MA: Jones & Bartlett.

Haines, S. T., Ammann, R. R., Beehrle-Hobbs, D., & Groppi, J. A. (2010). Protected professional practice evaluation: a continuous quality-improvement process. *American Journal of Health-System Pharmacy: AJHP: Official Journal of the American Society of Health-System Pharmacists, 67*(22), 1933–1940.

Hardy, R., & Smith, R. (2001). Enhancing staff development with a structured preceptor program. *Journal of Nursing Care Quality, 15*, 9–17.

Institute of Medicine. (2010) The future of nursing: Leading change, advancing health. www.iom.edu/Reports/2010/The-Future-of-Nursing-Leading-Change-Advancing-Health.aspx%20.

Jambunathan, J. (1992). Planning a peer review program. *Journal of Nursing Staff Development, 8*(5), 235–239.

Pan, H., Hsu, G., Yang, T., Huang, J., Chou, C., Liang, H., & Wong, K. (2013). Peer reviewing of screening mammography in Taiwan: its reliability and the improvement. *Chinese Medical Journal, 126*(1), 68–71.

Schmalenberg, C., Kramer, M., Brewer, B., Burke, R., Chmielewski, L., Cox, K., & Waldo, M. (2008). Clinically competent peers and support for education: structures and practices that work. [Article 3 in a series of 8]. *Critical Care Nurse, 28*(4), 54.

The Joint Commission. (2019). *Joint Commission Standards. The Joint Commission.* Terrace, IL: Oakbridge.

Group Management for Effective Outcomes

OUTLINE

OBJECTIVES

- Discuss nurse leader responsibility regarding group management.
- Review techniques for working with groups.
- Review techniques for leading groups and meetings.
- Differentiate between functional and dysfunctional groups.
- Review the different methods used to evaluate staff performance.
- Identify the difference between supervising and evaluating the work of others.
- Review the importance of supervising and leading groups, task forces, and patient care conferences.

KEY TERMS

cohesiveness degree to which the members are attracted to the group and wish to retain membership in it

committee group that deal with specific issues involving several service areas

competing groups groups in which members compete for resources or recognition

group aggregate of individuals who interact and mutually influence each other; several individuals assembled together or who have some unifying relationship

real (command) groups groups that accomplish tasks in an organization and are recognized as legitimate organizational entities

task group several individuals who work together to accomplish specific time-limited assignments

teams real groups in which people work cooperatively with each other to achieve a goal

GROUPS AND TEAMS

Nurses work as part of a team on the unit where they are employed. This does not necessarily mean that they are all practicing team nursing, but they are part of a larger group that is responsible for the overall delivery of care on the unit. As a team member it is important to know how to work within a team, how to manage teams, and how to evaluate the performance of others.

A group consists of individuals who interact and influence each other. Groups exist in organizations. According to Sullivan and Decker, 2009, group members include:

- Individuals from a single work group, such as a unit-based council
- Individuals at similar job levels from more than one work group, such as a nursing retention council
- Individuals from different job levels, such as the "night council"
- Individuals from different work groups and different job levels in the organization, such as interdisciplinary groups composing a service excellence committee

As can be seen from this definition, there are a number of groups that function within a nursing unit. Some of these groups will be:

- *Interdisciplinary teams:* These are sometimes called collaboratives, which are composed of the different functions caring for a patient. An example would be an ambulatory chemotherapy collaborative, in which the team composition includes the nurse, the pharmacist, the dietician, the admission clerk, and the intravenous therapist.
- *Patient care team:* This may be similar to the group of individuals actually providing actual care to the patient. It may be composed of all individuals responsible for care per shift or over 24 hours.
- *Performance improvement team:* It may include individuals from various disciplines and from various levels of the organization (e.g., department head, staff nurse, environmental services member, etc.).
- *Discharge management team:* It may include case manager, home care nurse, physical therapist, social worker, etc.

The nurse and nurse manager are also part of a much larger group called the patient care (or nursing) department. As a member of this larger group, it is important to support the overall goals of the patient care department and be a functional valued member of this team.

The differences between groups and teams are described in Box 15.1. Teams are real groups in which individuals must work cooperatively with each other to achieve some overarching goal (Sullivan and Decker, 2009).

One of the first rules for any team, committee, or council is the development of the charge of the group. This is often called the bylaws or rules of the group. The development of such bylaws focuses the work of the group to the expected outcomes or committee rules stated in the bylaws.

An example of a Nursing Council Bylaw is given here.

ACTIVE LISTENING

The first rule for dealing with individuals and with teams is to be a good listener. As a good listener, you must listen actively. This is when the person listening is

---

BOX 15.1   Differences Between Groups and Teams

Groups
1. Members have a common purpose, but work independently, sometimes competitive with one another
2. Individuals may have limited knowledge about one another
3. Meetings serve as a forum to receive reports and coordinate activity
4. Meetings follow an agenda with set time constraints
5. Attendance is not essential; the group can function with absent members and substitutes
6. The composition of the group may vary
7. Individuals rather that the group are recognized for effectiveness

Teams
1. Members are interdependent, collaborating for a common mission or project, never competitive with one another
2. Trust develops from learning about one another; how to anticipate behavior
3. Meetings serve to evaluate team effectiveness
4. Meetings are often unstructured, allowing time for strategic planning and team development.
5. Attendance and participation of each member are essential
6. Team members may not appoint substitutes
7. Individual performance is secondary to team effectiveness

(From Nees, T. (2010). *Seven characteristics of groups and teams.* http://leadingtoserve.com/?p=172.)

completely focused and tuned in to the individual who is speaking. The active listener is nonjudgmental and comprehends the full conversation. See Box 15.2 for guidelines on active listening.

CONDUCTING MEETINGS

Nurse managers are often asked to lead group or team meetings. Many of these may be staff meetings for the review of issues of importance to the unit, performance improvement teams, patient care teams, or other shared governance teams. Table 15.1 outlines some guidelines for leading group meetings (Sullivan and Decker, 2009).

These guidelines can be further adapted to delineate guidelines for leading teams (Table 15.2), such as patient care teams.

EFFECTIVE AND INEFFECTIVE TEAMS

Parker, 1990 states that a team is a group of people with a high degree of interdependence geared toward the achievement of a goal or a task. Not all teams function well, and there are times when even the most qualified team has a dysfunctional day. If a team has a "bad day," it is important for the team member or leader to evaluate the reasons for the poor performance. If the reasons can be understood, it is important to alter the way the team works to increase functionality, efficiency, and patient outcomes.

An effective team is able to move the agenda forward with clear decision making, a level of understanding of the goals and actions, and the willingness of the team members to participate in the decision-making process.

The original work done by McGregor, 1960 has stood the test of time and continues to show significant differences between effective and ineffective teams (Table 15.3).

Not all teams are functional! And it is very difficult for members who are working within the team to realize their level of effectiveness. If you feel the team is not working and it should, you may want to evaluate a team's effectiveness using a team assessment questionnaire tool.

BOX 15.2 Guidelines for Active Listening

1. Slow down your internal processes and seek data. Do not interrupt the speaker.
2. The more information you acquire through listening, the less interpretation you do (making up the missing pieces or motivations). The less information you have, the more interpretation you do.
3. Realize that the first words from the other person are not necessarily representative of inner thoughts and feelings. Be patient.
4. When listening, suspend your own beliefs and views and judgments, at least temporarily. Attempt to understand the perspective of the other person, particularly if it is different from yours.
5. Realize that any judgments or "labels" strongly influence the manner in which you listen to the other person.
6. Appreciate the difference between understanding other people's perspectives and agreeing with them. First strive to understand. Then you may agree or disagree.
7. Effective listening is based on an inner desire to learn about another's unique experience of the world.

(Modified from Olen, D. (1992). *Communicating speaking and listening to end misunderstanding and promote friendship.* Germantown, WI: JODA Communications.

TABLE 15.1 Guidelines for Leading Group Meetings

- Begin and end on time
- Start with the agenda and stick to it
- Create a warm, accepting, and nonthreatening climate
- Arrange seating to minimize differences in power, maximize involvement, and allow visualization of all meeting activities (a U-shape is optimal)
- Use interesting and varied visuals and other aids
- Clarify all terms and concepts; avoid jargon
- Foster cooperation in the group
- Establish goals and key objectives
- Keep the group focused
- Focus the discussion on one topic at a time
- Facilitate thoughtful problem solving based on evidence
- Allocate time for all problem-solving steps
- Promote involvement
- Facilitate integration of material and ideas
- Encourage the exploration of implications of ideas
- Facilitate the evaluation of the quality of the discussion
- Elicit the expression of dissenting opinions
- Summarize discussion
- Finalize the plan of action for implementing decisions
- Arrange for follow-up

These guidelines can be further adapted to delineate guidelines for leading teams (see Table 15.2), such as patient care teams.

TABLE 15.2 Guidelines for Leading Teams

- Do not waste staff time
- Create a warm, accepting, and nonthreatening climate
- Be knowledgeable of all team members' abilities and values
- Communicate in clear terms that are understood by all team members
- Clarify all terms and concepts; avoid jargon
- Foster cooperation in the group
- Establish goals and key objectives for the day
- Routinely check on the performance of the group and patient outcomes to determine whether changes in the plan are needed

- Facilitate thoughtful problem solving based on evidence
- Allocate time for all changes in the delivery of care
- Promote involvement of all members
- Facilitate the integration of work and ideas of all team members
- Assist other team members if needed
- Evaluate work at the end of the shift
- Thank all team members for the work done
- Assist any members who need improvement

TABLE 15.3 Attributes of Effective and Ineffective Teams

Attribute	Effective Team	Ineffective Team
Working environment	Informal, comfortable, relaxed	Indifferent, bored, tense, stiff
Discussion	Focused	Frequently unfocused
	Shared by almost everyone	Dominated by a few
Objectives	Well understood and accepted	Unclear, or many personal agendas
Listening	Respectful; encourages participation	Judgmental; much interruption and "grandstanding"
Ability to handle conflict	Comfortable with disagreement	Uncomfortable with disagreement
	Open discussion of conflicts	Disagreement usually suppressed, or one group aggressively dominates
Decision making	Usually reached by consensus	Often occurs prematurely
	Formal voting kept to a minimum	Formal voting occurs frequently
	General agreement is necessary for action; dissenters are free to voice	Simple majority is sufficient for action; minority is expected to go along with opinion
Criticism	Frequent, frank, relatively comfortable, constructive	Embarrassing and tension-producing, destructive
	Directed toward removing obstacle	Directed personally at others
Leadership	Shared; shifts from time to time	Autocratic; remains clearly with committee chairperson
Assignments	Clearly stated	Unclear
	Accepted by all despite disagreements	Resented by dissenting members
Feelings	Freely expressed, open for discussion	Hidden, considered "explosive" and inappropriate for discussion
Self-regulation	Frequent and ongoing, focused on solutions	Infrequent, or occurs outside meetings

(Modified from McGregor, D. (1960). *The human side of enterprise.* New York: McGraw-Hill.)

TEAM ASSESSMENT QUESTIONNAIRE

Instructions: Use the following scale to indicate how each statement applies to your team. Evaluate the statements honestly and without overthinking your answers.

3 = Usually
2 = Sometimes
1 = Rarely

_____1. Team members are passionate and unguarded in their discussion of issues.

_____2. Team members call out one another's deficiencies or unproductive behaviors.

_____3. Team members know what their peers are working on and how they contribute to the collective good of the team.

_____4. Team members quickly and genuinely apologize to one another when they say or do something inappropriate or possibly damaging to the team.

_____ 5. Team members willingly make sacrifices (such as budget, turf, head count) in their departments or areas of expertise for the good of the team.

_____ 6. Team members openly admit their weaknesses and mistakes.

_____ 7. Team meetings are compelling, not boring.

_____ 8. Team members leave meetings confident that their peers are completely committed to the decisions that were agreed on, even if they were in initial disagreement.

_____ 9. Morale is significantly affected by the failure to achieve team goals.

_____ 10. During team meetings, the most important and difficult issues are put on the table to be resolved.

_____ 11. Team members are deeply concerned about the prospect of letting down their peers.

_____ 12. Team members know about one another's personal lives and are comfortable discussing them.

_____ 13. Team members end discussions with clear and specific resolutions and action plans.

_____ 14. Team members challenge one another about their plans and approaches.

_____ 15. Team members are slow to seek credit for their own contributions, but quick to point out those of others.

Scoring

Combine your scores for the preceding statements as indicated in the following table.

Dysfunction 1: Absence of Trust	Dysfunction 2: Fear of Conflict	Dysfunction 3: Lack of Commitment	Dysfunction 4: Avoidance of Accountability	Dysfunction 5: Inattention to Results
Statement 4: ___	Statement 1: ___	Statement 3: ___	Statement 2: ___	Statement 5: ___
Statement 6: ___	Statement 7: ___	Statement 8: ___	Statement 11: ___	Statement 9: ___
Statement 12: ___	Statement 10: ___	Statement 13: ___	Statement 14: ___	Statement 15: ___
Total: ___	Total: ___	Total: ___	Total: ___	Total: ___

A score of 8 or 9 is a probable indication that the dysfunction is not a problem for your team.
A score of 6 or 7 indicates that the dysfunction could be a problem.
A score of 3 to 5 is probably an indication that the dysfunction needs to be addressed.
Regardless of your scores, it is important to keep in mind that every team needs constant work, because without it, even the best ones deviate toward dysfunction.
(From Lencioni, P. (2002). *The five dysfunctions of a team: a leadership fable.* San Francisco: Jossey-Bass.)

POWER AND CONTROL

Whenever there is a team effort, power and control usually come into play. When a person reacts to a situation at the "feeling" level, there are often blame and judgment calls. People normally would like to believe that their input and contributions are respected and used by the group. For a team to be effective, each member of the group must be able to effectively communicate, offer constructive criticism, and acknowledge the positive at every chance (Box 15.3) A "just" culture throughout an organization will assist with such freedom in communication (see Chapter 8).

RECOGNIZE AND REWARD SUCCESS

Rewards are listed as one important principle of high-performing organizations. The Studer Group (2007, 2012) has defined nine principles of high-performing organizations. The ninth principle is to recognize and reward success. Everyone makes a difference! Start creating legends in your organization. A legend is an example of those who live the organizational values. By creating legends we establish real-life examples for others to follow. Create win-win situations for your staff. Never let great work go unnoticed! The first step in creating a legend in your organization is to reward

---

BOX 15.3   Guidelines for Acknowledgment

1. Acknowledgments must be specific. The specific behavior or action that is appreciated must be identified in the acknowledgment; for example, "Thank you for taking notes for me when I had to go to the dentist. You identified three key points that appeared on the test."
2. Acknowledgments must be "eye to eye."
3. Acknowledgments must be sincere, that is, from the heart. Each of us recognizes insincerity. If you do not truly appreciate a behavior or action, do not say anything. Insincerity often makes people angry or upset, thus defeating the goal.
4. Acknowledgments are more powerful when they are given in public. Most people receive pleasure from public acknowledgment and remember these occasions for a long time. For people who are shy and may prefer no public acknowledgment, this is an opportunity to work on a personal growth issue with them. Public acknowledgment is an opportunity to communicate what is valued.
5. Acknowledgments need to be timely. The less time that elapses between the event and the acknowledgment, the more powerful and effective it is and the more the acknowledgment is appreciated by the recipient.

(From Yoder-Wise, P. (2011). *Leading and managing in nursing* (p. 353). St. Louis: Elsevier.)

team members for a job well done. Much of the work in creating legends in your organization will be communicated through the various committees and team meetings. Such award and recognition has been documented to be related to increased nurse satisfaction (Guyton, 2012).

QUALITIES OF A TEAM PLAYER

Nurses work in a collaborative environment, yet many nurses have concerns about the lack of ability of some individuals to work as part of a team: "They just don't support us!"

Maxwell, 2002 has identified the following 17 characteristics that make a good team player:

1. *Adaptability:* Inflexibility does not work in teams. Being rigid in thinking or behavior is destructive to both the individual and to the team.
2. *Collaboration:* Collaboration is more than cooperation. It means each person brings something to the project that adds value to the team and supports the creation of synergy.
3. *Commitment:* This is the passion in the face of adversity to take action and make things happen. It is the passion to do whatever it takes to accomplish the team objectives.
4. *Communicate:* Communication should happen early and often. Frequency of interaction with other team members and talking with them and sharing thoughts, ideas, and experiences are the activities that support teamwork.
5. *Competence:* Competence translates as someone who is capable, highly qualified, and does the job well.
6. *Dependable:* Team members who are dependable follow through and do what they have agreed to do, and do it well, without prodding or delay.
7. *Disciplined:* Discipline is doing what you really do not want to do so you can accomplish the goals you really want. It includes paying attention to detail in thinking, in emotions, and in the actions you take.
8. *Adding value:* Helping a teammate advance or grow into a better person or team player, helping teammates advance the team, and believing in your teammates before they believe in themselves are all examples of adding value.
9. *Enthusiastic:* Enthusiasm focuses on becoming a highly energetic team member who has a positive attitude and believes that the team, together, can be better than anyone dreamed they could be.
10. *Intentional:* The team and its members have a purpose for themselves and for the team. Every action counts and is meaningful including focusing on doing the right things in each moment and following through with these actions to their logical conclusion.
11. *Awareness of the mission:* Each team member has a sense of purpose and mission that drives all thoughts, ideas, and actions to do what is best for their team and their cause.
12. *Prepared:* Being prepared translates as being ready for every meeting and event and begins with a thorough assessment of what is needed, aligning the appropriate work with the appropriate effort, addressing the mental aspects of the right attitude, and being ready to take action.

13. *Relationship oriented:* The ability to be connected to other members of the team and to be in a relationship with them is the core of being relationship oriented. These relationships and the mutual respect on which they are built create cohesiveness on the team.
14. *Improve yourself:* As a team member, you strive to continually grow and reflect, both routinely and periodically, on how well each venture or assignment went and what you could have done better. This is a process of self-reflection.
15. *Selflessness:* Putting others on the team ahead of yourself by being generous to team members, avoiding "playing politics," showing loyalty toward team members, and valuing interdependence among team members over the American value of being independent are all examples of selflessness.
16. *Solution focused:* Do not be consumed with all of the problems associated with the endeavor; instead, focus on finding the solutions. Think about what is possible.
17. *Tenacious:* Being tenacious means giving your all, with determination, and refusing to stop until the goal has been accomplished.

Strong patient and nurse outcomes depend on the work of the entire team, so it is important for all staff members to understand their significance and value within the larger organizational and team structure.

INTERDISCIPLINARY TEAMS

- Highly functional interdisciplinary teams are essential in today's health care system. The following are some of the different team members who work with nurses:
- Physicians
- Dieticians
- Case managers
- Social workers
- Teachers
- Respiratory therapists
- Physical therapists
- Occupational therapists
- Psychologists
- Pharmacists

Having a team composed of members from varied disciplines often creates a more challenging team function in that everyone is attempting to protect their own "turf" and assume power. In the early stages of these groups, there may be some turf wars until the team forms a single identity.

Durskat and Wolf, 2001 believed that three major components of smoothly functioning teams must be created:
1. Mutual trust among the members
2. A strong sense of team identity (that the team is unique and worthwhile)
3. A sense of team efficacy (that the team performs well and its members are synergistic in their manner of working together)

One area of particular concern in today's health care environment is the outcome measure of readmission. Hospitals are being penalized through penalties in reimbursement for heart failure readmission rates above the nationwide average. Interdisciplinary/interorganizational teams have been formed to oversee the development of protocols that transverse the multiple organizations that take care of the patient through the multitude of transitions of care during the chronic disease care process. In the bundle payment system, the efficiency of such teams are important in terms of reimbursement. Such teams need to be highly effective, organized, and outcome driven.

SUPERVISING THE WORK OF OTHERS

Nurses continuously supervise the work of others. This may include the nursing assistant, licensed practical nurse/licensed vocational nurse (LPN/LVN), other registered nurses, patient care technicians, and the unit clerk. Many conversations occur among these groups with various purposes such as
- To orient, teach, and guide coworkers according to their individual learning styles and needs, consistent with their backgrounds, experience, and assignments
- To stimulate desire for self-improvement in supervisees
- To encourage supervisees to use their unique talents and develop special skills
- To model desired attitudes, skills, interests, and work habits

TYPES OF CONVERSATIONS

In the evaluation of team members, some organizations are defining team members as high-medium-low (H-M-L) performers. Essentially, high performers are people who deliver solutions. Middle performers can identify the problem, but may lack the experience or self-confidence to bring solutions. Low performers tend to blame others for the problem; they act like renters instead of owners. The Studer Group, 2007, 2011; The Studer Group, 2012 suggested that leaders rate themselves. The best leaders are always willing to perform an honest self-assessment. Are you a high, middle, or low performer? What actions will you take as a result?

Often, leaders using this exercise to rank their employees ask, "What if I have an employee who is technically excellent, but nobody wants to work with them?" To qualify as a high performer, an individual must be excellent both technically and as a team member. In fact, the Studer Group (2007, 2011) even suggested terminating the employment of those who get results, but do not role model the organization's standards of behavior because they are so damaging to overall employee morale.

According to the Studer Group (2007, 2011), after the ranking of an employee as an H-M-L performer, an employee tracking log should be used to track the name, rating (H-M-L), initial meeting date, and follow-up date/comments. Always hold meetings with high performers first, middle performers next, and low performers last. Ordering the meetings in this way accomplishes several things. High performers, for example, can dispel fear about the meetings when other employees ask why the boss wanted to meet with them. Perhaps most importantly, leaders report that they feel energized and fortified for those difficult low-performer conversations once they have enjoyed so many positive conversations with employees they value.

H-M-L conversations are not evaluations tied to pay, so they should not take place at evaluation time. However, by repeating these meetings twice a year, conversations can complement staff evaluations so employees get the more frequent feedback they seek from managers. Leaders can help employees, especially middle performers, understand that these 15-minute meetings are opportunities for recognition, coaching, and professional development.

The objectives and outcomes are distinct for each type of conversation.

High-performer conversations: Re-recruit the best performers by giving specific positive feedback about what they do well, their accomplishments, and examples of positive attitude. Share information about where the organization is going, and ask if there is anything you can do for them to make their job better.

Middle-performer conversations: Use a support coach technique. The overall tone of the meeting must be positive. Begin by reassuring these individuals that you value their contributions and that your goal is to retain them as valuable employees. Thank them for what they do well. Then identify and discuss one specific area for development; something you would like them to improve. Complete the conversation by reaffirming their good qualities and expressing your appreciation.

Low-performer conversations: Do not start the meeting out on a positive note. Use the DESK approach:

- **D**escribe what has been observed.
- **E**valuate how you feel.
- **S**how what needs to be done.
- **E**nsure that employees **K**now the consequences of the continued poor performance.

Because low performers are so skilled at excuses, guilt, and indignation, these conversations can be difficult for managers. The manager needs to remain calm, objective, and clear about consequences if performance does not improve by a specified date. If the behavior has not improved, the nurse manager needs to follow through and take action. Refer to Chapter 14 for Performance Appraisal.

Table 15.4 gives an example of a differentiating staff worksheet.

TABLE 15.4 Differentiating Staff Worksheet

	High	Medium	Low
Definition	Comes to work on time	Good attendance	Points out problems in a negative way
	Good attitude	Loyal most of the time	Positions leadership poorly
	Problem solves	Influenced by high and low performers	Master of we/they
	You relax when you know they are scheduled	Wants to do a good job	Passive aggressive
	Good influence	Could just need more experience	Thinks they will outlast the leader
	Use for peer interviews	Helps manager be aware of problems	Says manager is the problem
	Five-pillar ownership		
	Brings solutions		
Professionalism	Adheres to unit policies concerning breaks, personal phone calls, leaving the work area, and other absences from work	Usually adheres to unit policies concerning breaks, personal phone calls, leaving the work area, and other absences from work	Does not communicate effectively about absences from work areas
			Handles personal phone calls in a manner that interferes with work
			Breaks last longer than allowed
Teamwork	Demonstrates high commitment to making things better for the work unit and organization as a whole	Committed to improving performance of the work unit and organization	Demonstrates little commitment to the work unit and the organization
		May require coaching to fully execute	
Knowledge and competence	Eager to change for the good of the organization	Invested in own professional development	Shows little interest in improving own performance or the performance of the organization
	Strives for continuous professional development	May require some coaching to fully execute	Develops professional skills only when asked
Communication	Comes to work with a positive attitude	Usually comes to work with a positive attitude Occasionally gets caught up in the negative attitude of others	Comes to work with a negative attitude
			Has a negative influence on the work environment
Safety awareness	Demonstrates the behaviors of safety awareness in all aspects of work	Demonstrates the behaviors of safety awareness in most aspects of work	Performs work with little regard to the behaviors of safety awareness

(From *The Studer Group. The nine principles. (2007). Retrieved December 9, 2007, from* <www.studergroup.com/dotCMS/knowledgeAssetDetail?inode=217849>.)

SUMMARY

Once you have worked on a specific unit for a period of time the culture of the hospital and the unit will become clear. Positive attitudes foster positive attitudes; negative work habits foster negative work habits. The nurse manager is charged with creating an environment conducive to high-quality patient care and staff satisfaction. The interactions within the team environment set the tone. Supervision and evaluation are part of a process of continuous improvement and staff development.

CLINICAL CORNER

Supporting a Culture of Communication at a Unit-Based Level

Maintaining a culture of communication at the unit level is of utmost importance in health care settings. It is the responsibility of every member of the unit team to support communication initiatives that may influence patient safety, continuity of care, planning of care, and optimal patient outcomes. At Hackensack University Medical Center, communication guides our professional nursing practice and the delivery of patient care.

One of the most critical times of communication at the unit level is during shift-to-shift handoff. It is essential that this report is standardized and all information is shared with a common goal of maintaining patient safety. On our 16-bed pediatric oncology/hematology/blood and marrow transplant (BMT) unit, shift-to-shift handoff is communicated face to face with the oncoming nurse. To guide patient report, we use a Kardex to communicate important information including the patient's weight, allergies, diagnosis, chemotherapy regimen, nursing orders, type of intravenous (IV) line and fluid, dressing changes, recent blood transfusions, and lab results. More recently, our institution has added an additional resource to our electronic medical record to standardized shift-to-shift report across all units. This new resource, known as IPASS (illness severity, patient summary, action list, situation awareness, and synthesis), brings information from the electronic medical record into one organized flowsheet. This report format supports our organization's safety initiatives to ensure communication is standardized and key patient information is not missed.

Our unit also supports our institution's mission of bedside shift report and safety checks. Communicating at the bedside has several benefits for the nurse and the patient and family. It creates an opportunity to involve the patient and family in the discussion of the plan of care and clarify any questions or concerns they may have. As the oncoming nurse, bedside shift report is very beneficial in ensuring our patient is safe and stable. Safety checks are completed to ensure emergency equipment is set up appropriately, the patient's ID band is on and intact, the IV site does not have any complications, and medication is infusing as per the orders in the medication administration record. When the nurse can complete a quick initial assessment of their patient during bedside report and safety check, it can also assist in making prioritization decisions at the beginning of the shift.

An additional way to support communication at the unit level is through a team huddle at change of shift. Team huddles are led by the charge nurse at change of shift and gives an opportunity for each outgoing nurse to discuss important information about their patients to all of the oncoming nurses. Pertinent information is shared so that every member of the team is informed about all patients on the unit. Written communication among charge nurses is also beneficial to ensure essential patient information is shared to guide future decisions about patient assignments and unit staffing needs. Our unit uses an assignment sheet, which includes a detailed synopsis of the unit. It includes a brief description of every patient's plan including information such as procedures, blood transfusions, chemotherapy infusions, isolation, and bone marrow transplants. Further information about the patient's plan of care is discussed during our daily multidisciplinary rounds. Our team consists of nurses, physicians, advance practice nurses, residents, a dietician, social worker, child life specialist, research coordinators, and an education liaison. The team meets daily to discuss each patient and then visits each patient and family for further assessment and discussion of the plan of care. Our staff nurses are integral members of the multidisciplinary team and make every effort to be part of these daily rounds.

An additional way that our children's hospital facilitates communication among all members of the health care team is through the initiation of unit-based safety huddles. When these huddles first started, they were conducted at change of shift with the day/night charge nurse, the senior resident, and a member from the hospital safety team. Staff communicated "gaps in the system," such as near miss errors, supply shortages, critical patients, or staffing needs. Staff were encouraged to communicate openly and honestly. The issues addressed at the safety huddle were then relayed to the appropriate leaders or departments. Recently the unit-based safety huddles have emerged to include all units of our children's hospital including inpatient and outpatient units, nurse managers, and administrators. The format of these huddles is a 15-minute conference call beginning at 8 a.m. This change has promoted communication at all levels of the institution, providing our units with the opportunity to discuss important patient care issues including safety, staffing, supply, or equipment issues and capacity management updates. The huddles allow an opportunity for all units to communicate any concerns from the previous day, ensuring that all members of our team are on the same page, working together to provide safe care and the best patient experience possible. After our children's hospital huddle, an institution-wide safety huddle is held in a face-to-face setting to further allow for open communication about issues that may be affecting patient safety and optimal care.

CLINICAL CORNER—Cont'd

Supporting communication at the unit level also entails organization-wide communication about new or revised policies, updates from committee meetings, information from unit-based council meetings, results of quality data, and results from patient surveys. Every member of the unit team has an email address supplied by the institution and is responsible for checking e-mail on a regular basis. Managers and other leaders use email to communicate important information that affects nurses and patient care. Other methods that have been used on our unit to communicate important information include bulletin boards and newsletters. Bulletin boards in the unit hallways display important changes to practice, not only to staff but to patients as well, providing the patient with knowledge and understanding of the care they receive. Our unit also uses bulletin boards in the staff lounge to display educational opportunities such as, "Journal Article of the Month" and patient case studies.

At the hospital-wide level, shared governance-based nursing councils allow for information to be shared among units. One such council is the Staff Advisory Council. This council consists of representatives from every unit-based council throughout the medical center. The purpose of this council is to "facilitate collaboration of staff nurses for the pursuit of excellence in patient care." At each monthly meeting, different units report on their yearly goals, the actions taken to meet the goals, and their outcomes. Unit representatives are responsible for communicating the information shared at this council with their own unit. Additionally, minutes from this council and the other nursing councils are available on the hospital intranet. It has become an expectation that all staff nurses are aware of information discussed at council meetings because much of the information shared affects patient care and ultimately patient outcomes.

At Hackensack University Medical Center, communication is part of the care delivery model and the professional practice model. Within both of these models, the patient is at the center and guides our nursing practice. Communication at the unit level will always be essential between staff nurses, the multidisciplinary team, and the entire health care organization to ensure all patients are treated with the best care possible and have the opportunity to achieve the best outcomes.

Gina M. Dovi, MSN, RN, CPHON
Karen Madigan, BSN, RN, CPON

EVIDENCE-BASED PRACTICE

(From Fowler, K. (2018) Communicating in a culturally diverse workforce. *Nursing Management, 49*(9), 50–54.)

As the Latino population continues to grow in the United States, the need for a culturally diverse workforce heightens. The current registered nurse (RN) workforce does not reflect the increasing diversity of the population. Demands of nurse leaders include the ability to retain a skilled, engaged, and diverse staff. The leader's communication style directly influences the nurse-leader RN relationship, coordination of work, and RN satisfaction with the work environment. Ensuring that nurse leaders have competence in communication will position an organization for success in an increasingly diverse environment.

This descriptive correlational study collected data using a survey tool (the Supervisor Leadership and Communication Inventory, and the Utrecht Work Engagement Scale) and retrospective hospital turnover and retention statistics to investigate the effect of nurse communication on RN turnover, retention, and job engagement. Respondents consisted of 247 RNs in an acute care hospital near the United States/Mexico border, with a population that is 82.27% Latino.

The surveys were linked to 13 nurse leaders who were in the nurses' direct chain of command. The data were analyzed for turnover, nurse leader communication competence, leadership characteristics, and engagement.

The 53-item Supervisor Leadership and Communication Inventory codes score into one of three zones: red, yellow, or green. Leaders in the green zone communicate proactively, providing meaningful feedback and effective mentoring. Yellow zone communication is highlighted by misaligned objectives, firefighting of issues, and ineffective explanations, whereas red zone communication is one-way, micromanaged, and task based. Of the 13 leaders included in the analysis, 7.7% were communicating from the red zone, 53.8% from the yellow zone, and 38.5% from the green zone.

RN engagement correlated positively with all variables measured by the Supervisor Leadership and Communication Inventory (supervisor communication supervisor leadership, employee behavior, and organizational outcomes). The analysis demonstrates medium strengths of association between job engagement and supervisor communication skill ($r = .464$, $P < .001$),

Continued

EVIDENCE-BASED PRACTICE—Cont'd

supervisor leadership (r = .394, P < .001), and employee behavior (r = .315, P < .001). The strength of the association between job engagement and organizational outcomes was high (r = .60, P < .001). There is a positive relationship, indicating that higher supervisor communication/leadership scores and employee behavior scores lead to higher organizational outcomes scores.

Data analysis also showed that leadership was positively correlated with job engagement (r = .394, P < .001). Organizational outcomes were also positively associated with RN engagement (r = .491, P < .001).

Taking into consideration that leader communication competence and RN engagement are positively correlated, recommendations consist of a three-pronged approach. First, organizations need to evaluate their current leaders' communication by asking staff. Often, senior leaders have a different view of nurse leaders than the staff. Nursing staff members should be considered major stakeholders when evaluating the communication and leadership style of their nurse leaders. The second recommendation is to prioritize individualized communication training plans for nurse leaders, which must include enhanced diversity training. Last, nurse leaders should build leadership capacity through training to devise purposeful activities focused on developing engaged employees.

▮ NCLEX® EXAMINATION QUESTIONS

1. A group consists of individuals who interact and influence one another. Groups exist in organizations. Group members usually do not include individuals from:
   A. A single work group
   B. Different job levels
   C. The same job levels
   D. A different facility

2. Today, patients are very interested in their health outcomes. Usually items are viewed online even before they see their physician for a visit. In an effort to prepare the patient/family when the patient is discharged, the plan should be done:
   A. On admissions to the facility
   B. The day before discharge
   C. The day of discharge
   D. When the physician writes the order for discharge

3. The degree to which the members are attracted to the group and wish to retain membership in it is:
   A. Cohesiveness
   B. Cooperation
   C. Control
   D. Team support

4. As a team member it is important to know:
   A. How to work within a team
   B. How to manage teams
   C. How to evaluate the performance of others
   D. All are correct

5. There are a number of groups that function within a nursing unit. Some of these groups will be:
   A. Interdisciplinary teams
   B. Patient care team
   C. Performance improvement team
   D. All are correct

6. As a new nurse, you should be aware that one of the first rules for any team, or council is to:
   A. Evaluate the bylaws or rules of the group
   B. Dismiss any group member to disagrees with the bylaws
   C. Develop a plan that another unit of the hospital uses
   D. Inform the group that there will only be a total of three meetings

7. When an individual in the group does not start the meeting out on a positive note, the conversations of the individual are considered to be:
   A. Low-performer
   B. Middle-performer
   C. High-performer
   D. Mediocre performer

8. Because low performers are so skilled at excuses, guilt, and indignation, these conversations can be difficult for:
   A. Managers
   B. Team members
   C. Group members
   D. High-performing members

9. Once you have worked on a specific unit for a period of time the _____ of the hospital and the unit will become clear.
   A. Culture
   B. Mission
   C. Vision
   D. Values

10. In your first position as a registered nurse, it is important to know that:
    A. Positive attitudes foster positive attitudes

B. Negative attitudes foster negative work habits.
C. Creating an environment conducive to high-quality patient care and staff satisfaction is key
D. All of the above are correct

Answers: 1. D 2. A 3. A 4. D 5. D 6. A 7. A
8. A 9. A 10. D

BIBLIOGRAPHY

Durskat, V., & Wolf, S. (2001). Building the emotional intelligence of groups. *Harvard Business Review, 79*, 81–91.

Guyton, N. (2012). Nine principles of successful nursing leadership. *American Nurse Today. August, 7*(8).

Lencioni, P. (2002). *The five dysfunctions of a team: A leadership fable.* San Francisco: Jossey-Bass.

Maxwell, J. (2002). *The 17 essential qualities of a team player.* Nashville, TN: Thomas Nelson Publishers.

McGregor, D. (1960). *The human side of enterprise.* New York: McGraw-Hill.

Parker, G. M. (1990). *Team players and teamwork.* San Francisco: Jossey-Bass.

Sullivan, E. J., & Decker, P. J. (2009). *Effective leadership and management in nursing* (6th ed.). Upper Saddle River, NJ: Pearson Prentice Hall.

The Joint Commission. (2019). Joint Commission Standards for Healthcare. Chicago, IL.

The Studer Group. (2007, 2011). The nine principles. www.studergroup.com/dotCMS/knowledgeAssetDetail?inode=217849.

The Studer Group. (2012). It's not rocket science: Strategies to blast your hospital into the highest patient experience stratosphere. https://programs.gha.org/Portals/5/documents/societies/GSHHRA/2012/HANDOUT%20Rocket%20Science%20(Otten).pdf.

Ethical and Legal Issues in Patient Care

OBJECTIVES

- Differentiate between ethics and bioethics.
- Identify ethical dilemmas in nursing.
- Discuss the role of the nurse in advance directives.
- Review the principles of ethical decision making.
- Identify interventions designed to protect patients' rights.
- Discuss the responsibility of the ethics committee.

- Differentiate between negligence and malpractice.
- Explain why the nurse is at risk for legal issues.
- Identify issues of importance for patient charting.
- Discuss potential risk factors in health care settings.
- Identify issues of importance in the Nurse Practice Act.
- Explain why nurses must be aware of each state's Nurse Practice Act.

KEY TERMS

advance directive document that allows the competent patient to make choices regarding health care before it is needed

autonomy provides for the privilege of self-determination in deciding what happens to one's body in health care

beneficence duty to do good to others; to maintain a balance between benefits and harm; to provide all patients, including the terminally ill, with caring attention; and to treat every patient with respect and courtesy; requires that care providers contribute to the health and welfare of the patient and not merely attempt to avoid harm to the patient or client

bioethics ethics specific to health care

corporate liability responsibility of an organization for its own wrongful conduct

durable power of attorney for health care decisions document that permits an individual to give a surrogate or proxy the authority to make decisions for that person in the event that they become incompetent

ethics science that deals with the principles of right and wrong and of good and bad, and governs our relationships with others. It is based on personal beliefs and values

informed consent consent for treatment given by a patient after three requirements are met: the patient has the capacity to consent, consent is voluntary, and the patient receives information regarding treatment in a manner that is understandable

Institutional Review Board (IRB) a group that has been formally designated to approve, monitor, and review biomedical and behavioral research involving humans with the alleged aim to protect the rights and welfare of the subjects. This group performs critical oversight functions for research conducted on human subjects that are scientific, ethical, and regulatory. They are research review panels that determine the legal and ethical protection of subjects participating in medical research

justice principle of fairness in which an individual receives what is due, owed, or legitimately claimed; the treating of all parties equally, regardless of

economic or social background, and learning the state's and organization's laws for reporting abuse; requires that individuals be given what they deserve or can legitimately claim

living will advance directive that indicates what an individual dictates regarding treatment or life-saving measures in the future

morality behavior in accordance with custom or tradition that usually reflects personal or religious beliefs

nonmaleficence principle of doing no harm: observing safety rules and precautions and keeping skills-up-to date; prohibits deliberate harm and demands weighing risks with the benefits of treatment

Omnibus Budget Reconciliation Act (OBRA) of 1987 one provision of this act provides patients with the right to be free from any physical or chemical restraint imposed for the purpose of discipline or convenience and not required to treat medical symptoms

Patient Self-Determination Act federal law requiring every health care facility receiving Medicare or Medicaid to provide written information to adult patients concerning their right to make health care decisions

personal liability responsibility and accountability of individuals for their own actions or inactions

policies and procedures written standardized protocol that is authorized by the health care organization

restraint direct application of physical force to a patient, with or without the patient's permission, to restrict freedom of movement; the physical force may be human, via mechanical devices, or a combination thereof

risk management clinical and administrative activities that organizations undertake to identify, evaluate, and reduce the risk of injury to patients, staff, and visitors, and the risk of loss to the organization itself

tort private or civil wrong or injury, including action of bad faith breach of contract, for which the court will provide a remedy in the form of an action for damages

ETHICAL DECISION MAKING

Today's nurses are in the public eye in the discussion of many different ethical issues and dilemmas, such as technology that maintains life for severely premature infants, technology that advances the life of severely brain-damaged patients, stem cell research, the issues of what constitutes brain death, transplant and donor programs, and end-of-life decisions. Concern for ethics has also moved beyond the clinical arenas to the business of health care, with the potential for Medicare fraud, suspect business decision making, and the protection of patient information. Ethical decision making will have an effect on your clinical professional role, your leadership role, and your research role. Professions are defined in part by the ethics that define their practice. One of the hallmarks of a profession is the existence of a code of ethics that governs the practice of the members of the profession. Nursing and nurses have long been recognized for their commitment to high ethical standards; it has been named the "most ethical profession" the last few years.

Ethical decision making is required when there is an ethical dilemma. Ethical dilemmas occur when there is a conflict between two or more ethical principles.

Common Ethical Principles and Their Rules

1. *Beneficence:* Duty to do good and to protect the patient's welfare. An example is carefully adhering to infection-control principles for all patients.
2. *Nonmaleficence:* Principle of doing no harm. Nurses who maintain their skills are practicing the principle of "doing no harm."
3. *Justice:* Principle of fairness in which an individual receives what is owed. All patients receiving the same level of culturally competent care is an example.
4. *Autonomy:* Respect for individual liberty and the person's right to self-determination. Informed consent is an example of adherence to the principle of autonomy.
5. *Fidelity:* Duty to keep one's word. Senior leaders adhering to all contracts is an example of leadership fidelity.
6. *Respect for others:* Right of people to make their own decisions, such as not telling a patient what he "should do" but allowing him to make his own decision.

7. *Veracity:* Obligation to tell the truth. As a professional, this would be a requirement to admit mistakes promptly or to not lie to a patient about bad news.
(List adapted from Little, 2003, p. 269.)

Such a conflict comes into place with the conflict between (1) the principle of autonomy (the duty to respect the patient's choice) and the duty to do only what the patient wants and (2) the principle of beneficence (the duty to protect the patient's welfare) and the duty to do only what the patient needs. An example would be the conflict that arises when a patient refuses dialysis that will prolong their life. Another example would be the situation in which the family does not want their frail elderly mother given the news that her grandson has been hospitalized with a life-threatening injury. The conflict here is between veracity and self-respect. The decision of what to do is guided by beneficence. Often there is no correct decision. There are many questions that arise in clinical care, such as the following (Schroeder, 1995):

- When do we refrain from using technology?
- When do we stop using technology, once it is started?
- Who is entitled to technology? Those who can pay? Those who are uninsured? Everyone, no matter what?

During the COVID-19 pandemic, questions also arose with the potential of rationing ventilators.

In addition to the clinical situations that cause ethical conflicts, nurses and health care personnel bring their own values and beliefs into the dilemma. There are times when the beliefs of the health care personnel are the dilemma. An individual with a strong religious belief in the sanctity of life may have ethical conflicts about do-not-resuscitate (DNR) orders, abortions, and genetic engineering. Cultural values and traditions may also be at the center of ethical dilemmas. Nurses and patients may believe that talking about death invites death to the door. It is important to be aware of your beliefs and to not let them interfere with the legal and professional requirements of your position. If you have beliefs that will prevent you from performing some of the requirements of your position, it is necessary to inform your supervisor so that the patient needs can always be met.

TRADITIONAL ETHICAL THEORIES

The study of ethics has resulted in different theories that are used to guide decision making. Box 16.1 provides traditional ethical theories.

As a nurse, you will be guided by both ethical theories and your own personal values and beliefs and professional expectations (American Nurses Association [ANA], 2015; (International Council of Nurses 2009). The fundamental values of nursing are expressed in the Code of Ethics for Nurses. They are the values, such as respect for patient autonomy, acting in the patient's best interest, and maintaining professional competence, that all nurses commit to uphold when they enter the profession.

AMERICAN NURSES ASSOCIATION'S CODE OF ETHICS FOR NURSES

Nurses must always act as patient advocates. The Nightingale Pledge in 1893 was viewed as the first code of ethics for nurses. The ANA approved the most recent Code of Ethics for Nurses in 2015.

BOX 16.1   Traditional Ethical Theories

Utilitarianism
- Decisions based on what will provide the greatest good for the greatest number of people.
- For example, the decision to force people with pulmonary tuberculosis into treatment is ethical, according to this theory, because it protects the greater population from infection.

Teleology (or Consequentialist Theory)
- The value of a situation is determined by its consequences.
- Thus, the outcome not the action itself is what counts; sometimes referred to as the "all's well that ends well" ethical approach.

Deontology (or Formalism)
- An act is good only if it springs from goodwill.
- This ethical theory does not allow for actions based on the concept of "the end justifies the means" (Little, 2003).

(From Kelly-Heidenthal, P. (2004). *Essentials of nursing leadership and management.* Clifton Park, NY: Thomson Delmar Learning.)

Revised Code of Ethics for Nurses

1. The nurse practices with compassion and respect for the inherent dignity, worth, and unique attributes of every person.
2. The nurse's primary commitment is to the patient, whether an individual, family, group, community, or population.
3. The nurse promotes, advocates for, and protects the rights, health, and safety of the patient.
4. The nurse has the authority, accountability, and responsibility for nursing practice; makes decisions; and takes action consistent with the obligation to promote health and to provide optimal care.
5. The nurse owes the same duties to self as to others, including the responsibility to promote health and safety, preserve wholeness of character and integrity, maintain competence, and continue personal and professional growth.
6. The nurse, through individual and collective effort, establishes, maintains, and improves the ethical environment of the work setting and conditions of employment that are conducive to safe, quality health care.
7. The nurse, in all roles and settings, advances the profession through research and scholarly inquiry, professional standards development, and the generation of both nursing and health policy.
8. The nurse collaborates with other health professionals and the public to protect human rights, promote health diplomacy, and reduce health disparities.
9. The profession of nursing, collectively through its professional organizations, must articulate nursing values, maintain the integrity of the profession, and integrate principles of social justice into nursing and health policy (ANA, 2015).

INTERNATIONAL COUNCIL OF NURSES' INTERNATIONAL CODE OF ETHICS FOR NURSES

The ICN International Code of Ethics for Nurses, most recently revised in 2012, is a guide for action based on social values and needs. The code has served as the standard for nurses worldwide since it was first adopted in 1953. The code is regularly reviewed and revised in response to the realities of nursing and health care in a changing society. In 2020 the ICN launched a consultation for the code expecting a newly revised code to be launched in 2021. The code makes it clear that inherent in nursing is respect for human rights, including the right to life, the right to dignity, and the right to be treated with respect. The ICN International Code of Ethics for Nurses guides nurses in everyday choices and supports their refusal to participate in activities that conflict with caring and healing.

International Council of Nurses' International Code of Ethics for Nurses

1. *Nurses and people:* The nurse's primary professional responsibility is to people requiring nursing care. In providing care, the nurse promotes an environment in which the human rights, values, customs, and spiritual beliefs of the individual, family, and community are respected. The nurse ensures that the individual receives sufficient information on which to base consent for care and related treatment. The nurse holds in confidence personal information and uses judgment in sharing this information. The nurse shares with society the responsibility for initiating and supporting action to meet the health and social needs of the public, in particular those of vulnerable populations. The nurse also shares responsibility to sustain and protect the natural environment from depletion, pollution, degradation, and destruction.
2. *Nurses and practice:* The nurse carries personal responsibility and accountability for nursing, practice, and maintaining competence by continual learning. The nurse maintains a standard of personal health such that the ability to provide care is not compromised. The nurse uses judgment regarding individual competence when accepting and delegating responsibility. The nurse at all times maintains standards of personal conduct that reflect well on the profession and enhance public confidence. The nurse, in providing care, ensures that uses of technology and scientific advances are compatible with the safety, dignity, and rights of people.
3. *Nurses and the profession:* The nurse assumes the major role in determining and implementing acceptable standards of clinical nursing practice, management, research, and education. The nurse is active in developing a core of research-based professional knowledge. The nurse, acting through the professional organization, participates in creating and maintaining equitable social and economic working conditions in nursing.
4. *Nurses and coworkers:* The nurse sustains a cooperative relationship with coworkers in nursing and other fields. The nurse takes appropriate action to safeguard individuals when their care is endangered by a coworker or any other person (ICN, 2012a,b; copyright © 2012).

One mark of a profession is the establishment of determination of ethical behavior for its members. In addition to the ANA and ICN codes, specialty nursing organizations and hospitals have developed codes of ethical behavior.

To assist you in dealing with the complex ethical issues that exist, hospitals have formed ethics committees. These committees are interdisciplinary and include representatives from clinical nursing, administration, medicine, social work, pharmacy, legal, and clergy. The work of ethics committees lies in three areas (Agich & Younger, 1991; Dalgo & Anderson, 1995):

- Education (seminars and workshops for committee members)
- Policy and guideline recommendations (specific hospital policies)
- Case review (analyzes patient cases and provides clear options)

As a nurse, you have the right to call on the ethics committee for a referral. Cases are often referred to the ethics committee for discussion. Issues commonly addressed by ethics committees are end-of-life issues, organ donation, and futility-of-care issues.

A systematic approach to the identification and meaning of ethical issues has been suggested by the University of Washington School of Medicine. The recommended "workup" includes review of medical indications, patient preferences, quality of life, and contextual issues. This workup describes "what is." Then the decision making moves to the next phase and involves questions such as:

- What is the issue?
- Where is the conflict?
- What is this case about? Is it similar to other cases encountered? What is known about them?
- Is there a precedent? Is there a paradigm case (e.g., Karen Ann Quinlan, Nancy Cruzan, Terri Schiavo, Jahi McMath)?

- Who is involved and what roles do they play?
Another model to address ethical issues is to:
- Identify the problem
- Tease out the ethical dilemma
- Gather objective and subjective data
- Look at alternatives
- Study the consequences of the alternatives
- Select the most appropriate alternative
- Compare the selected alternative with the clinician's or executive's value system
(Rundio et al., 2016, p. 127)

END-OF-LIFE ISSUES

End-of-life issues frequently revolve around the issue of advance directives. An advance directive is an end-of-life decision made by a patient in advance of the actual need. Many individuals confuse an advance directive with a DNR order, but they are not the same.

The Patient Self-Determination Act of 1990 requires that all individuals receiving medical care must be given written information about their rights under state law to make decisions about their care, including the right to accept medical or surgical treatment. This information needs to include information about their rights to formulate advance directives.

An advance directive instructs health care personnel on the patient's desires for care in certain circumstances. An advance directive, sometimes called a "living will," is a set of instructions documenting a person's wishes regarding medical care intended to sustain life. It is used if a patient becomes terminally ill, incapacitated, or unable to communicate or make decisions. Everyone has the right to accept or refuse medical care. A living will protects the patient's rights and removes the burden for making decisions from family, friends, and physicians. The ethical dilemma exists if the patient's family refuses to allow the advance directive to be used or if a health care professional refuses to implement the directives.

ORGAN DONATION

Although organ donation is a personal choice, there may be times when an ethical dilemma may ensue with carrying out this wish. For example, if a person has decided to be an organ donor and has made this clear on their driver's license, at the time of death the family may strongly disagree with this decision. Some other ethical questions surrounding organ donation include:

- Do people have the right to petition for organs across the Internet?
- If someone purchases an organ, is the health care system under any obligation to perform the transplant?
- Is it acceptable to purchase organs?
- Should healthier transplant candidates be given preference for organs?
(Adapted from Rundio et al., 2016, p. 130.)

Some states have mandated that a request be made for organ or tissue donation at the time of a patient's death. In hospitals where organ transplantations are done, there is usually a full-time organ donation coordinator. Nurses may be called on to request organ donations if the facility where they are employed charges nurses with this responsibility. Again, the nurse should be very direct in making these requests so there are no miscommunications, saying, for example, "Have you considered organ donation for your loved one?"

Written consent and hospital policies and procedures must be strictly followed. There is no cost to the donor family. The usual funeral expenses still apply.

Facts: Did You Know?

As of February 2021 more than 107,000 people in the United States were on the waiting list for a lifesaving organ transplant.

- A name is added to the national transplant waiting list every 9 minutes.
- Seven percent of people on the waiting list, more than 6500 each year, die before they are able to receive a transplant.
- On average, 17 people die every day from the lack of available organs for transplant.
- 39,000 transplants were performed in 2020.
- One deceased donor can save up to eight lives through organ donation and can save and enhance more than 100 lives through the lifesaving and healing gift of tissue donation.
- Organ recipients are selected based primarily on medical need, location, and compatibility.
- Organs that can be donated after death are heart, liver, kidneys, lungs, pancreas, and small intestines. Tissues include corneas, skin, veins, heart valves, tendons, ligaments, and bones.

- The cornea is the most commonly transplanted tissue. More than 40,000 corneal transplants take place each year in the United States.
- A healthy person can become a "living donor" by donating a kidney, or a part of the liver, lung, intestine, blood, or bone marrow.
- More than 6000 living donations occur each year. One in four donors is not biologically related to the recipient.
- The buying and selling of human organs is not allowed for transplants in the United States, but it is allowed for research purposes.
- In most countries, it is illegal to buy and sell human organs for transplants, but international black markets for organs are growing in response to the increased demand around the world.

(The American Transplant Foundation, 2021 https://www.organdonor.gov; The American Transplant Foundation 2014)

Organ Procurement Organizations

Organ procurement organizations (OPOs) are a unique component of health care. By federal law, they are the only organizations that can recover organs from deceased donors for transplantation. There are 58 federally designated OPOs throughout the United States and its territories. OPOs are generally structured to include clinical services, hospital development, donor family services, and public education.

The federal conditions of participation for organ donation, adopted in 1998, require hospitals to refer all deaths to OPOs for evaluation and to work collaboratively with the OPO on an approach for consent (New Jersey Sharing Network, 2014a).

Religious Views

The following are the views of various religious groups on organ donation and transplantation (American Council on Transplantation, 2007).

African Methodist Episcopal (AME) and African Methodist Episcopal Zion (AME Zion)

Organ and tissue donation is viewed as an act of neighborly love and charity by these denominations. These groups encourage all members to support donation as a way of helping others.

Amish

The Amish will consent to transplantation if they know that it is for the health and welfare of the recipient. They would be reluctant to donate their organs if the outcome was known to be questionable; however, nothing in the Amish understanding of the Bible forbids them from using modern medical services.

Baptists

Organ and tissue donation is advocated as an act of charity. In 1988 the Southern Baptist Convention passed a resolution supporting donation as a way to alleviate suffering and to have compassion for the needs of others.

Buddhists

Buddhists believe that organ and tissue donation is a matter of individual conscience.

Catholics

Catholics view organ donation as an act of charity, fraternal love, and self-sacrifice. Transplants are ethically and morally acceptable to the Vatican.

The Church of Christ Scientist

The Church of Christ Scientist takes no specific position on transplants or organ donation as distinct from other medical or surgical procedures. Church members usually rely on spiritual rather than medical means of healing. They are free to choose the form of medical treatment they desire, including organ transplantation. The decision of organ donation is left to the individual.

Hindus

Hindus are not prohibited by religious law from donating; it is considered an individual decision.

Jehovah's Witnesses

Jehovah's Witnesses do not encourage organ donation, but believe it is a matter for individual conscience according to the Watch Tower Bible and Tract Society, the legal corporation for the religion. The group does not oppose donating or receiving organs; however, all organs and tissue must be completely drained of blood before transplantation.

Judaism

Judaism teaches that saving a human life takes precedence over maintaining the sanctity of the human body.

Latter-Day Saints (Mormons)

According to church leaders, Latter-Day Saints (Mormons) are not prohibited by religious law from donating their organs or receiving transplants. The decision is a personal one.

Mennonites

Mennonites have no prohibition against organ donation and transplantation. Church officials state such decisions are individual ones.

Muslims

The Muslim Religious Council initially rejected organ donation by followers of Islam in 1983, but it has since reversed its position provided that donors consent in writing in advance. The organs and tissues of Muslim donors must be transplanted immediately and not be stored in organ banks.

Protestants

Protestantism encourages and endorses organ donation. Protestants respect the individual's conscience and a person's right to make decisions regarding their own body.

Quakers

Quakers do not oppose organ donation and transplantation. The decision is an individual one.

Seventh-Day Adventists

Seventh-Day Adventist officials have stated organ donation and transplantation to be acceptable practices for members. The decision is an individual one.

FUTILITY OF CARE

Ethical dilemmas often arise in patient care situations where there are concerns about the futility of care. The ethical conflict arises when the principle of beneficence ("do not harm") is called into question. Will further treatment benefit the patient? This is a time when a consultation with the ethics committee may be appropriate.

Some hospitals are offering a more humane approach to the DNR request. Families often misinterpret the DNR order as an order to do nothing. The intent of the order is to "allow a natural death". It is also important to understand that a decision not to receive "aggressive

2 medical treatment" is not the same as withholding all medical care. A patient can still receive antibiotics, nutrition, pain medication, and other interventions when the goal of treatment becomes comfort rather than cure. This is called palliative care, and its primary focus is helping the patient remain as comfortable as possible.

Physician Orders for Life-Sustaining Treatment (POLST) is a form that gives seriously ill patients more control over their end-of-life care, including medical treatment, extraordinary measures (such as a ventilator or feeding tube), and cardiopulmonary resuscitation. The National POLST Paradigm is an approach to end-of-life planning based on conversations between patients, loved ones, and health care professionals designed to ensure that seriously ill or frail patients can choose the treatments they want, or do not want, and that their wishes are documented and honored. Unlike other documents, such as an advance directive, a completed POLST form is an actual medical order that becomes a part of the individual's medical record. It also is valid in all health care settings (Fig. 16.1).

ORGANIZATIONAL ETHICS

A hospital's behavior toward its patients and its business practices has a significant effect on the patient's experience of, and response to, care. Thus, access, treatment, respect, and conduct affect patient rights. Access to hospital care is a major ethical issue in health care. Does a hospital have the right to refuse to care for a patient who does not have adequate insurance?

As a manager, you will be responsible for setting the ethical tone on your unit and guaranteeing that all patient and employee rights are respected. You will also have to practice ethically in all leadership and managerial actions. This will mean protecting the rights of your staff and providing a professional work environment. Staff members need to be able to work in an environment where they are free to report issues of concern. Hospitals have created departments of corporate compliance to oversee the reporting, documentation, and continued improvement of areas of organizational ethical concern. Senior leaders of the organization are responsible for the safe stewardship of the organization in both business practices and all areas of clinical care.

Combined Advance Directive for Health Care
(Combined Proxy and Instruction Directive)

I understand that as a competent adult, I have the right to make decisions about my health care. There may come a time when I am unable, due to physical or mental incapacity, to make my own health care decisions. In these circumstances, those caring for me will need direction concerning my care and will turn to someone who knows my values and health care wishes. I understand that those responsible for my care will seek to make health care decisions in my best interests, based upon what they know of my wishes. In order to provide the guidance and authority needed to make decisions on my behalf:

I, _____, hereby declare and make known my instructions and wishes for my future health care. This advance directive for health care shall take effect in the event I become unable to make my own health care decisions, as determined by the physician who has primary responsibility for my care, and any necessary confirming determinations. I direct that this document become part of my permanent medical records.

In completing Part One of this directive, you will designate an individual you trust to act as your legally recognized health care representative to make health care decisions for you in the event you are unable to make decisions for yourself.

In completing Part Two of this directive, you will provide instructions concerning your health care preferences and wishes to your health care representative and others who will be entrusted with responsibility for your care, such as your physician, family members and friends.

Part One: Designation of a Health Care Representative

A) Choosing a Health Care Representative:

I hereby designate:

name _____

address _____

city_____ state _____

telephone _____

as my health care representative to make any and all health care decisions for me, including decisions to accept or to refuse any treatment, service or procedure used to diagnose or treat my physical or mental condition, and decisions to provide, withhold, or withdraw life-sustaining measures. I direct my representative to make decisions on my behalf in accordance with my wishes as stated in this document, or as otherwise known to him or her. In the event my wishes are not clear, or a situation arises I did not anticipate, my health care representative is authorized to make decisions in my best interests, based upon what is known of my wishes.

Fig. 16.1 Combined advance directive for health care. (From NJ Commission on Legal and Ethical Problems in the Delivery of Health Care: NJ Bioethics Commission, March 1991.)

I have discussed the terms of this designation with my health care representative and he or she has willingly agreed to accept the responsibility for acting on my behalf.

_____

B) Alternate Representatives: If the person I have designated above is unable, unwilling, or unavailable to act as my health care representative, I hereby designate the following person(s) to act as my health care representative, in order of priority stated:

1. name _____   2. name _____
address _____   address _____
city_____ state_____   city_____ state_____
telephone _____   telephone _____

Part Two: Instruction Directive

In Part Two, you are asked to provide instructions concerning your future health care. This will require making important and perhaps difficult choices. Before completing your directive, you should discuss these matters with your health care representative, doctor, and family members or others who may become responsible for your care.

In **Sections C and D,** you may state the circumstances in which various forms of medical treatment, including life-sustaining measures, should be provided, withheld, or discontinued. If the options and choices below do not fully express your wishes, you should use **Section E,** and/or attach a statement to this document that would provide those responsible for your care with additional information you think would help them in making decisions about your medical treatment. **Please familiarize yourself with all sections of Part Two before completing your directive.**

C) General Instructions. To inform those responsible for my care of my specific wishes, I make the following statement of personal views regarding my health care.

Initial ONE of the following two statements with which you agree:

1. _____I direct that all medically appropriate measures be provided to sustain my life regardless of my physical or mental condition.

2. _____There are circumstances in which I would not want my life to be prolonged by further medical treatment. In these circumstances, life-sustaining measures should not be initiated and if they have been, they should be discontinued. I recognize that is likely to hasten my death. In the following, I specify the circumstances in which I would choose to forgo life-sustaining measures.

If you have initialed statement 2, on the following page please initial each of the statements (a, b, c) with which you agree:

Fig. 16.1 Continued

a. _____ I realize that there may come a time when I am diagnosed as having an incurable and irreversible illness, disease, or condition. If this occurs, and my attending physician and at least one additional physician who has personally examined me determine that my condition is **terminal,** I direct that life-sustaining measures that would serve only to artificially prolong my dying be withheld or discontinued. I also direct that I be given all medically appropriate care necessary to make me comfortable and relieve pain.

In the space provided, write in the bracketed phrase with which you agree:

To me, terminal condition means that my physicians have determined that:

_____

[I will die within a few days] [I will die within a few weeks]
[I have a life expectancy of approximately _____ or less (enter 6 months or 1 year)]
b. _____ If there should come a time when I become **permanently unconscious,** and it is determined by my attending physician and at least one additional physician with appropriate expertise who has personally examined me, that I have totally and irreversibly lost consciousness and my capacity for interaction with other people and my surroundings, I direct that life-sustaining measures be withheld or discontinued. I understand that I will not experience pain or discomfort in this condition, and I direct that I be given all medically appropriate care necessary to provide for my personal hygiene and dignity.

c. _____ I realize that there may come a time when I am diagnosed as having an **incurable and irreversible** illness, disease, or condition that may not be terminal. My condition may cause me to experience severe and progressive physical or mental deterioration and/or a permanent loss of capacities and faculties I value highly. If, in the course of my medical care, the burdens of continued life with treatment become greater than the benefits I experience, I direct that life-sustaining measures be withheld or discontinued. I also direct that I be given all medically appropriate care necessary to make me comfortable and to relieve pain.

(Paragraph **c.** covers a wide range of possible situations in which you may have experienced partial or complete loss of certain mental or physical capacities you value highly. If you wish, in the space provided below you may specify in more detail the conditions in which you would choose to forgo life-sustaining measures. You might include a description of the faculties or capacities, which, if irretrievably lost would lead you to accept death rather than continue living. You may want to express any special concerns you have about particular medical conditions or treatments, or any other considerations, that would provide further guidance to those who may become responsible for your care. If necessary, you may attach a separate statement to this document or use **Section E** to provide additional instructions.)

Examples of conditions that I find unacceptable are:

_____
_____
_____
_____

Fig. 16.1 Continued

D) Specific Instructions: Artificially Provided Fluids and Nutrition; Cardiopulmonary Resuscitation (CPR). On page 3 you provided general instructions regarding life-sustaining measures. Here you are asked to give specific instructions regarding two types of life-sustaining measures—artificially provided fluids and nutrition and CPR.

In the space provided, write in the bracketed phrase with which you agree:

1. In the circumstances I initialed on page 3, I also direct that artificially provided fluids and nutrition, such as feeding tube or intravenous infusion,

_____

[be withheld or withdrawn and that I be allowed to die]
[be provided to the extent medically appropriate]

2. In the circumstances I initialed on page 3, if I should suffer a cardiac arrest, I also direct that cardiopulmonary resuscitation (CPR)

_____

[not be provided and that I be allowed to die]
[be provided to preserve my life, unless medically inappropriate or futile]

3. If neither of the above statements adequately expresses your wishes concerning artificially provided fluids and nutrition or CPR, please explain your wishes below.

_____

_____

_____

E) Additional Instructions: You should provide any additional information about your health care preferences that is important to you and that may help those concerned with your care to implement your wishes. You may wish to direct your health care representative, family members, or your health care providers to consult with others, or you may wish to direct that your care be provided by a particular physician, hospital, nursing home, or at home. If you are or believe you may become pregnant, you may wish to state specific instructions. If you need more space than is provided here you may attach an additional statement to this directive.

_____

_____

_____

F) Brain Death: The state of New Jersey recognizes the irreversible cessation of all functions of the entire brain, including the brain stem (also known as whole brain death), as a legal standard for the declaration of death. However, individuals who cannot accept this standard because of their personal religious beliefs may request that it not be applied in determining their death.

Fig. 16.1 Continued

Initial the following statement only if it applies to you:

_____To declare my death on the basis of the whole brain death standard would violate my personal religious beliefs. I therefore wish my death to be declared solely on the basis of the traditional criteria of irreversible cessation of cardiopulmonary (heartbeat and breathing) function.

G) After Death-Anatomical Gifts: It is now possible to transplant human organs and tissue in order to save and improve the lives of others. Organs, tissues, and other body parts are also used for therapy, medical research, and education. This section allows you to indicate your desire to make an anatomical gift and if so, to provide instructions for any limitations or special uses.

Initial the statements that express your wishes:

1. _____ **I wish** to make the following anatomical gift to take effect upon my death:

A. _____ any needed organs or body parts.
B. _____ only the following organs or parts

_____

for the purposes of transplantation, therapy, medical research or education, or

C. _____ my body for anatomical study, if needed.
D. _____ special limitations, if any;

_____

If you wish to provide additional instructions, such as indicating your preference that your organs be given to a specific person or institution, or be used for a specific purpose, please do so in the space provided below.

_____
_____
_____

2. _____ **I do not wish** to make an anatomical gift upon my death.

Part Three: Signature and Witnesses

H) Copies: The original or a copy of this document has been given to the following people (Note: If you have chosen to designate a health care representative, it is important that you provide him or her with a copy of your directive):

1. name _____   2. name _____

address _____   address _____

city _____ state _____   city _____ state _____

telephone_____   telephone _____

Fig. 16.1 Continued

I) Signature: By writing this advance directive, I inform those who may become entrusted with my health care of my wishes and intend to ease the burdens of decision making that this responsibility may impose. I have discussed the terms of this designation with my health care representative and he or she has willingly agreed to accept the responsibility for acting on my behalf in accordance with this directive. I understand the purpose and effect of this document and sign it knowingly, voluntarily, and after careful deliberation.

Signed this _____ day of _____, 20 _____ .

signature _____

address _____

city_____ state _____

J) Witnesses: I declare that the person who signed this document, or asked another to sign this document on his or her behalf, did so in my presence, that he or she is personally known to me, and that he or she appears to be of sound mind and free of duress or undue influence. I am 18 years of age or older, and am not designated by this or any other document as the person's health care representative.

1. witness _____

address _____

city_____ state _____

signature _____

date _____

2. witness _____

address _____

city_____ state _____

signature _____

date _____

**New Jersey Commission on Legal and Ethical
Problems in the Delivery of Health Care
(The New Jersey Bioethics Commission)
March 1991**

Fig. 16.1 Continued

Hospitals are legally and ethically obligated to uphold the following patient rights to:

- Participate in treatment decisions,
- Provide informed consent to treatment,
- Receive considerate and respectful care,
- Review records,
- Be informed of hospital policies, and
- Expect reasonable and appropriate continuity of care after hospitalization.

The Patient Care Partnership of the American Hospital Association replaced what was originally named the Patients' Bill of Rights (Box 16.2). The partnership informs patients about what they should expect during their hospital stay with regard to their rights and responsibilities.

RESEARCH

As a nurse, you will participate in clinical research during your career. The ethical requirements of research should be well understood and be part of your work. Hospitals and other workplaces participating in research involving human subjects have Institutional Review Boards (IRBs) that set guidelines for the research and approve all research studies that occur in the institution. Although the regulations for IRBs are federal law (U.S. Code of Federal Regulations, Department of Health and Human Services [DHHS] Title 45, Part 46, titled *Protection of Human Subjects*, and the U.S. Food and Drug Administration [FDA] Title 21, Part 50 and Title 21, Part 56), they have arisen in light of ethical violations of the rights of patients.

The IRB's primary concerns are to determine that:

- The rights and welfare of the human subjects are protected adequately,
- The risks to subjects are outweighed by the potential benefits of the research,
- The selection of subjects is equitable, and
- Informed consent will be obtained and documented.

LEGAL ISSUES

State Board of Nursing

As a nurse you are well aware that you are held accountable for all of your actions both as an individual nurse and as the nurse managing the care of others. It is important, therefore, to have an understanding of legal

---

BOX 16.2   Patient Bill of Rights

The Patient Care Partnership: Understanding Expectations, Rights, and Responsibilities
The American Hospital Association's Patient Care Partnership states that the patient has the following rights.

High-Quality Hospital Care
Patients have the right to be provided with the care needed, with skill, compassion, and respect.

A Clean and Safe Environment
There are hospital policies and procedures in place to ensure that patients have an environment free from errors, abuse, and neglect.

Involvement in Your Care
Patients are entitled to be made aware of the benefits and risks of treatments, whether treatments are experimental or part of a research study, what can be expected from treatment and any long-term effects it might have on quality of life, what should be done after discharge, and the financial consequences of uncovered services or out-of-network providers. Patients should inform health

care providers of any past illnesses, surgeries, hospital admissions, allergies, and all medications and dietary supplements taken. Patients should also inform health care providers of any health care goals and values or spiritual beliefs that are important to the well-being of the patient. It should be made clear who the power of attorney is, if the patient has a living will, or advance directives in place.

Protection of Your Privacy
Patients' privacy must be protected at all times once in the health care system. Patients will receive a Notice of Privacy Practices that describes the specific hospital privacy plan and means of accomplishing this.

Help When Leaving the Hospital
The hospital personnel will identify sources of follow-up care such as home care or ordering equipment needed for home.

Help With Your Billing Claims
The hospital billing department will file health care claims and assist the patient with any questions regarding the bill and patient coverage.

(Adapted from *American Hospital Association. Patient bill of rights.* (2015). Retrieved September 21, 2021, from < www.aha.org/content/00-10/pcp_english_030730.pdf.>)

issues and their effect on the profession. The first contact that you will have will be the state licensing authority and the laws of that authority. The first thing you will do after graduation is pass the NCLEX® examination. On passing this milestone, you will receive your license to practice professional nursing. This license is given by the individual state where you are practicing and the license is governed by the statutory regulations of that particular state.

State boards of nursing in each state define those actions and duties of a nurse that are allowable by the profession guided by the state's practice act and common law. Nurse practice acts affect all areas of nursing practice. Nurse practice acts set educational standards, examination requirements, and licensing requirements and regulate the nursing profession in each particular state. State boards of nursing exist to foster public protection, to ensure consumer protection from fraud and abuse, and to respond to changes in the health care practice environment. The National Council of State Boards of Nursing serves as a central clearinghouse, ensuring that individual state actions are enforced in all states in which an individual nurse may hold licensure.

Because each state has its own practice act and regulations, all nurses need to know the provisions of the practice act of the state in which they are licensed. This is especially important in the areas of diagnosis and treatment that differ from state to state. The addresses and web addresses of the various state boards are listed in Chapter 20.

If you are a nurse licensed in one state while practicing telenursing or giving telephone triage in another state, it is imperative you know the nursing regulations of the state in which your care is being delivered. With the advent of multistate licensures, nurses licensed in one state may legally practice in some other states without obtaining additional licensure. The state in which you practice is the state under whose regulations you are accountable. Not all states have multistate licenses, so again it is imperative that you know about the practice requirements of your state.

Disciplinary Action by the State Board of Nursing

As a nurse manager, you are also responsible for the monitoring of the practice of employees under your supervision and ensuring that they remain current with their licensure. A list of all individuals who hold nursing licenses, registered nurses, and licensed practical nurses is maintained by the vice president of nursing. The nurse must show the original state license to the vice president of nursing or his or her designee when the new nursing license has been issued. Many state boards of nursing now have online licensee directories that give you the status of an individual's license.

The nurse and the nurse leader are responsible for protecting the license of nurses in the organization. Disciplinary actions by the state board of nursing will occur if a complaint about a nurse's action triggers an investigation. Potential situations that may trigger an investigation include the following:
- Impaired nursing practice (see Chapter 9)
- Negligence
- Incompetence
- Abuse
- Fraud
- Practicing beyond the scope of the license

Corporate Liability

Corporate liability is the responsibility of an organization for its own wrongful conduct. The health care facility must maintain an environment conducive to quality patient care. Corporate liability includes (1) the duty to hire, supervise, and maintain qualified, competent, and adequate staff; (2) the duty to provide, inspect, repair, and maintain reasonably adequate equipment; and (3) the duty to maintain safety in the physical environment (Sullivan & Decker, 2009).

Malpractice

In the delivery of patient care, there is always a potential for malpractice and negligence. Malpractice refers to "any misconduct or lack of skill in carrying out professional responsibilities" (Sullivan & Decker, 2009). It is also defined as failure of a professional person to act as other prudent professionals with the same knowledge and education would act under similar circumstances. Four elements must be present for malpractice to occur:
1. *Duty:* How would a reasonable and prudent provider behave under the same circumstances?
2. *Breach of duty:* Did the provider breach the standard of care in this particular situation?
3. *Causation:* Was the unreasonable, careless, or inappropriate behavior on the part of the provider the proximate cause of the injury or insult?
4. *Injury:* Did injury to the client occur?
   (From Rundio et al., 2016, pg. 65)

This is one of the reasons nurses need to maintain personal malpractice insurance. The employing organization maintains blanket malpractice coverage for all employees, but it is highly recommended that individuals purchase their own personal nursing liability insurance. Most commonly, nurses are subject to legal liability arising from malpractice and negligence. Nursing negligence malpractice occurs when the nurse's actions do not meet the standard of care, when the nurse's actions are unreasonable, or when the nurse fails to act and causes harm. Harm related to nursing clinical practice commonly arises from negligent acts and omissions (unintentional torts) and a variety of intentional acts (intentional torts) such as invasion of privacy, assault and battery, or false imprisonment (Aiken, 2004). See Box 16.1 for reasons that nurses should have personal malpractice insurance.

Tort Law

A **tort** is a "private or civil wrong or injury, including action of bad faith breach of contract, for which the court will provide a remedy in the form of an action for damages" (*Black's Law Dictionary*, 2019, cited in Martin & Cain, 2003).

A tort can be any of the following (Carroll, 2006, p. 279):

1. Denial of person's legal rights
2. Failure to comply with public duty
3. Failure to perform private duty that harms another person

A tort can be unintentional, such as malpractice or neglect, or intentional, such as assault and battery or invasion of privacy. For malpractice to exist, the following elements must be present (Carroll, 2006, p. 280):

1. *A duty exists:* This is automatic when a patient is in a health care facility.
2. *A breach of duty occurs:* The nurse did something that should not have been done or did not do something that should have been done.
3. *Causation:* The nurse's action directly led to a patient injury.
4. *Injury:* Harm comes to the patient.
5. *Damages:* Compensate the patient for injury.

Negligence

Negligence refers to the failure of an individual to perform an act (omission) or to perform an act (commission) that a "reasonable, prudent person would not perform in a similar set of circumstances" (Sullivan & Decker, 2009; Rundio et al., 2016). Negligence is also defined as the failure to exercise the proper degree of care required by the circumstance.

Common negligence allegations in nursing include the following:

- Medication errors
- Patient falls
- Use of restraints
- Equipment injuries
- Failure to take appropriate nursing action
- Failure to follow hospital procedure
- Failure to supervise treatment

An institution's policies and procedures describe the performance expected of nurses. Deviation from this expected performance can result in liability for negligence or malpractice. A nurse failing to adhere to institutional policy runs the risk of the employer denying the nurse defense in a lawsuit.

Charting

Most malpractice/negligence lawsuits take place years after the actual event. When a nurse is named in a lawsuit, it is likely that the memory of the event will have greatly diminished. The documentation in the patient care record may be the most reliable source of information. Therefore, a nurse's charting ability serves a double purpose of reminding of the care delivered to that particular patient. Documentation on an electronic medical record has become standardized in many facilities. Such electronic documentation is usually standard driven, making it easier for the nurse to document appropriately. But if the nurse needs to document in a nonelectronic record it is important to remember the rules of nursing documentation (Box 16.3).

Review Table 16.1 to determine FLAT charting (factual, legible, accurate, timely).

Standard of Care

Box 16.3 shows a standard of care for pain management. This standard of care would form the basis for the expectation of care delivered to all patients within an institution. Deviation from this care can be defined as malpractice. As stated earlier, the clinical problems that most commonly lead to malpractice/negligence lawsuits are restraints, medication errors, patient falls, privacy violations, and other adverse events. Therefore,

BOX 16.3 Memorial Sloan-Kettering Cancer Center

The Standard of Care For the Patient with Pain
Nursing Diagnosis
Pain, acute and/or chronic related to:
- Disease
- Treatment
- Procedure
- Other, specify

General Outcomes
1. Patient will report adequate pain relief.
2. Patient will have minimal side effects from analgesic regimen.
3. Patient will be satisfied with his/her pain management.

Outcome Criteria
The patient will:
1. Be assessed for pain at least every 12 hours and PRN (pro re nata) in the inpatient setting and at each outpatient visit
2. Report pain intensity (e.g., using 0-to-10 scale or categorical)
3. Report satisfaction of relief of pain
4. Experience minimal side effects from analgesic regimen

The patient/family/caregiver will:
1. Describe the pain management plan including rationale, drug, route, dose, frequency, and potential side effects and whom to notify for questions or problems
2. Notify the physician or nurse if pain is not adequately controlled or if questions, problems, or concerns about pain management arise in either the inpatient, outpatient, or home setting
3. Participate with the interdisciplinary team to determine the most effective and cost-efficient pain management program
4. Describe their responsibilities in pain management

Assessment
Pain assessment is the cornerstone of all effective pain management. A thorough assessment leads clinicians to the etiology of the pain itself and to other new diagnoses that may be treatable. The choice of a specific treatment depends on a full assessment and the identification of specific pain syndromes. The assessment assists the clinician in more fully understanding the patient's pain problem and how the pain affects daily life. Also, repetitive assessments are necessary for the evaluation of the current pain treatment plan.
1. Assess and document pain intensity and satisfaction with relief regularly, at least every 12 hours for inpatients and with each clinic visit for outpatients

2. Assess and document pain systematically including location(s), intensity, quality, onset, duration, precipitating and relieving factors (including use of analgesics and proper analgesic history), occurrence of breakthrough pain, satisfaction with relief and presence and severity of side effects (especially constipation)
3. Consider effect of pain on sleep, mood, appetite, activity, usual functioning in self-care and job, and role in family and community
4. Assess and document the patient's knowledge of his or her pain along with attitudes and values regarding pain and its meaning
5. Assess and document the presence of factors that affect patient suffering, such as anxiety, depression, anger, attitude toward disease, attitude toward treatment
6. Assess for the presence of social, practical, and financial supports that affect the plan for pain management
7. Review current disease state and extent of disease, results of recent imaging studies, current therapy, future therapy, and coexisting conditions

Interventions
1. Collaborate with multidisciplinary team and advocate for pain control options most appropriate for the patient, family, caregiver, and setting
2. Administer prescribed analgesics and deliver interventions in a timely, logical, and coordinated manner
3. Review with patient how to describe the severity of his or her pain (e.g., 0-to-10 scale or categorical scale), satisfaction with relief, and presence and severity of side effects
4. Monitor ongoing effectiveness of analgesic regimen and other interventions; document medication administration and effectiveness of analgesic regimen in accordance with policy
5. Consult with MD/nurse practitioner (NP)/physician assistant (PA), or advanced practice nurse (APN) of primary service about:
   - Appropriate modifications in analgesic regimen
   - Treatment of analgesic-related side effects (*refer to following nursing diagnosis related to side effects of analgesics*)
6. Ensure that conversions from opioid to opioid and route to route are accurate
7. Alter environment to provide comfort (e.g., decrease lighting and noise, provide privacy, limit visitors as patient wishes)
8. Facilitate use of nonpharmacologic interventions (e.g., relaxation, focused breathing, distraction) when appropriate

BOX 16.3   Memorial Sloan-Kettering Cancer Center—cont'd

9. Provide patient/family/caregiver with information about medication, dose, route, frequency, and potential side effects (refer to specific nursing diagnosis related to individual side effects as appropriate)
10. Explore patient/family/caregiver concerns about the use of opioids
11. Provide information to allay fears and correct misconceptions (specifically in relation to addiction, tolerance, physical dependence)
12. Review with patient, family, and caregiver their responsibility in pain management:
    * Understanding the nature of the pain, treatment, and expected response to treatment
    * Understanding the rationale, drug, dose, frequency, and side effects of prescribed analgesics
    * Obtaining medications, renewing prescriptions, and monitoring medication supply
    * Reporting to MD/NP/PA or registered nurse any new or unrelieved pain, change in pain location, quality or intensity, and side effects from analgesic regimen
13. Consult with advanced practice pain management nurses as needed
14. Discuss with MD/NP/PA regarding consult with anesthesiology pain management group or neurology pain service
15. Include pain management in discharge plan, identify need for home assessment and intervention, and communicate plan to ambulatory office practice nurse
16. Document plan, interventions, and outcomes

   Aspects of the pain management are specific to certain patient populations. To provide as comprehensive a standard as possible without redundancy, population-specific concerns will be covered at the end of the nursing diagnosis section. There information will be found related to the following groups: patients with acute pain, chronic pain, and chronic pain with acute pain episodes; pediatric and geriatric patients; patients with altered communication, and those with a history of substance abuse.

Nursing Diagnosis

Lack of knowledge of patient/family/caregiver related to aspects of pain management which may include but are not limited to:
* Pain/etiology of pain
* Understanding of principles and methods of pain management
* Analgesics (nonopioid, opioid, and adjuvant analgesics)
* Equipment/devices used to provide analgesics
* Potential side effects of analgesics

* Potential for physical dependence/tolerance/addiction
* Nonpharmacologic interventions
* Expected participation in the analgesic regimen

   Lack of knowledge is based on nursing assessment that the patient/family/caregiver lacks the information necessary to enable them to be active, informed participants in the plan of care. Knowledge deficit encompasses all dimensions of learning: cognitive, psychomotor, and affective. In relation to pain management, patients, their families, and caregivers need information about pain and the medications and the regimens ordered. For those who need special equipment to deliver their pain medication, it is important to provide opportunities to practice with that equipment. They also need information and reassurance to allay fears and concerns about opioid use, specifically, addiction, tolerance, and physical dependence.

   A knowledge deficit does not apply if the individual is unable to understand the information or change behavior because of cognitive or physical impairments that may be related to medications such as opioids or other organic causes. To apply the concept of knowledge deficit, the nurse must assess and recognize the patient's, families' and caregivers' basic knowledge about the cause of pain and its treatment and plan to **provide the right information, in the right way, at the right time**.

Outcome Criteria

In addition to the general outcomes listed in the pain, acute, and/or chronic section, the patient/family/caregiver will:
1. Notify the MD/NP/PA or RN of any new or unrelieved pain, change in pain location, quality or intensity, and side effects from analgesic regimen
2. Identify cause of pain
3. State the rationale of prescribed analgesic regimen
4. Identify the medications, doses, route, frequency, and potential side effects of prescribed analgesics
5. Use equipment related to pain management appropriately
6. Comply with the analgesic regimen
7. Use nonpharmacologic methods as appropriate
8. Express an understanding of the differences between physical dependence, tolerance, and addiction

Assessment

Assess and document patient, family and caregiver's knowledge regarding:
1. Nature of pain, treatment, and expected response to treatment
2. How to report pain intensity and relief
3. Specific prescribed analgesic regimen (drug, dose, route, frequency, and potential side effects [specifically constipation])

Continued

BOX 16.3   Memorial Sloan-Kettering Cancer Center—cont'd

4. Physical dependence, tolerance, addiction, and other concerns related to the use of opioids
5. Use of special equipment (if applicable)
6. The role and responsibility of patient, family, and caregiver in pain management
7. Availability of resources at Memorial-Sloan Kettering Cancer Center (MSKCC) and in the community

Interventions

1. Assist patient, family, and caregivers in understanding the pain and its causes
2. Teach the patient, family, and caregivers methods of reporting pain intensity and relief
3. Explain specific prescribed analgesic regimen (drug, dose, route, frequency, and potential side effects), concepts of physical dependence, tolerance, and addiction, and clarify any other misconceptions related to the use of opioids
4. Provide information (print, audio, video) about:
   • Analgesics and adjuvants, their action, dose, route, frequency, and potential side effects
   • Use of special equipment (if applicable)
   • Various nonpharmacologic interventions (if appropriate)
5. Review with patient, family, and caregivers information regarding route of administration:
   • *Neural blockade and neurolytic procedures:* Purpose of prognostic block (to predict the efficacy of a permanent ablating procedure); reinforce teaching initiated by anesthesia pain management (APMG)
   • *Epidural catheter:* Rationale for using the epidural route, basic concepts about the use of opioids and/or local anesthetics, possible side effects and their treatment, setting realistic goals/expectations concerning pain relief, and progression from epidural analgesia to oral medications (if applicable)
   • *Intravenous (IV), subcutaneous, or epidural patient-controlled analgesia (PCA):* Goals for PCA therapy, prescribed programmed analgesic regimen, how to give a PRN "rescue" dose for anticipated or breakthrough pain, and reasons for notifying the

nurse (e.g., increased pain, sleepiness, hallucinations, nausea, vomiting, itching, urinary retention)
   • *Discharge instructions for patients going home with IV, subcutaneous, or epidural PCA:* Home health care (hi-tech) agency follow-up; operation of PCA pump (e.g., changing batteries, start/stop); dressing change procedures; assessment of epidural catheter site, IV access site, or subcutaneous needle insertion site; universal precautions when handling and disposing of needles; method of needle disposal; delivery of supplies; follow-up appointments; and emergency phone numbers
   • *Additional information specific for patients discharged with a subcutaneous needle for intermittent or continuous infusions:* Changing subcutaneous needle every 5 days or more often if redness or other discoloration, tenderness, swelling, bleeding, or drainage occurs and use of proper technique when inserting the subcutaneous needle
6. Provide instructions and allow opportunity to practice using equipment (pumps, etc.) needed for the prescribed analgesic regimen
7. Allow time for patient/family/caregiver to express concerns, ask questions, discuss analgesic regimen, and demonstrate skills
8. Provide patient/family/caregiver with name and phone numbers of resources at Memorial-Sloan Kettering Cancer Center and in the community who will assist you with pain management
9. Review with patient and family their responsibility in pain management:
   • Understanding the nature of pain, treatment, and expected response to treatment
   • Understanding the rationale, drug, dose, frequency and potential side effects of prescribed analgesics
   • Obtaining medications, renewing prescriptions, and monitoring medication supply
   • Reporting to MD/NP/PA or RN any new or unrelieved pain, change in pain location, quality, intensity or side effects from analgesic regimen
10. Document plan, interventions, and outcomes.

(Note: This is taken from a more comprehensive document titled "Care of the Patient in Pain: Standard of Oncology Nursing Practice" by the Pain Standard Committee.)

---

it is important for the nurse and nurse manager to practice according to established policy and procedure.

Incident Reports

The filing of an incident report forms the basis of organization-wide reporting from a risk management perspective. The purpose of an incident report is to provide a factual account of an incident or an adverse event to ensure that all facts surrounding the incident are reported. The incident reporting system provides the risk manager with an opportunity to investigate all serious situations. Aggregated data from incident reports

TABLE 16.1   FLAT Charting

1. **F**actual: What you see, not what you think happened
2. **L**egible: No erasures; corrections should be made with a single line drawn through the error and initialed
3. **A**ccurate and complete: For example, color of tracheostomy secretions
4. **T**imely: Completed as soon after the occurrence as possible

(From Kelly-Heidenthal, P., & Marthaler, M. T. (2004). *Delegation of nursing care*. Clifton Park, NY: Thomson Delmar Learning. p. 145)

are used by management to improve health care processes within the organization and for the early identification of emerging problems. Refer to your agency for the process for incident reporting. In general, incident report forms should be completed by the following:

1. Staff member involved in the occurrence
2. Staff member who discovered the incident
3. Staff member to whom the incident was reported

Incident reports should be completed as soon after the occurrence as possible. Accurately record all details of the incident and objectively describe the description of the incident and actions taken in response to it. It is important not to provide subjective information stating what should or could have been done to avoid the incident. If a document includes this information, the nurse can be asked in court why he or she did not take those actions to avoid the incident. The report also needs to include patient assessment and monitoring after the incident (Carroll, 2006).

Nurses can also be mentioned as parties in medical malpractice. In such situations, a nurse's liability is determined by the state's nurse practice act and the institution's policies and procedures. Above and beyond personal liability for personal clinical practice, nurses also have accountability and liability for their acts of delegation and supervision. As a primary care coordinator, the nurse manages the environment of care delivery. Ensuring staff competence and reporting incompetent practice are key. The nurse manager can also be held accountable for the negligence of contract employees (agency nurses) even though they are not employees of a particular institution. This is why it is important that the nurse managers are aware of skills, competencies, and knowledge of all staff working with them. Nurse managers also need to be aware of legal issues in the area of human resources. They will need to be aware of hiring standards, performance review standards, management of employees with problems, compliance with union contract, and terminations.

Health Care Information

Invasion of privacy and confidentiality is a tort violation. The Health Insurance Portability and Accountability Act (HIPAA) was enacted in 1996 to give people control over their personal information. It also made organizations that create or receive personal information accountable for protecting it. Information disclosed by patients is confidential and should be available only to authorized personnel. Nurses must obtain permission to release information to family members and close friends, and to others. This makes it difficult when nurses attempt to release information over the telephone. The nurse must identify the caller as an appropriate receiver of such information. Also, photographs, research information, or videos of the patient may not be used without specific signed releases. Computerized information also needs to be protected. Nurses charting on a hallway computer must not leave information visible on the computer screen to individuals in the hallway. Of particular concern is the increasing use of social media. Many employer policies do not address nurses' use of social media to discuss workplace issues on personal devices. A nurse may face serious consequences for inappropriate use of social media. Instances of inappropriate use of social and electronic media may be reported to the board of nursing. Depending on the laws of jurisdiction, the board of nursing may investigate reports of inappropriate disclosures on social media sites on the grounds of unprofessional conduct, unethical conduct, mismanagement of patient records, and breach of confidentiality (from *A Nurse's Guide to Social Media*. www.ncsbn.org/NCSBN_SocialMedia.pdf). Some tips in dealing with social media are included in Box 16.4.

INFORMED CONSENT

Nurses will often be called on to witness patient consent. There are three elements of informed consent (Nathanson, 1996, cited in Rowland & Rowland, 1997, p. 188):

BOX 16.4   How to Avoid Disclosing Confidential Patient Information

With awareness and caution, nurses can avoid inadvertently disclosing confidential or private information about patients. The following guidelines are intended to minimize the risks of using social media:

- Nurses must recognize that they have an ethical and legal obligation to maintain patient privacy and confidentiality at all times.
- Nurses are strictly prohibited from transmitting by way of any electronic media any patient-related image. In addition, nurses are restricted from transmitting any information that may be reasonably anticipated to violate patient rights to confidentiality or privacy, or otherwise degrade or embarrass the patient.
- Nurses must not share, post, or otherwise disseminate any information or images about a patient or information gained in the nurse/patient relationship with anyone unless there is a patient-care–related need to disclose the information or other legal obligation to do so.
- Nurses must not identify patients by name or post or publish information that may lead to the identification of a patient. Limiting access to postings through privacy settings is not sufficient to ensure privacy.
- Nurses must not refer to patients in a disparaging manner, even if the patient is not identified.
- Nurses must not take photos or videos of patients on personal devices, including cell phones. Nurses should follow employer policies for taking photographs or videos of patients for treatment or other legitimate purposes using employer-provided devices.

- Nurses must maintain professional boundaries in the use of electronic media. Similar to in-person relationships, the nurse has an obligation to establish, communicate, and enforce professional boundaries with patients in the online environment. Use caution when having online social contact with patients or former patients. Online contact with patients or former patients blurs the distinction between a professional and personal relationship. The fact that a patient may initiate contact with the nurse does not permit the nurse to engage in a personal relationship with the patient.
- Nurses must consult employer policies or an appropriate leader within the organization for guidance regarding work-related postings.
- Nurses must promptly report any identified breach of confidentiality or privacy.
- Nurses must be aware of and comply with employer policies regarding use of employer-owned computers, cameras, and other electronic devices, and use of personal devices in the workplace.
- Nurses must not make disparaging remarks about employers or coworkers. Do not make threatening, harassing, profane, obscene, sexually explicit, racially derogatory, homophobic, or other offensive comments.
- Nurses must not post content or otherwise speak on behalf of the employer unless authorized to do so, and must follow all applicable policies of the employer.

(From *A Nurse's Guide to Social Media.* .Retrieved September 21, 2021, from < www.ncsbn.org/NCSBN_SocialMedia.pdf.>)

---

1. *Information and knowledge:* For any patient to make a valid decision regarding a treatment, they must have adequate information to consider. Health care providers are responsible for informing patients of the diagnosis, prognosis, available alternatives to treatment recommended, risks and benefits of treatment options, and the risks of not accepting treatment. This information must be presented to a patient in understandable terms. Both The Joint Commission (2020) and the American Hospital Association require that hospitals meet a patient's communication needs.

2. *Competence:* Adults over 18 years of age in most states are legally competent and capable of giving valid consent for medical treatment. The patient must be of sound mind and free from any legal or mental impediments from making a binding decision regarding health care. Therefore, a patient who has a legal guardian or is a minor may not be legally competent to give consent. Each state has different rules about age of competence; it is therefore necessary to be mindful of the states' legalities.

3. *Voluntariness:* For a patient's consent to be voluntary, the patient must freely elect to undergo the treatment without any sort of physical or psychological coercion. If the person is intimidated, threatened, or coerced by health care personnel, there could be a lack of valid consent.

Regarding the physician's responsibility in the communications process, the physician providing or performing the treatment and/or procedure (not a delegated representative) should disclose and discuss the following with the patient:

- The patient's diagnosis, if known
- The nature and purpose of a proposed treatment or procedure
- The risks and benefits of a proposed treatment or procedure
- Alternatives (regardless of their cost or the extent to which the treatment options are covered by health insurance)
- The risks and benefits of the alternative treatment or procedure
- The risks and benefits of not receiving or undergoing a treatment or procedure

In turn, the patient should have an opportunity to ask questions to elicit a better understanding of the treatment or procedure, so that they can make an informed decision to proceed or to refuse a particular course of medical intervention (American Medical Association, 2021).

The consent for treatment is given by a patient after three requirements are met: the individual has the capacity to consent, consent is voluntary, and the individual receives information regarding treatment in a manner that is understandable to him or her (Sullivan & Decker, 2009).

Individual capacity to consent is determined by age and competence. The legal age is determined by state laws. Competency is determined when an individual has the ability to make choices and understands the consequences of their choices. When individuals make choices without force, fraud, deceit, or duress, they are acting voluntarily. And the information must contain all of the following (Sullivan & Decker, 2009):

1. An explanation of the treatment to be performed and the expected results
2. A description of the anticipated risks and discomforts
3. A list of potential benefits
4. A disclosure of possible alternatives
5. An offer to answer the patient's questions
6. A statement that the patient may withdraw his or her consent at any time

Nurses are often asked to witness a patient's informed consent. In signing the document, the nurse is witnessing the patient's signature, not validating the patient's complete understanding. A nurse has a right to refuse to sign if they think that any of the previously listed information is not met.

Patient Restraints

Basic human rights are not forfeited on entry into a health care facility. A competent patient has the right to refuse restraints unless he or she is at risk of harming others. Improper use of restraints may constitute assault or false imprisonment. If a patient has to be restrained, the patient has a right to the least restrictive restraint use at all times. Injuries resulting from improper use of restraints often are a cause of legal complaints.

The Omnibus Budget Reconciliation Act (OBRA) of 1987 gives patients the right to be free from any physical or chemical restraint imposed for the purpose of discipline or convenience and not required to treat medical symptoms.

Restraint use must meet the following requirements:

1. There is a physician's order for specific duration and circumstances for use.
2. PRN orders are not permitted.
3. There is continuous assessment and reassessment of patient as per hospital policy.
4. Informed consent for use must be given (if the patient is unable to give consent, proxy consent is necessary).

Patient Self-Determination Act

The Patient Self-Determination Act provides legislative support to the expression of a patient's consent to or refusal of medical treatment, even when the patient is no longer able to verbalize them. Patients who can verbalize refusal of care are allowed to sign out "against medical advice". Health care organizations have policies and procedures surrounding patients signing out against medical advice. In this situation the nurse documents in detail the events leading to the refusal of care and documents patient awareness of the consequences of refusal. Patients who are unable to verbalize consent or refusal can do so with the following documents:

1. Advance medical directive
2. Durable power of attorney
3. Health care proxy
4. Living will
5. POLST

Advance Medical Directive

Advance medical directives are written instructions expressing an individual's health care wishes in the event of incapacitation. A sample is shown in Fig. 16.1.

Durable Power of Attorney

These are legal instructions enabling an individual to act on another's behalf. In health care, it is often part of an advance medical directive. Fig. 16.2 is an example of such instructions.

Durable Power of Attorney for Health Care Decisions
■ *Take a copy of this with you whenever you go to the hospital or on a trip* ■

It is important to choose someone to make healthcare decisions for you when you cannot make or communicate decisions for yourself.   Tell the person you choose what healthcare treatments you want. The person you choose will be your agent. He or she will have the right to make decisions for your healthcare. If you DO NOT choose someone to make decisions for you, write NONE on the line for the agent's name.

I,_____, SS# _____ (optional), appoint the person named in this document to be my agent to make my healthcare decisions.

This document is a Durable Power of Attorney for Healthcare Decisions, My agent's power shall not end if I become incapacitated or if there is uncertainty that I am dead. This document revokes any prior Durable Power of Attorney for Healthcare Decisions. My agent may not appoint anyone else to make decisions for me. My agent and my care-givers are protected from any claims based on following this Durable Power of Attorney for Healthcare. My agent shall not be responsible for any costs associated with my care. I give my agent full power to make all decisions for me about my healthcare, including the power to direct the withholding or withdrawal of life-prolonging treatment, including artificially supplied nutrition and hydration/tube feeding. My agent is authorized to:

• Consent, refuse or withdraw consent to any care, procedure, treatment, or service to diagnose, treat or maintain a physical or mental condition, including artificial nutrition and hydration;
• Permit, refuse, or withdraw permission to participate in federally regulated research related to my condition or disorder
• Make all necessary arrangements for any hospital, psychiatric treatment facility, hospice, nursing home, or other healthcare organization; and, employ or discharge healthcare personnel (any person who is authorized or permitted by the laws of the state to provide healthcare services) as he or she shall deem necessary for my physical, mental, or emotional well-being;
• Request, receive, review and authorize sending any information regarding my physical or mental health, or my personal affairs, including medical and hospital records; and execute any releases that may be required to obtain such information;
• Move me into or out of any state or institution;
• Take legal action, if needed;
• Make decisions about autopsy, tissue and organ donation, and the disposition of my body in conformity with state law; and
• Become my guardian if one is needed.

In exercising this power, I expect my agent to be guided by my directions as we discussed them prior to this appointment and/or to be guided by my Healthcare Directive (*see reverse side*).

If you DO NOT want the person (agent) you name to be able to do one or other of the above things, draw a line through the statement and put your initials at the end of the line.

Agent's name _____ Phone _____ Email _____
Address _____

*If you do **not** want to name an alternate, write "none."*

Alternate Agent's name _____ Phone _____ Email _____
Address _____

Execution and Effective Date of Appointment
My agent's authority is effective immediately for the limited purpose of having full access to my medical records and to confer with my healthcare providers and me about my condition. My agent's authority to make all healthcare and related decisions for me is effective when and only when I cannot make my own healthcare decisions.

SIGN HERE for the *Durable Power of Attorney* and /or *Healthcare Directive* forms. Many states require notarization. It is recommended for the residents of all states. Please ask two persons who are not related to you or financially connected to your estate to witness your signature.

Signature _____ Date _____

Witness_____ Date _____ Witness _____ Date _____

Notarization:
On this_____ day of _____ , in the year of _____, personally appeared before me the person signing, known by me to be the person who completes this document and acknowledged it as his/ her free act and deed.

IN WITNESS WHEROF, I have set my hand and affixed my official seal in the Court of _____ ,

State of _____ , on the date written above.

Notary Public_____

Commission expires_____

Fig. 16.2 Sample durable power of attorney. (Reprinted with permission from the Center for Practical Bioethics.)

Healthcare Treatment Directive

■ *If you only want to name a Durable Power of Attorney for Healthcare Decisions, draw a large X through this page.* ■

I, _____, SS# _____, want everyone who cares for me to know what
healthcare I want.   (optional)

I always expect to be given care and treatment for pain or discomfort even if such care may affect how I sleep, eat, or breathe.

I would consent to, and want my agent to consider my participation in federally regulated research related to my disorder or condition.

I want my doctor to try treatments/interventions on a time-limited basis when the goal is to restore my health or help me experience a life in a way consistent with my values and wishes. I want such treatments/interventions withdrawn when they cannot achieve this goal or become too burdensome to me.

I want my dying to be as natural as possible. Therefore, I direct that no treatment (including food or water by tube) be given just to keep my body functioning when I have

  • a condition that will cause me to die soon, or

  • a condition so bad (including substantial brain damage or brain disease) that I have no reasonable hope of achieving a quality of life that is acceptable to me.

An acceptable quality of life to me is one that includes the following capacities and values. (Describe here the things that are most important to you when you are making decisions to choose or refuse life-sustaining treatments.)

_____

_____

_____

_____

| Examples: | • recognize family or friends | • make decisions | • communicate |
| | • feed myself | • take care of myself | • be responsive to my environment |

If you do not agree with one or other of the above statements, draw a line through the statement and put your initials at the end of the end of the line.

In facing the end of my life, I expect my agent (if I have one) and my caregivers to honor my wishes, values, and directives.

For further clarification, please refer to my *Caring Conversations* Workbook, which is located at _____.

**Be sure to sign the reverse side of this page even if you do not wish
to appoint a Durable Power of Attorney for Healthcare Decisions**

**Talk about this form and your ideas about your healthcare with the person you have chosen to make decisions for you,
your doctors, family, friends, and clergy. Give each of them a completed copy.**

You may cancel or change this form at any time. You should review it often. Each time you review it, put your initials and the date here. _____

This document is provided as a service by the Center for Practical Bioethics.
For more information, call the Center for Practical Bioethics at 816-221-1100
Email – *bioethic@practicalbioethics.org* • Website – *www.practicalbioethics.org*

Fig. 16.2 Continued

Health Care Proxy

Documents delegate the authority to make health care decisions to another when the patient has become incapacitated.

Living will and POLST documents were discussed earlier in this chapter.

Nurse's Responsibility in Advance Directives

Most health care organizations have policies for the documentation of patient self-determination documents. Nurses are required to ask patients and families if there are advance directives on initial assessment. These documents are then placed in the chart for future reference if necessary. State statutes regarding advance directives vary from state to state, so it is important to know state practice.

Good Samaritan Laws

Although nurses are legally covered for professional actions within the workplace, there are often concerns about professional actions in times of emergency outside of the health care institution. Good Samaritan laws have been enacted to encourage professionals to render help in an emergency or accident situation. The Hawaii Good Samaritan Act reads: "Any person who in good faith renders emergency care, without remuneration or expectation of remuneration, at the scene of an accident or emergency to the victim of the accident or emergency shall not be liable for any civil damages resulting from the person's acts or omission, except for such damages as may result from the person's gross negligence or wanton acts or omissions" (U.S. Legal Definitions, 2008).

SUMMARY

As a nurse, you will be confronted with ethical and legal dilemmas throughout your career. The nature of these dilemmas will change as science and technology advance. It is important, however, to recognize that as a nurse and nurse leader, you are responsible for the following:

- Creating an ethically and legally principled environment
- Upholding standards of conduct established by the profession
- Being committed to bringing about any changes needed
- Being dedicated to ethical and legal principles

- Role-modeling the ethical, legal, and professional behavior of those working under your supervision; this governs:
  - Interactions with people requiring nursing care
  - Responsibility for maintaining competence in nursing practice
  - Responsibility for meeting the health needs of the public
  - Maintaining cooperative relationships with members of the interdisciplinary health care team
  - Determining and implementing desirable standards of nursing practice and education (ICN, cited in Little, 2003; Carroll, 2006).

CLINICAL CORNER

The Nurse's Role in Medical Aid-in-Dying Laws

Advances in modern medicine have fundamentally changed the trajectory of many diseases, resulting in longer life expectancies. Many patients have benefited from innovative modalities and modern treatments that have resulted in cure, amelioration of distressing symptoms, or increased life spans. Nevertheless, mortality is an inescapable reality of the human experience and all patients with life-limiting illnesses will eventually succumb to their disease.

In recent years, there has been increasing recognition of the importance of end-of-life planning for patients with terminal illnesses. This is due, in large part, to the work of hospice and palliative care nurses and physicians who work tirelessly to assist patients and their families confronting a terminal illness. Hospice and palliative care professionals understand the importance of discussing end-of-life care as these discussions are requisite to fully understand patients' preferences. Unfortunately, it is not uncommon for patient preferences to be overlooked (Keating et al., 2018). In many instances, patients receive treatments that are misaligned with their preferences and wishes, often without a corresponding medical benefit. Research clearly demonstrates that patients with terminal illnesses experience a myriad of symptoms, both physical and psychological, that negatively affect their quality of life (Temel et al., 2017). Distress is a common end-of-life symptom that can leave patients confused and ambivalent about their end-of-life choices and decisions (Chochinov et al., 2016).

👤 CLINICAL CORNER—cont'd

The Nurse's Role in Medical Aid-in-Dying Laws

Patients, now more than ever, have increased awareness of end-of-life options, in particular medical aid in dying. With medical aid-in-dying laws, patients with terminal illness can request medication from their physician with the intent of hastening their death. This end-of-life option continues to expand in the United States and has become an option for patients with unrelieved suffering. This complicated option has sparked numerous debates. As discussions surrounding medical aid in dying continue, nurses will undoubtedly be looked to for guidance and support. Consequently, nurses from all clinical settings will need to be knowledgeable of all end-of-life options, including current medical aid-in-dying legislation, to be able to offer compassionate and nonjudgmental care with patients' requests for a hastened death.

Medical Aid in Dying in the United States: A Growing Trend

Medical aid-in-dying laws have dramatically changed the landscape of end-of-life care in the United States. Medical aid in dying provides a legal avenue for patients to end their lives by the self-administration of medication that will hasten their death. This differs from euthanasia in which someone other than the patient administers medication with the intent of hastening the patient's death. United States federal law prohibits euthanasia and is, therefore, an illegal practice. Although both practices have sparked intense debate over the complex issue of death and dying in the United States, euthanasia is inconsistent with the core values of the nursing profession (ANA, 2019). Moreover, euthanasia violates the trust of both patients and the general public. For some, medical aid-in-dying is seen as a compassionate, welcome, and long awaited end-of-life option. Others view the intentional and purposeful ending of a patient's life as morally abhorrent. How one views medical aid-in-dying is deeply personal, which is an issue that both patient and provider must come to terms with. Regardless of a nurse's personal position on medical aid-in-dying, it is imperative that all nurses understand their ethical obligation within the context of the patient's voluntary choice to pursue medical aid-in-dying.

Medical aid-in-dying laws are regulated at the state level; legislation must be passed to allow it. Under these laws, which are increasing in a number of U.S. jurisdictions, patients with a life expectancy of 6 months or less can request a prescription from their physician to legally end their lives. Currently, nine states (California, Colorado, Hawaii, Maine, Montana, New Jersey, Oregon, Vermont, and Washington State) and the District of Columbia have such legislation. Most of these laws are heavily based on the Oregon Death with Dignity Act that became law in 1998 (State of Oregon, 2019). According to Oregon's Death with Dignity 2018 Data Summary, 2216 prescriptions have been written with 1459 individuals having died from legally ingesting the prescribed drugs from 1998 through 2018 (State of Oregon, 2019). Approximately one-third of prescriptions were not used. The differential between prescriptions written and patient deaths is caused by either patient expiration or patient change of mind.

Under the medical aid-in-dying laws, the following requirements must be met to allow a physician to prescribe lethal medication:

- Patients must be age 18 years or older and deemed capable to give informed consent and not suffering from a psychiatric or psychological disorder or depression causing impaired judgment.
- Two physicians must confirm that the patient has a terminal illness with less than 6 months to live.
- Patients will then have to make 2 verbal and 1 written request for the medication over a period of at least 15 days. The written request must be witnessed by at least two individuals who must attest that the patient is making a voluntary choice and is capable of making an informed choice.
- Physicians must inform patients of feasible alternatives including hospice and palliative care.
- The patient must take the medication themselves; it cannot be administered by others (State of Oregon, 2019).

Nursing and End-of-Life Care

The unique role of contemporary nursing in the care of the terminally ill can be traced back to Florence Nightingale's work with dying soldiers in the Crimean War in 1854 (Ellis, 2019). Later in the 20th century, Dame Cicely Saunders continued Nightingale's work of improving the care of the dying, which eventually provided the foundation for modern hospice care (Kelley & Morrison, 2015). The specialty of hospice nursing spread from England to the United States during the 1970s sparking a national movement of hospice care in the American health care system. Decades later, palliative care later evolved from hospice into a medical subspecialty, caring for patients with chronic and life-limiting illnesses throughout the disease trajectory up to and including end-of-life. Both hospice and palliative care aim to improve the quality of life for patients and their families. Palliative care can be delivered at any point in the trajectory of a chronic or life-limiting illness, whereas hospice is typically reserved for those with a life expectancy of 6 months or less (Kelley & Morrison, 2015).

Continued

CLINICAL CORNER—cont'd

The Nurse's Role in Medical Aid-in-Dying Laws

The Nurse's Role in Aid in Dying

End-of-life care is an essential and important component of nursing care. Nurses must provide a comfortable environment for patients when discussing end-of-life options, including requests for a hastened death. Nurses should be keenly aware of pertinent aid-in-dying laws, as they attempt to fully understand the meaning behind a request for medical aid-in-dying. Furthermore, nurses should also be comfortable discussing all options available to patients with life-limiting illnesses including hospice and palliative care. Research has demonstrated that there are misconceptions of hospice and palliative care (Shalev et al., 2019). Therefore, nurses should be knowledgeable of the role each plays in the care of patients with life-limiting illnesses to address and debunk any misconceptions. When it comes to the nurse's role in medical aid-in-dying, "nurses are ethically prohibited from administering medical aid-in-dying medications" (ANA, 2019, p. 2). Additionally, "nurses should reflect on personal values related to medical aid-in-dying and be aware of how those values inform one's ability to provide information in response to a patient's request" (ANA, 2019, p. 2). The following are recommendations from the ANA designed to assist nurses on ethical decision making when patients inquire and/or seek medical aid-in-dying:

- Remain objective when discussing end-of-life options with patients who are exploring medical aid-in-dying.
- Have an ethical duty to be knowledgeable about this evolving issue.
- Be aware of their personal values regarding medical aid-in-dying and how these values might affect the patient-nurse relationship.
- Have the right to conscientiously object to being involved in the aid-in-dying process.
- Never abandon or refuse to provide comfort and safety measures to the patient.
- Project the confidentiality of the patient who chooses medical aid-in-dying.
- Remain objective and protect the confidentiality of health care professionals who are present during the aid-in-dying process, and the confidentiality of those who choose not to be present.
- Be involved in end-of-life policy discussion on local, state, and national levels, including advocating for palliative and hospice care services (ANA, 2019, p. 2).

Conclusion

Confronting a terminal illness poses many challenges for patients and their families and the providers who care for them. Nurses have always been on the frontlines when it comes to providing end-of-life care. Patients and families trust nurses and expect to be able to discuss all options when it comes to end-of-life care.

As technology and societal mores change, end-of-life considerations will also change. As the main providers of care, nurses must continue to strive to be at the forefront of the evolving landscape of end-of-life care. Having an understanding of the ethical issues surrounding medical aid-in-dying laws will assist nurses in clarifying their personal values and views. Only then can nurses provide a compassionate and nonjudgmental approach to discussions with patients requesting a hastened death. It is our duty; it is our obligation. We must always endeavor to provide exceptional physical, psychological, and spiritual care at very phase of life, especially at end-of-life.

David Liguori DNP, NP-C, ACHPN
Assistant Professor of Nursing
Ramapo College of New Jersey

References

American Nurses Association. (ANA). (2019). *The nurse's role when a patient requests medical aid in dying [Position statement].* Silver Spring, MD: ANA.

Chochinov, H., Johnston, W., McClement, S., Hack, T., Dufault, B., Enns, M.,... Kredenster, M. (2016). Dignity and distress towards the end of life across four non-cancer populations. *PLoS One, 11*(1), e0147606.

Ellis, H. (2019). Florence Nightingale: creator of modern nursing and public health. *Journal of Perioperative Practice, 30*(5), 145–146.

Keating, N., Huskamp, H., Kouri, E., Schrag, D., Hornbrook, M., Haggstrom, D., & Landrum, M. (2018, July). Physicians belief may override cancer patients wishes for end-of-life care. *Health Affairs, 37*(7). Retrieved September 21, 2021, from <https://www.healthaffairs.org/doi/abs/10.1377/hlthaff.2018.0015>.

Kelley, A., & Morrison, S. (2015). Palliative care for the seriously ill. *New England Journal of Medicine, 373*, 747–755.

Shalev, A., Phongtankeul, V., Kozlov, E., Shen, M., Adelman, R., & Reid, M. (2019). Awareness and misperceptions of hospice and palliative care: a population-based survey study. *American Journal of Palliative Care, 35*, 431–439.

State of Oregon Public Health Division, Center for Health Statistics. *Oregon Death With Dignity Act 2018 Data Summary.* (2019). Retrieved September 21, 2021, from <https://www.oregon.gov/oha/PH/PROVIDERPARTNERRESOURCES/EVALUATION-RESEARCH/DEATHWITHDIGNITYACT/Documents/year21.pdf>.

Temel, J., Greer, A., El-Jawahri, W., Pirl, E., Park, V., Ryan, D. (2017). Effects of early integrated palliative care in patients with lung and GI cancer: a randomized clinical trial. *Journal of Clinical Oncology, 35*(8), 834–841.

EVIDENCE-BASED PRACTICE

Abstract

Nursing turnover is a problem not only in the United States, but worldwide.

There is a direct correlation between a facility's ethical climate and the nurses' commitment. This study was to determine the correlation between nurses' perception of ethical climate and organizational commitment in teaching hospitals in the southeastern region of Iran. It was a descriptive study. The sample size was 275 nurses working in four teaching hospitals in the southeastern region of Iran. The Ethical Climate Questionnaire and the Organizational Commitment Questionnaire were used. The study found a positive correlation among professionalism, caring, rules, independence climate, and organizational commitment.

The nursing shortage exists in other countries, not just in the United States. This article is focused on the nursing shortage in Iran.

The Importance of the Study

There is no published research, before this study, to evaluate the correlation between ethical climate and nurses' organizational commitment.

Review of the Literature

The authors reviewed a study by Tsai and Huang (2008) on Taiwanese nurses, a study by Filipova (2007), a study by Cullen et al. (2003), and a study by Shafer (2009).

Organizational Commitment

This is when an employee is positive about the institution where they work, accepting the values of the workplace and would like to remain an employee at the facility.

Ethical Climate

Victor and Cullen (1987) stated there are five distinct types of organizational ethical climate: caring, professionalism, rules, independence, and instrumental:

Caring: A caring climate may be based on the utilitarianism ethical criterion in which the most important concern is what is best for others and people look out for each other's interests, whereas the primary goal is to offer the greatest good for the greatest number of people.

Professionalism: This dimension is related to the deontology ethical criterion. In this climate, the first consideration is whether a decision violates law and codes. People are expected to strictly follow legal or professional standards, and the law or ethical code of the profession is the major consideration. People are expected to comply with legal and professional standards over and above all other considerations.

Rules: The rules climate is related to the deontology ethical criterion. Based on this climate, it is very important to follow the organization's rules and procedures strictly, and everyone is expected to do so. People in facilities with this climate follow organization policies to the letter.

Independence: The independence dimension is associated with the deontology ethical criterion. In this climate people are expected to follow their own personal and **moral beliefs**. Each person decides for themselves what is right or wrong; in other words, people are guided by their own personal ethics.

Instrumental: This dimension is associated with the egoistic criterion, and its primary goal is to provide personal benefits. In this climate, people protect their own interests above all else and are mostly out for themselves.

Method

This was a descriptive analytical study done in 2011. The sample size was 88 people. It was then upgraded to include 185 people, then up to 300 people. The questionnaires were done.

Results

Approximately 275 nurses from city hospitals in the southeastern region of Iran participated in the study. It was found that the climate has a direct and significant correlation only with affective commitment. In addition, a caring climate has a direct and significant correlation with affective and normative commitments. The same was also found to apply to a climate of independence. An instrumental climate has no significant correlation with affective commitment.

Discussion

The study found that there was a correlation between ethical climate and organizational commitment. Ethical climate causes employees to have a positive correlation with job satisfaction.

Conclusion

The results of this study showed a positive and significant correlation between hospital climate and organizational commitment of nurses.

References

Borhani, F., Jalali, T., Abbaszadeh, A., & Haghdoost, A. (2014). Nurses' perception of ethical climate and organizational commitment. *Nursing Ethics, 21*(3), 278–288.

Continued

EVIDENCE-BASED PRACTICE—cont'd

Cullen, J. B., Parboteeah, K. P., & Victor, B. (2003). The effect of ethical climate on organizational commitment: a two study analysis. *Journal of Business Ethics, 46,* 127–141.

Filipova, A. (2007). *Perceived organizational support and ethical work climates as predictors of turnover intention of licensed nurses in skilled nursing facilities. PhD Thesis.* Kalamazoo, MI: Western Michigan University.

Shafer, W. E. (2009). Ethical climate, organizational-professional conflict and organizational commitment: a study of Chinese

auditors. *Accounting, Auditing & Accountability Journal, 22*(7), 1087–1110.

Tsai, M. T., & Huang, C. C. (2008). The relationship among ethical climate types, facets of job satisfaction, and the three components of organizational commitment: a study of nurses in Taiwan. *Journal of Business Ethics, 80,* 565–581.

Victor, B., & Cullen, J. B. (1987). A theory and measure of ethical climate in organizations. *Research in Corporate Social Performance & Policy, 9,* 51–71.

NCLEX® EXAMINATION QUESTIONS

1. You are the nursing supervisor and there is a patient that will be going to the operating room for a kidney transplantation. It is the ultimate responsibility of the _____ to check and ensure that the organ donor and recipient are correct.
   A. Surgeon
   B. Anesthesiologist
   C. Registered nurse and surgeon
   D. Surgeon and anesthesiologist

2. Another name is added to the organ donation list every _____ minutes.
   A. 5
   B. 6
   C. 7
   D. 12

3. Issues that are commonly addressed by ethics committees are:
   A. End-of-life issues, organ donation, futility-of-care issues
   B. End-of-life issues, organ donation, change in the durable power of attorney
   C. Organ donation, futility-of-care issues, pediatric patient issues
   D. Organ donation, do not resuscitate order, Jehovah's Witness issues

4. The American Nurses Association approved the revised code of ethics in 2015. There are _____ codes.
   A. 9
   B. 10
   C. 12
   D. 20

5. What is the document that permits an individual to give a surrogate or proxy the authority to make decisions for that person in the event that they become incompetent?
   A. Living will
   B. Durable power of attorney for health care decisions
   C. Advance directive
   D. Informed consent

6. Care providers have the duty to do good to others; to maintain a balance between benefits and harm; to provide all patients, including terminally ill, with caring attention; and to treat every patient with respect and courtesy. What is the requirement that care providers contribute to the health and welfare of the patient and not merely attempt to avoid harm to the patient or client?
   A. Beneficence
   B. Nonmaleficence
   C. Personal liability
   D. Corporate liability

7. Which of the following sets educational standards, examination requirements, and licensing requirements and regulates the nursing profession in each particular state?
   A. The National League for Nursing
   B. Nurse practice acts
   C. State board of nursing
   D. The National Council of State Boards of Nursing

8. Hospitals are legally and ethically obligated to uphold patient rights, which include the right to:
   A. Review records; family can also review records
   B. Participate in treatment decisions and to provide consent to treatment
   C. Be informed of hospital bylaws and hospital attorneys' names and telephone numbers
   D. Expect reasonable care after hospitalization

9. The Organ Procurement and Transplantation Network is a(n) _____ network.
   A. State
   B. Local
   C. National
   D. International

10. The difference between bioethics and ethics is:
    A. Bioethics is specific to health care; ethics deals with the principles of right and wrong
    B. Bioethics is specific to health care; ethics deals with the g, good and bad
    C. Bioethics is specific to health care; ethics deals with the principles of right and wrong and good and bad with no issues of beliefs and values
    D. Bioethics is specific to health care; ethics is the science that deals with the principles of right and wrong and good and bad, and governs our relationships with others. It is based on personal beliefs and values

Answers: 1. C   2. D   3. A   4. A   5. B   6. A   7. B   8. B   9. C   10. D

REFERENCES

Agich, G. J., & Younger, S. J. (1991). For experts only? Access to hospital ethics committees. *Hastings Center Report*, *21*(5), 17–25.

American Council on Transplantation. (2007). Religious concerns about transplantation. Retrieved September 21, 2021, from <www.sharenj.org/religiou.html.>

American Nurses Association. (2015) *Code of ethics for nurses with interpretive statements*. Silver Spring, MD: American Nurses Publishing. Retrieved September 21, 2021, from www.nursingworld.org/ethics/chcode.htm.

American Medical Association. (2021). *Code of medical ethics opinion 2.1*. AMA. Retrieved September 20, 2021, from<https://www.ama-assn.org/delivering-care/ethics/informed-consent.>

American Hospital Association. (2015) Patient bill of rights. Retrieved September 21, 2021, from <www.aha.org/content/00-10/pcp_english_030730.pdf.>

American Transplant Foundation. (2014). *Transplant Facts and Myths*. Retrieved September 21, 2021, from <www.americantransplantfoundation.org/about-transplant/facts-and-myths/.>

Carroll, P. (2006). *Nursing leadership and management: A practical guide*. Clifton Park, NY: Delmar Thomson Learning.

Dalgo, J. T., & Anderson, F. (1995). Notes from the field: developing a hospital ethics committee. *Nursing Management*, *26*(9), 104–106.

International Council of Nurses. (2009) *International Code of Ethics for Nurses*. Geneva, SW: ICN.

International Council of Nurses. (2016) *ICN Code of Ethics for Nurses*. Geneva, Switzerland: ICN.

International Council of Nurses [ICN]. (2012a) *The ICN code of ethics*. Switzerland: Geneva.

International Council of Nurses [ICN]. (2012b). www.icn.ch/icncode.pdfwww.icn.ch/ethics.htm

Kelly-Heidenthal. P. (2004). *Essentials of nursing leadership and management* (p. 295). Clifton Park, NY: Thomson Delmar Learning.

Little, C. (2003). Ethical dimensions of patient care. In P. Kelly-Heidenthal (Ed.), *Nursing leadership and management* (pp. 266–279). Clifton Park, NY: Thomson Delmar Learning.

Memorial Sloan Kettering. *Standard of care pain management*. (2015). Retrieved September 21, 2021, from <http://prc.coh.org/html/standard%20of%20care-Memorial%20Sloan.asp.>

Nathanson, M. (1996). *Home Health Care Law Manual*. Gaithersberg, MD: Aspen Publishers.

New Jersey Sharing Network. (2014a). *Health care professionals*. Retrieved September 21, 2021, from <www.sharenj.org/.>

New Jersey Sharing Network. (2014b). *Fast facts*. Retrieved September 21, 2021, from <www.sharenj.org/.>

NJ Hospital Association. (2014). *POLST*. Retrieved September 21, 2021, from < www.njha.com/media/201361/POLSTWhite.pdf.>

Rowland, H., & Rowland, B. (1997). *Nursing administration handbook* (4th ed.). Gaithersberg, MD: Aspen Publishers, Inc.

Rundio, A., Wilson, V., & Meloy, F. (2016). *Nurse executive review and resource manual*. Silver Spring, MD: ANCC.

Schroeder, S. (1995). Cost containment in US healthcare. *Academic Medicine*, *70*, 861–866.

Sullivan, E., & Decker, P. (2009). *Effective leadership and management in nursing*. Upper Saddle River, NJ: Prentice-Hall.

The American Transplant Foundation. (2021) *Organ donation facts*. HRSA. Retreived from <https://www.organdonor.gov> September 20, 2021.

The Joint Commission. (2020). *Comprehensive accreditation manual*. Oakbrook Terrace, IL: TJC.

Tomey, A. M. (2004). *Guide to nursing management and leadership* (7th ed, p. 75). St. Louis: Mosby.

U.S. Legal Definitions. (2008) *Good Samaritan laws & legal definition*. Retrieved September 21, 2021, from <http://definitions.uslegal.com/g/good-samaritans/.>

WEBSITES

The Joint Commission. www.jointcommission.org/.
National Council of State Boards of Nursing. www.ncsbn.org.
American Nurses Association. www.nursingworld.org.
www.optn.org/.
U.S. Department of Health & Human Services: Health Resources & Services Administration. www.organdonor.gov/.

Case Scenario: A master's-prepared nurse with advanced knowledge and skills in the care of older adults serves as the primary coordinator of care in a facility that uses a model of care that enables continuity throughout acute episodes. One of the facility's overriding missions is to improve transitions to more at-home care for clients with a history of recent hospitalizations and multiple chronic conditions. As part of the nurse's trajectory along the clinical ladder, he maintains active and ongoing professional involvement in improving nursing through evidenced-based practices, including research activities and writing a published nursing article. He has currently taken on the role of one-on-one mentorship with a new RN who has just joined the team. This new nurse is an advanced beginner with enough experience to recognize patterns in work, but he continues to need help in setting priorities and relies heavily on rules and protocols to guide his work. The APN is in the process of setting up a meeting to review ethics in working with older adults in transitional care, and he invites the new RN to join him in planning meetings as part of his onboarding exposure to the goals of his new team.

ITEM TYPE: EXTENDED DRAG & DROP

1. In mentoring the new RN, the APN encourages him to take an interest in advancing on the clinical ladder for himself. **Place a check mark next to each area of clinical practice and professional excellence that are commonly recognized in a clinical ladder program.** (Chapter 10).

Clinical Practice and Professional Excellence	Recognized in Clinical Ladder Program
A. Evidence-based practice in nursing	
B. Volunteer nursing/health service outside the hospital	

Clinical Practice and Professional Excellence	Recognized in Clinical Ladder Program
C. Shared governance participation on hospital or unit committees	
D. Volume of patients treated	
E. Health education for staff, patients, and others	
F. Acuity of patients' conditions	

ITEM TYPE: EXTENDED DRAG & DROP

2. Well into his second week on the job, the RN asks the APN for guidance. "I have a patient who is suddenly refusing all medical treatment. He says he's lived a good life and doesn't want to linger anymore. He's pulled out his IV!" When the APN and RN arrive back in the patient's room, another nurse is scolding the patient to hold still. As she inserts the IV back into his arm, the patient is shaking his head, crying now, and calling for his son. The APN stops the process, saying that the patient has the right to refuse. The other RN argues that on admission he gave informed consent. **Place a check mark next to each condition that must be met to establish informed consent.** (Chapter 16).

Condition	Required to Establish Informed Consent
A. Purpose of treatment is delivered using standard, accepted medical terminology.	
B. Patient must have no medical or legal impediments to making informed decisions.	

Condition	Required to Establish Informed Consent
C. Patient must agree voluntarily, without physical or psychological coercion.	
D. Patient has right of refusal after court proceedings establish competence.	
E. The responsibility rests on medical staff to present complete information in terms that the patient can fully understand.	
F. Medical professionals have a duty to reject treatment refusal if they know that treatment is in the best interests of the patient.	

ITEM TYPE: MATRIX

3. Use an X to indicate which nursing practices illustrate each of these common ethical principles used by nurses in the course of their work. Each practice will apply to only one principle, and each practice will be used. (Chapter 16).

Nursing Practices	Autonomy	Fidelity	Veracity
A. Admits mistakes promptly			
B. Instructs patient on informed consent			
C. Refuses to lie to patient regarding bad news			
D. Does not tell a patient what to do but respects the patient's right to decide			
E. Keeps one's word			
F. Adheres to all contracts			
G. Offers only the level of care that the patient agrees to			

ANSWERS

1. ABCE
2. BCE
3. **Autonomy:** BDG; **Fidelity:** EF; **Veracity:** AC

New Knowledge, Innovations, and Improvements

SECTION OUTLINE

Magnet-recognized institutions conscientiously integrate evidence-based practice and research into clinical and operational processes. Nurses are educated about evidence-based practice and research, enabling them to appropriately explore the safest and best practices for their patients and practice environment and to generate new knowledge. Published research is systematically evaluated and used. Nurses serve on the board that reviews proposals for research, and knowledge gained through research is disseminated to the community of nurses. There are established evolving programs related to evidence-based practices, and research that supports and improves practice. Such work environments continually support the advancement of patient care and the clinical inquiry of the nurses supporting high-quality patient care. (American Nurses Credentialing Center [ANCC], 2019, p. 59)

Innovations in patient care, nursing, and the practice environment are the hallmark of organizations receiving Magnet recognition. Establishing new ways of achieving the triple aim of the Institute of Medicine (IOM) of high-quality patient-centered, effective, and efficient care is the outcome of transformational leadership, empowering structures and processes, and exemplary professional practice in nursing (ANCC, 2013, 2019).

This section will deal with the outcomes of practice environments that support quality care. It will deal with the responsibility of the nurse in the continuing improvements in practice, the use of evidence in delivery of care, and the nursing role in research.

Improving Organizational Performance

OBJECTIVES

- Identify the key focus of performance improvement.
- Discuss trends in quality improvement.
- List three drivers of quality.
- Outline two models of performance improvement.
- Identify three clinical outcome measures.

- Identify major patient safety goals.
- Describe four nursing outcomes specific to desired specialty.
- Relate a clinical activity to a performance model.

KEY TERMS

lean culture performance improvement model dealing with minimization of waste in processes

National Patient Safety Goals set of nationwide goals set by The Joint Commission to focus performance in areas of patient safety

outcome measurable result related to a strategic objective

retrospective review analysis of past events, usually through a chart audit

risk management organized program to prevent the incidence of preventable accidents, injuries, and errors

root-cause analysis retrospective review of the event to evaluate potential causes of the problem or sources of variation in the process

sentinel event unexpected occurrence involving death or serious physical or psychological injury

Six Sigma performance improvement model based on the idea of minimal defects and concerns

IMPROVING ORGANIZATIONAL PERFORMANCE

The year 1998 was pivotal in the quest for improvement in health care. In that year, the IOM issued a report, "To Err Is Human: Building a Safer Health System," detailing the problem of medical errors in health care. The Advisory Commission on Consumer Protection and Quality also released a report calling for a national commitment to improve quality, concluding that "there is no guarantee that any individual will receive high quality care for any particular health problem … the health care industry is plagued … with errors in health care" (Advisory Commission on Consumer Protection and Quality in the Health Care Industry, 1998). It was found that these quality concerns occur typically because of ways in which care is organized. Health care organizations were challenged to ensure that services were safe, effective, patient-centered, timely, efficient, and equitable.

Performance improvement (PI) has been shown to be a powerful tool to help health care organizations become safer and more efficient and patient centered. Total quality management, which is also referred to as PI or quality improvement, has been used in industry since the 1950s, and it has been related to improvements in productivity and quality. It is usually process oriented, with process improvements made to improve efficiency and effectiveness.

HISTORICAL PERSPECTIVES

In the 1950s, The Joint Commission on Accreditation of Healthcare Organizations was formed, and the evaluation of care delivered in health care institutions began. During the 1960s, the American Nurses Association began to develop standards of nursing practice, which became the basis for early quality assurance programs. In the 1970s, the U.S. Congress established Professional Standards Review Organizations to review the quality and cost of care delivered to Medicare and Medicaid recipients. Quality assurance required audits of care. These audits measured basic compliance, emphasizing what was done "wrong," but did little to advance a philosophy of learning from performance.

Health care costs became a major issue in the 1980s, and society began to question the efficiency and effectiveness of health care (Phelps, 1997). Health care administrators turned to industry for lessons learned in managing efficiency. Industry had adopted quality management techniques in the 1950s. An early proponent was W. Edwards Deming, who worked with the Japanese automotive industry after World War II. His 14-point management philosophy is the underpinning of total quality management:

1. Create constancy of purpose toward improvement of product and service, with the aim to become competitive and to stay in business, and to provide jobs.
2. Adopt the new philosophy. We are in a new economic age. Western management must awaken to the challenge, must learn their responsibilities, and take on leadership for change.
3. Cease dependence on inspection to achieve quality. Eliminate the need for inspection on a mass basis by building quality into the product in the first place.
4. End the practice of awarding business on the basis of the price tag. Instead, minimize total cost. Move toward a single supplier for any one item, on a long-term relationship of loyalty and trust.
5. Improve constantly and forever the system of production and service, to improve quality and productivity, and thus constantly decrease costs.
6. Institute training on the job.
7. Institute leadership. The aim of supervision should be to help people and machines and gadgets to do a better job. Supervision of management and production workers is in need of an overhaul.
8. Drive out fear, so that everyone may work effectively for the company.
9. Break down barriers between departments. People in research, design, sales, and production must work as a team to foresee problems of production and in use that may be encountered with the product or service.
10. Eliminate slogans, exhortations, and targets for the workforce asking for zero defects and new levels of productivity. Such exhortations only create adversarial relationships, as the bulk of the causes of low quality and low productivity belong to the system and thus lie beyond the power of the workforce.
11. Eliminate work standards (quotas) on the factory floor. Substitute leadership. Eliminate management by objective. Eliminate management by numbers and numerical goals. Substitute leadership.
12. Remove barriers that rob hourly paid workers of their right to pride in workmanship. The responsibility of supervisors must be changed from sheer

numbers to quality. Remove barriers that rob people in management and engineering of their right to pride in workmanship. This means the abolishment of the annual or merit rating and management by objective.

13. Institute a vigorous program of education and self-improvement.

14. Put everybody in the company to work to accomplish the transformation. The transformation is everybody's job (Deming, 2000a).

Deming believed that an industry consists of multiple processes and decisions, which are interrelated, and developed a "system of profound knowledge" (Deming, 2000b):

- All work consists of multiple processes.
- Differences in work are the result of the system of work, not individual worker performance.
- New work designs are based on our understanding of how work processes relate to one another.
- An understanding of what motivates people.

His model for improvement was the Plan–Do–Check–Act (PDCA) cycle, which remains in widespread use today. Juran (1989) elaborated on Deming's work in total quality management. He believed that quality "did not happen by accident," but was the result of a quality trilogy: planning, control, and improvement. In 1960 Crosby defined quality as the extent to which processes were in conformance with the requirements of the customer. He was known for believing that things should be done "right the first time" and for the philosophy of "zero defects" (Nielsen, Merry, Schyve, & Bisognano, 2004). Although these three proponents of QI focused on work processes, Donabedian (1992) contributed the idea of outcome as part of the overall quality structure. Outcomes involve the results achieved, and they reflect the effectiveness of the process components. The focus of these outcomes allows institutions to measure themselves against the standards and the competition. A comparison of traditional QA and improvement processes is shown in Table 17.1.

KEY FOCUS OF PERFORMANCE IMPROVEMENT

This focus on outcomes has moved health care from a compliance model toward one of "best practice." Although accrediting bodies and federal regulators set minimum standards of compliance, many hospitals are

TABLE 17.1   Comparison of Traditional Quality Assurance and Quality Improvement Processes

Attribute	Key Points
Commitment to a better way	Excited about designing a better future
Courage to challenge power bases and norms	Closest to the work
Go beyond role, take initiative, think outside the box	Assurance of change happening
Persona	Self-motivated, generate enthusiasm
Caring	Commitment to patients and their welfare
Humility	About the change, not about "me"
Sense of humor	Self-support through challenges

(From Yoder-Wise, P. (2015). *Leading and managing in nursing* (6th ed.) [Table 20.2]. St. Louis, MO: Elsevier. Data from Katzenbach, J. R., Beckett, F., Dichter, S., Feigen, M., Gagnon, C., Hope, Q., & Ling, T. (1996). *Real change leaders*. New York, NY: Random House.)

now moving toward a model of "best in class." Examples of organizations that recognize such best practice are the American Nurses Association and its Magnet Award for Nursing, and the Malcolm Baldrige National Quality Award for performance excellence. Hospitals winning the Magnet Award are listed at https://www.nursingworld.org/organizational-programs/magnet/find-a-magnet-organization. The hospitals that have been recognized by receiving the Malcolm Baldrige National Quality Award are listed at https://www.nist.gov/baldrige/award-recipients.

The key focus of PI includes:

- Meeting and exceeding the needs of the customer/stakeholder
- Building organizational learning into each work process
- Continually evaluating and improving work processes
- Assessing all customer requirements and needs
- Being data driven

- Continually looking at current performance
- Constantly striving to "do it better"

It is vital to remember that all PI must be "data driven" and not based on anecdote.

DRIVERS OF QUALITY

The key focus of the quality movement is meeting the needs of the customer. In organizations striving for best practice, this may mean exceeding the needs of the customer. According to the IOM (1998), the key Domains of Quality are effectiveness, efficiency, equity, patient centeredness, safety, and timeliness. The Institute for Healthcare Improvement's (2015) triple aim focuses on improving the patient experience of care (including quality and satisfaction), improving the health of populations, and reducing the per capita cost of health care.

The key customers of health care are the patient and family; they are at the center of all drivers of quality. Other customers of the hospital include the physicians and the community. North Mississippi Health System defines patients and families as their key customers. They identify their key stakeholders as the members of the community, the active and referring physicians, local employers, and third-party payers. The key requirements of these customers and stakeholders are listed in Table 17.2

What is important is that each set of customers has specific requirements that need to be met by the health care organization. The degree to which these key requirements are met forms a base for the patient satisfaction measures of the institution. Other customers include regulators, partners, and payers.

Quality outcomes also are a key requirement of the patient and the community. How do hospitals measure quality outcomes? There are a variety of means.

OUTCOME MEASURES

The key to PI is the "result" of all actions taken to improve patient care. Although it is important to "do what we say we do," it is more important to "do it well." So just how well do we deliver patient care?

TABLE 17.2	Key Customer and Stakeholder Groups and Requirements	
Group	**Requirements**	**Outcome Measure[a]**
Customer group: Patients (including families)	Provide me with quality care	Various outcome measures, mortality rates, time on ventilator postcoronary artery bypass grafting, guidelines for stroke management, inpatient core measures, etc.
	Be nice to me	Patient satisfaction measures
	Do not keep me waiting	Emergency services wait time
	Be low cost	Labor costs, cost of care
Stakeholder groups: Community (health and wellness)	Provide me with community health programs	Proactive community prevention and wellness results, outpatient diabetes management outcomes
	Teach me more about nutrition and obesity	Nursing, Midwifery and Health Systems health plan cholesterol levels
Active and referring medical staff	Provide high-quality care to my patients	Quality of care outcomes
	Collaborate with me	Physician satisfaction
	Make it easy for me to practice/refer	Physician satisfaction
Local employers and third-party payers	Provide me with easy access to quality and cost-effective health care/plan solutions	Community health assessment indicator, not-for-profit health care ratings

[a]For specific measures, see The North Mississippi Baldrige application. [Section 7]. https://www.nist.gov/ba;drige/north-mississippi-health-services

(From North Mississippi Health System. (2012). *Baldrige application*. Retrieved January 4, 2022, from <https://www.nist.gov/baldrige/north-mississippi-health-services>)

Patient care units have an abundance of data available to them. One common outcome used by patient care units is patient satisfaction. A majority of health care organizations across the United States measure patient satisfaction. Two of the common vendor satisfaction measures are Press Ganey and Gallup. The data can be segmented to list the performance of specific units/shifts. The key requirements of the patient/family at North Mississippi Health System are listed in Fig. 17.1. They were identified as provision of quality care, being nice, no waiting, and low cost. The key requirements of other stakeholders are also listed.

Patient satisfaction surveys are customized to include information on the key requirements of the patients of an institution. With the use of nationwide surveys, hospitals can compare their performance with that of other local hospitals, of similar hospitals, and of best-in-class performers. Fig. 17.2 provides an example of a patient satisfaction data set. This graph shows that from 2009 to 2011 in six of the health facilities of the North

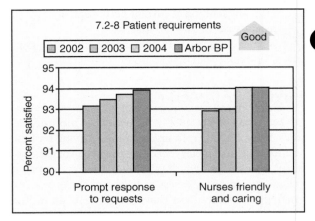

Fig. 17.1 Our nurses consistently score above the national and state TOP BOX comparisons. Our nurses validate that PEOPLE who provide a caring culture is a distinctive CC (core competency). (From North Mississippi Health System. (2012). Baldrige Application [Fig. 7.2-7]. Retrieved January 4, 2022, from <https://www.nist.gov/baldrige/north-mississippi-health-services>, p. 45.)

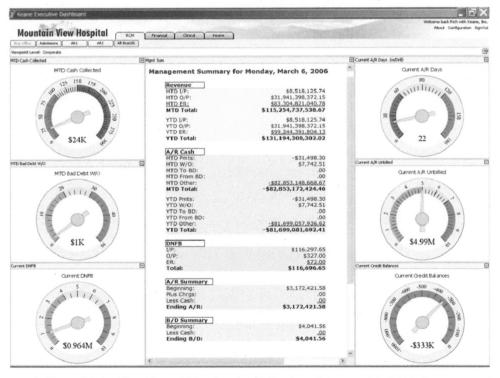

Fig. 17.2 Scorecard. (From Clinical Dashboard Metrics. (n.d.) Retrieved August 20, 2018, from www.dashboard-zone.com/hospital-dashboard-clinical-dashboard-metrics.>)

Mississippi Health System, patients felt that "nurses always communicated well" at a rate above the top box state mean and national top box national mean.

Other data sets available to the nurse include the National Database of Nursing Quality Indicators, which is a database owned by Press Ganey (2021) (https://www.pressganey.com). The database collects and evaluates unit-specific and nurse-sensitive data from hospitals in the United States and internationally. Participating facilities receive unit-level comparative data reports to use for QI purposes. Nursing-sensitive indicators reflect the structure, process, and outcomes of nursing care (Box 17.1) (American Nurses Credentialing Center, 2019).

Nurses will need to know outcomes that directly affect their unit. Common outcomes for all units are infection rates, patient satisfaction, and performance on The Joint Commission (TJC)'s Core Measures. The Core Measures are specific to the unit, so it is important to know which measure or indicator reflects your unit and your level of performance. The initial core measures include heart failure, acute myocardial infarction, pneumonia, surgical infection, and pregnancy. Others measures are pain management and children's asthma care. Participating hospitals collect data related to their performance on the specific measures, and these measures are then reported to TJC. This data set allows for nationwide comparison on performance. TJC's Core Measures are available at https://www.jointcommission.org/PerformanceMeasurement/PerformanceMeasurement/default.htm.

BOX 17.1   Menu of Indicators Currently Being Collected

The menu of indicators currently being collected:
- Nursing hours per patient day
  - Registered nurses (RN) hours per patient day
  - Licensed practical/vocational nurses (LPN/LVN) hours per patient day
  - Unlicensed assistive personnel (UAP) hours per patient day
- Nursing turnover
- RN education/certification
- RN survey
  - Job satisfaction scales
  - Practice environment scale
- Staff mix
  - RN
  - Licensed practical/vocational nurses
  - Unlicensed assistive personnel
  - Percent agency staff

Additional Data Elements Collected
- Patient population; adult or pediatric
- Hospital category (e.g., teaching, nonteaching, etc.)
- Type of unit (critical care, step-down, medical, surgical, combined med-surgical, rehabilitation, and psychiatric)
- Number of staffed beds designated by the hospital

In-Patient Care Organizations
- Falls with injury
- Hospital-acquired pressure injury stages 2 and above
- Central line–associated bloodstream infection

- Catheter-associated urinary tract infection
- *Clostridium difficile*
- Methicillin-resistant *Staphylococcus aureus*
- Venous thromboembolism
- Peripheral intravenous infiltrations
- Physical and sexual assault
- Device-related hospital-acquired pressure injury

Ambulatory Setting
- Falls with injury
- Ambulatory surgical center patient burns
- Adverse outcomes of care: wrong site, side, patient, procedure, implant, or device
- Return to acute care
- Hb A$_{1c}$ target levels
- Extravasation rate
- Door-to-balloon time
- Antibiotic stewardship
- Delay in treatment
- Telehealth appropriate disposition

National Comparison Groups and Reports
National comparison data for the indicators are grouped based on patient (adult/pediatric) and unit type: critical care, step-down, medical, surgical, combined med-surgical, rehabilitation, psychiatric, and staffed bed size. Teaching and Magnet status is identified as it relates to participating hospitals. The quarterly reports provide the national comparison along with unit performance data trended over eight quarters.

(From American Nurses Credentialing Center (2019). *2019 Magnet application manual* (pp. 51–54). American Nurses Credentialing Center: Silver Spring, MD.)

There are also a wide variety of other outcomes that are used by hospitals including financial measures (e.g., cash on hand, market share, and length of stay), human resource measures (e.g., employee satisfaction and productivity), and ethical measures (e.g., community service and financial audits). Hospitals determine the outcomes to be used as part of the strategic planning process. Reporting of the identified outcomes often occurs via a scorecard, which gives a visual representation of current performance on the key outcomes (see Fig. 17.2). The first rule of PI is that it must be data driven; therefore, based on information derived from some of the various data sets available to the institution, a "concern" or a variance in process will be identified. In reaction to this "concern," a PI project will be initiated. These projects usually follow one of the following models.

A second rule of PI is that PI activities should be based on what is important to the customers. Your energies should be concentrated on what is important to them.

MODELS OF QUALITY

FOCUS Method

F: Focus on an opportunity for improvement
O: Organize a team involved with the process
C: Clarify the current process
U: Understand the causes of variation in the process
S: Based on evidence, Select the improvement

Plan–Do–Study–Act (PDSA) Cycle

This model is based on Deming's PDCA model that was discussed earlier.

Plan: Plan a change, with activity aimed at improvement.
Do: Carry it out.
Check/Study: Study the results: What happened? What did you learn? Did the change work?
Act: Adopt the change; rework the change.

Many organizations combine these models into a PDCA-FOCUS model (Fig. 17.3).

As organizations have matured in the PI journey, a process, Six Sigma, is being used in conjunction with PDSA. The objective of Six Sigma quality is to reduce process variation to no more than 3.4 "defects" per 1 million. DMAIC (define, measure, analyze, improve, and control) (GE, 2014) is the acronym used in Six Sigma. It is a data-driven quality strategy for improving processes (Box 17.2).

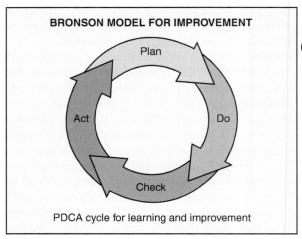

BRONSON MODEL FOR IMPROVEMENT

PDCA cycle for learning and improvement

Fig. 17.3 Plan–Do–Study–Act (PDCA) model. (From Bronson Methodist, 2007. *Baldrige application.* Retrieved August 20, 2018, from <http://baldrige.nist.gov/PDF_files/Bronson_Methodist_Hospital_Application_Summary.pdf>.)

EVIDENCE-BASED PRACTICE

This model describes the integration of research evidence with clinical experience to improve outcomes. The process for evidence-based practice includes (Sackett, Strauss, Richardson, Rosenberg, & Haynes, 2000) the following:

- Formulation of a question from current clinical concerns
- Access of relevant research
- Analysis of the evidence using established criteria
- Plan change in practice
- Implement change in practice
- Evaluate results

As a nurse, you will be asked to participate in process improvement teams. These teams are usually formed in reaction to a "concern" or variance in a process. These teams are usually interdisciplinary in nature and form the "O" of the PDCA-FOCUS model. You will receive team-based education as you join the team. You will also receive "just-in-time" training on the multiple data collection methods used by improvement teams. These include Pareto analysis, surveys, audits, cost-benefit analysis, decision matrix, and fishbone diagram. Some teams will have a certified Six Sigma member who is responsible for data interpretation. As you mature in improvement, you will receive education specific to the institution's model.

BOX 17.2 Six Sigma: DMAIC (Define, Measure, Analyze, Improve, and Control)

Six Sigma is a registered trademark and service mark of Motorola, Inc.

Define the customer, their critical to quality issues, and the core business process involved.
- Define who the customers are, their requirements for products and services, and their expectations
- Define project boundaries; the stop and start of the process
- Define the process to be improved by mapping the process flow

Measure the performance of the core business process involved.
- Develop a data collection plan for the process
- Collect data from many sources to determine types of defects and metrics
- Compare to customer survey results to determine shortfall

Analyze the data collected and process map to determine root causes of defects and opportunities for improvement.
- Identify gaps between current performance and goal performance
- Prioritize opportunities to improve
- Identify sources of variation

Improve the target process by designing creative solutions to fix and prevent problems.
- Create innovative solutions using technology and discipline
- Develop and deploy implementation plan

Control the improvements to keep the process on the new course.
- Prevent reverting back to the "old way"
- Require the development, documentation, and implementation of an ongoing monitoring plan
- Institutionalize the improvements through the modification of systems and structures (staffing, training, incentives)

LEAN CULTURE

The underlying principle of "lean" is that all processes contain waste. Womack and Jones (2003, p. 15) defined **lean** as a "way to do more and more with less and less— less human effort, less equipment, less time, and less space—while coming closer to providing customers with what they want."

One of the challenges of implementing lean in health care is that it requires people to identify waste in the work in which they are so invested (Table 17.3). All workers want to feel their work is valuable, perhaps most especially health care workers. Recognizing that much about their daily tasks is wasteful and does not add value can be difficult for health care professionals. A nurse who is hunting for supplies is doing it to serve the needs of patients. Nurses may not see this as wasted time and may not stop to wonder why those supplies are not where they need them every time they need them. If the supplies were always readily available, the time nurses spend hunting for them would instead be devoted to something more appropriate to their skills and expertise (Miller, 2005, p. 8).

RISK MANAGEMENT

Risk management can be defined as an organized program to prevent the incidence of preventable accidents, injuries, and errors (Kavaler & Spiegel, 2003). These errors, accidents, and injuries incur unintended cost to

TABLE 17.3 Value and Waste Examples in Health Care

Lean Thinking	Health Care
Value adding time	Diagnostic and care time
	Diagnostic time (collecting and analyzing clinical information)
	Active care time (clinical interventions)
	Passive care time (under observation, no interventions)
Nonvalue adding time (waste)	Diagnostic and care time
	Superfluous time (not needed diagnostics, observations or interventions)
	Administrative time

(From Joosten, T., et al. (2009). Application of lean thinking to health care: issues and observations. *International Journal of Health Care Quality, 21*, 341–347.)

the institution, and the risk management department is charged with defining the situations that place the health care institution at risk.

The National Patient Safety Goals further emphasize the importance of the risk management function (Box 17.3). These goals were formed based on the IOM 1998 report. This is a nationwide initiative with an overall goal of making specific improvements in patient safety of hospitals across the nation. The goals highlight problem areas and focus on system-wide solutions.

BOX 17.3   National Patient Safety Goals (2020)

2020 Joint Commission National Patient Safety Goals

Identify Patients Correctly

NPSG.01.01.01 NPSG.01.03.01

Use at least two ways to identify patients. For example, use the patient's name *and* date of birth. This is done to make sure that each patient gets the correct medicine and treatment.

Make sure that the correct patient gets the correct blood when they get a blood transfusion.

Improve Staff Communication

NPSG.02.03.01

Get important test results to the right staff person on time.

Use Medicines Safely

NPSG.03.04.01

NPSG.03.05.01 NPSG.03.06.01

Before a procedure, label medicines that are not labeled. For example, medicines in syringes, cups, and basins. Do this in the area where medicines and supplies are set up.

Take extra care with patients who take medicines to thin their blood.

Record and pass along correct information about a patient's medicines. Find out what medicines the patient is taking. Compare those medicines to new medicines given to the patient. Make sure the patient knows which medicines to take when they are at home. Tell the patient it is important to bring their up-to-date list of medicines every time they visit a doctor.

Use Alarms Safely

NPSG.06.01.01

Make improvements to ensure that alarms on medical equipment are heard and responded to on time.

Prevent Infection

NPSG.07.01.01

NPSG.07.03.01   NPSG.07.04.01   NPSG.07.05.01
    NPSG.07.06.01

Use the hand-cleaning guidelines from the Centers for Disease Control and Prevention or the World Health Organization. Set goals for improving hand cleaning. Use the goals to improve hand cleaning.

Use proven guidelines to prevent infections that are difficult to treat.

Use proven guidelines to prevent infection of the blood from central lines.

Use proven guidelines to prevent infection after surgery.

Use proven guidelines to prevent infections of the urinary tract that are caused by catheters.

Identify Patient Safety Risks

NPSG.15.01.01

Reduce the risk for suicide.

Prevent Mistakes in Surgery

UP.01.01.01

UP.01.02.01 UP.01.03.01

Make sure that the correct surgery is done on the correct patient and at the correct place on the patient's body.

Mark the correct place on the patient's body where the surgery is to be done. Pause before the surgery to make sure that a mistake is not being made.

Identify Patients Correctly

NPSG.01.01.01 NPSG.01.03.01

Use at least two ways to identify patients. For example, use the patient's name *and* date of birth. This is done to make sure that each patient gets the correct medicine and treatment.

Make sure that the correct patient gets the correct blood when they get a blood transfusion.

Use Medicines Safely

NPSG.03.04.01

NPSG.03.05.01 NPSG.03.06.01

Before a procedure, label medicines that are not labeled. For example, medicines in syringes, cups and basins. Do this in the area where medicines and supplies are set up.

Take extra care with patients who take medicines to thin their blood.

Record and pass along correct information about a patient's medicines. Find out what medicines the patient is taking. Compare those medicines to new medicines given to the patient. Make sure the patient knows which medicines to take when they are at home. Tell the patient it is important to bring their up-to-date list of medicines every time they visit a doctor.

Prevent Infection

NPSG.07.01.01 Use the hand cleaning guidelines from the Centers for Disease Control and Prevention or the World Health Organization. Set goals for improving hand cleaning. Use the goals to improve hand cleaning.

NPSG.07.05.01 Use proven guidelines to prevent infection after surgery.

Continued

BOX 17.3 National Patient Safety Goals (2020)—cont'd

Prevent Mistakes in Surgery

UP.01.01.01

UP.01.02.01 UP.01.03.01

Make sure that the correct surgery is done on the correct patient and at the correct place on the patient's body.

Mark the correct place on the patient's body where the surgery is to be done. Pause before the surgery to make sure that a mistake is not being made.

NPSG, National Patient Safety Goals.

(From *Ambulatory HealthCare National Patient Safety Goals*. (2020). Retrieved November 3, 2019, from <https://www.jointcommission.org/assets/1/6/2020_AHC_NPSG_goals_final.pdf>)

(From *Hospital National Patient Safety Goals*. (2020). Retrieved November 3, 2019, from <https://www.jointcommission.org/assets/1/6/2020_HAP_NPSG_goals_final.pdf.>)

BOX 17.4 Patient Handoffs

Patient handoffs occur thousands of times a day in hospitals. Patients are transferred from unit to unit, brought to surgery, from surgery to the postanesthetic care unit, and from postanesthetic care unit transferred to a unit. Many handoffs go off without a hitch, but devastating mistakes can happen during any of them.

"If you transfer a patient to the intensive care unit after surgery and the ventilator isn't ready, you're really riding on the edge" of patient safety, says Allan Goldman, head of the pediatric intensive care unit at Great Ormond Street Hospital and a chief architect of the hospital's collaboration with Ferrari.

A 2005 study in *The Wall Street Journal* found that nearly 70% of all preventable hospital mishaps occurred because of communication problems, and that many of these breakdowns occur during patient handoffs.

In 2003, the surgeons at London's Great Ormond Street Hospital noted the efficiency of the pit stops of the Ferrari race car team, and concluded that patient handovers were haphazard in comparison. The physicians traveled to Italy to meet with individuals at Ferrari headquarters and began to incorporate some of the lessons learned in their own processes. For instance, in a Formula One race, the "lollipop man" (with the paddle) ushers the car in and signals the driver when it is safe to go; it is not always clear in the hospital who is in charge.

Back in London, the physicians also sought the advice of two jumbo jet pilots and wrote a seven-page protocol for patient handoffs. After numerous improvements and changes, "information handover omissions" fell 49%, and the number of technical errors fell 42%.

(From Naik, G. (2006, November). Hospital races to learn lessons of Ferrari crew. *The Wall Street Journal*.)

Many health care institutions have integrated the risk management and PI activities. This relates to the process management nature of the risk management function. For example, Goal 2 (improve staff communication) integrates activities of both a risk management department and PI. Lessons are being learned from the aviation and race car industries in the area of handoffs, and processes are being designed to further enhance patient safety and reduce adverse events. The risk management department also investigates all identified accidents, injuries, errors, and adverse events. TJC requires all health care institutions to report sentinel events. A sentinel event includes the following:

- An unexpected occurrence involving death or serious physical or psychological injury, or the risk thereof. Serious injury specifically includes loss of limb or

function. The phrase "or the risk thereof" includes any process variation for which a recurrence would carry a significant chance of a serious adverse outcome.

- Such events are called "sentinel" because they signal the need for immediate investigation and response.
- The terms "sentinel event" and "medical error" are not synonymous; not all sentinel events occur because of an error, and not all errors result in sentinel events.

When a sentinel event is identified, a root-cause analysis is performed by a team that includes those directly involved in the process. This root-cause analysis is a retrospective review of the event done to evaluate potential causes of the problem or sources of variation in the process. In a root-cause analysis of the "handoff" procedure in the discussion of handoffs (Box 17.4), it was found that there was no systemized process for the handoff and that multiple failures of communication occurred because of this lack of process. This process was then changed and evaluated, and the outcomes were positive.

The major outcome of PI is the creation of a learning organization (Baldrige, 2014, p. 2). This means that learning:
- Is a regular part of daily work
- Is practiced at personal, unit, and organizational levels

- Results in solving problems at their source ("root cause")
- Is focused on building and sharing knowledge throughout the organization
- Is driven by opportunities to affect significant, meaningful change

This is the outcome of institution-wide PI.

SUMMARY

Nurses and organization administrators should continually learn from their performance. Health care organizations have a long history of collecting information on performance, but in the last 10 years, the emphasis on performance has changed as the health care environment has become more competitive. TJC requires organizations to collect information on the Core Measures and to determine how the individual hospital is performing. Nurses should know the levels of performance based on actual data. These results may be shown in dashboard form to allow the reader to make a quick determination of performance to target based on color. The use of data for PI is one means of continually learning about one's performance and making improvements based on reviews of performance. As a new nurse, it will be important to realize that as nurses in clinical practice, the review of data provides the opportunity to improve our practice to better meet the needs of the patient.

CLINICAL CORNER

The Nurse Leader Role in Quality

If you asked me 18 years ago, as a new bedside nurse, if I would be a nurse leader for the department of quality and performance improvement, I would have said no. The only reason I would have said no was because I had no idea a nurse leader in quality even existed. That was not something discussed in nursing school or during orientation to the nursing unit. Fast forward to present time and I cannot imagine myself working in another health care specialty role. As a bedside nurse, I quickly realized there were opportunities to improve processes and the patient experience but did not know how to get started. Nurses are busy carrying out multiple tasks to ensure patients' needs are met. This includes nursing assessments, documentation, administering medications, preparing the patient for exams, partnering with patients and families to optimize care, admissions, discharges ... the list goes on and on. These tasks are the focus of every nurse, every shift, every day. As a nurse, I wanted to make changes and understand more about organization culture and process change so I began to search for other opportunities. I would offer to work on projects just to get exposure to how things were done in the organization. After several years of project hopping and holding various positions, I advanced to a quality leadership role, which was a game-changer for me. I knew right away this was the career path to pursue. Because health care demands are growing, many new career opportunities have evolved, including nursing leadership in quality. Quality departments always existed, but in today's health care world quality is key. This is an ideal leadership role for nurses because it requires clinical skills, critical thinking, and innovation. Bedside nurses are fortunate to have programs such as shared governance structures and unit-based performance improvement teams to make improvements in their own processes yet often do not have the time to dedicate to these activities, and not because leadership does not afford the opportunities, but because patient care comes first. Most nurses do not fully understand the extent of organizational dynamics and how care is continuously being monitored and improved. In the quality role, I can take my years of bedside nursing experience and use my leadership skills to help make those changes.

The role of the nurse leader in quality is one that is diverse, challenging, and fulfilling. The nurse leader in quality has become a vital role in the health care industry. As a nurse, providing safe, high quality, and compassionate care is the ultimate goal in the profession. As a nurse leader in quality, the goal remains the same and is carried out through inspiration, influence, vision, and

Continued

teamwork. The role of the nurse leader in quality is to ensure high-quality patient outcomes and actively seek ways to improve care. Quality in health care encompasses continuous improvement, patient safety, infection control, regulatory compliance, cost-savings, clinical variation, technology integration, patient experience, and evidence-based practice. Over the last several years, the need for quality leaders has increased because of regulations and requirements set forth by many governing agencies. This holds true for inpatient and outpatient services, rehabilitation facilities, physician practices, and long-term care facilities. Health care organizations are required to provide data to these governing agencies and are held accountable to demonstrate high-quality outcomes. This transparency in the data has become the catalyst for how organizations manage quality outcomes and make changes to processes that may not have been previously optimal. Furthermore, outcome data are publicly reported allowing consumers to choose a health care facility based on quality outcomes.

Quality attracts consumers as consumers seek high-quality services and products whether at a restaurant, car dealership, or in a health care system. This means a patient who received services from Hospital A may now choose Hospital B because they have better patient experience scores or lower surgical site infection rates. For this reason, the nurse leader's role in quality is data-driven wherein they leverage that data to identify areas of opportunity. Nurses are also attracted to organizations that have high standards for quality, the tools needed for safe care, and a culture to speak up when experiencing safety concerns. Nurses want to be employed by an organization that puts quality and safety first. Similarly, organizations want to employ top-notch nurses making these things that much more important. At the end of the day, nurses and organizations have the same goal of providing the best possible care to patients and their families. This helps drive organizations to take a deep dive into processes and the overall culture of quality and safety.

There is no limit on what can be improved within a health care system. Just like any other business or corporation, quality needs to be at the forefront of organizations. The quality leader advocates for the nursing profession by ensuring processes are efficient with safe and reliable outcomes. This includes partnering with the clinical staff to facilitate change. The quality nurse leader is an advocate for improvement and values the relationship with the clinical staff. The clinical staff is the driving force behind what needs to be improved and the quality leader ensures resources are available to facilitate the change. This leadership role does go beyond nursing and generally has responsibility for the entire organization. Organizations face many challenges and having the appropriate governance structure for quality maximizes the chance for outcome sustainability.

Clinical nursing leadership serves as the bridge between the clinical staff and the desired outcomes. This role promotes the proactive approach to managing system issues or process failures. As health care continues to grow and evolve, the nurse leader in quality will need to stay abreast of new regulations to serve the needs of patients. This includes identifying new health care trends and applying evidence-based practice. Leadership in quality requires a working relationship with all areas within an organization as this role is a partnership to those closest to the bedside. Quality leaders have an understanding of the many competing priorities and projects on the clinical units and work with the local leadership staff to help prioritize activities. Quality and process improvement require a readiness for change and the quality nurse leader is the driver. As nurses, whether in a bedside or leadership role, we want to ensure the best services are provided with the highest-level quality to the patients and families we are privileged to care for.

Melissa Tunc, DNP, RN, HN-BC, CPHQ, PMCP
Lean Six Sigma Black Belt

EVIDENCE-BASED PRACTICE

(From Hancock, K. *Nursing and the journey to high reliability: nurses are the key to interprofessional collaborative practice.* Cleveland Clinic Blog. Retrieved January 4, 2022, from https://consultqd.clevelandclinic.org/nursing-and-the-journey-to-high-reliability/.)

High reliability concepts are tools that a growing number of hospitals are using to help achieve their safety, quality, and efficiency goals. These concepts are not an improvement methodology such as Six Sigma or lean. Instead, they are insights into how to think about and change the vexing quality and safety issues you face. Hospitals do most things right, much of the time. But even very infrequent failures in critical processes can have terrible consequences for a patient. Creating a culture and

EVIDENCE-BASED PRACTICE—cont'd

processes that radically reduce system failures and effectively respond when failures do occur is the goal of high reliability thinking.

At the core of high reliability organizations (HROs) are five key concepts, which we believe are essential for any improvement initiative to succeed:

1. *Sensitivity to operations:* This preserves constant awareness by leaders and staff of the state of the systems and processes that affect patient care. This awareness is key to noting risks and preventing them.
2. *Reluctance to simplify:* Simple processes are good, but simplistic explanations for why things work or fail are risky. Avoiding overly simple explanations of failure (unqualified staff, inadequate training, communication failure, etc.) is essential to understand the true reasons patients are placed at risk.
3. *Preoccupation with failure:* When near misses occur, these are viewed as evidence of systems that should be improved to reduce potential harm to patients. Rather than viewing near misses as proof that the system has effective safeguards, they are viewed as symptomatic of areas in need of more attention.
4. *Deference to expertise:* If leaders and supervisors are not willing to listen and respond to the insights of staff who know how processes really work and the risks patients really face, you will not have a culture in which high reliability is possible.
5. *Resilience:* Leaders and staff need to be trained and prepared to know how to respond when system failures do occur.

As more health care organizations like the Cleveland Clinic work on the journey to high reliability, exceptional nursing has never been more imperative. Nurses are the key to two of the foundational components of high reliability environments, quality and safety. As part of the Cleveland Clinic's Solutions for Value Enhancements (SolVE) program, nurses have been involved in innovative projects of this HRO.

Although many of their nurse managers admit that the thought of participation in these programs was overwhelming at first, those who have completed them agree the reward was well worth it.

Across the health system, nurse-led relationship-based improvement projects have affected caregiver teams in welcoming ongoing quality improvement, achieving excellence in quality and safety, and improving patient-centered care delivery. The following are two examples of this.

Willoughby Family Health Center Pediatrics

Standing up as one of the first nurse-led SolVE projects, nurses in the pediatric department at Willoughby Family Health Center knew they needed to improve transitions of care processes from pediatric to adult care. They also knew interprofessional collaboration was going to be imperative to their work.

To begin, they obtained leadership support, evaluated survey data, researched national data and best practices, and created and worked through process maps. They worked closely with numerous physicians, registered nurses, advanced practice registered nurses and health unit coordinators, and information technology, billing and coding, and call center caregivers.

Their work revealed several findings, including that providers were sometimes reluctant to let go of patients or they were not fully aware of national guidelines for transition. By collaborating and communicating with the entire caregiver team, the nurses leading the project initiated a new process for transition based on the 6 Core Elements of Transition from the national organization Got Transition.

They have since been working to evolve the transition process, address hidden challenges, and collect data. Pilots are currently in place in several Cleveland clinic family health center locations.

Pediatric Postanesthesia Care Unit

In 2015, nurses in the pediatric postanesthesia care unit were encountering noticeable delays in pain medication orders for postoperative patients. They knew they needed to find the root cause of the issue to properly keep their patients safe and minimize patient pain.

Turning their challenge into a SolVE project, they began building research and relationships. They looked at hundreds of patient charts; called on other children's hospitals across the nation for advice; collaborated with anesthesia caregivers, quality directors, nurses, pharmacists, and other caregivers; and created a process map that identified barriers to patient care. They used a fishbone diagram to help determine potential solutions.

Some of the team's most significant findings came from newfound collaboration with their anesthesia colleagues. They learned that the pharmacy department had its own stipulations and regulations for medication delivery. They also learned anesthesiologist caregivers did not have access to computers in the operating rooms to immediately enter orders. They also learned there were often technology delays between order entry and the medication-dispensing machine.

As a result, there was an average 17-minute delay for placement of pain medication orders once a patient was in the postanesthesia care unit.

Continued

EVIDENCE-BASED PRACTICE—cont'd

The team devised and implemented simple changes, such as adding a direct link for order entry by anesthesiologists in the computer system. They also made not-so-simple changes like creating a new "no transfer without orders" policy, which was a significant culture change on the unit.

The enhanced interprofessional collaborative practice paid off. Very quickly, the 17-minute delay in pain medication orders became a zero-minute delay.

Additionally, since the project ended and the new interventions have been incorporated into daily patient care, average length of stay has decreased by 42.9 minutes, unit costs have been reduced by roughly $80,000 annually, and both employee engagement and patient/parent satisfaction have improved.

A New Age of Care

Without question, interprofessional collaborative practice is an important part of becoming a HRO. When caregivers communicate, they can see opportunities and challenges through the "lens" of other care professionals. They can better recognize the value each caregiver brings to the table, remove silos, enhance teamwork, solve challenges, and improve patient care.

To help attain cultures of high reliability, nurse leaders should encourage nursing caregivers to pursue work that affects interprofessional collaboration and communication to propel team-based care and help deliver sustainability and structure to care delivery.

NCLEX® EXAMINATION QUESTIONS

1. As a new RN you will be attending in-service requirements prior to placement on your unit. An organized program to prevent incidence of preventable accidents, injuries, and errors is referred to as:
   A. Risk management
   B. Retrospective review
   C. Route cause analysis
   D. Sentinel event

2. Which of the following has been shown to be a powerful tool to help health care organizations become safer and more efficient and patient centered?
   A. Total quality management (TQM)
   B. Process improvement (PI)
   C. Quality improvement (QI) and PI
   D. All of the above are correct

3. The new RN should seek out health care facilities that are driven to provide safe quality patient care, always keeping the patient/families at the forefront. Which of the following should the RN keep in mind when applying for a first nursing position?
   A. Seek out Magnet-recognized institutions
   B. Seek out facilities that conscientiously integrate evidence-based practice into practice and research into clinical and operational processes.
   C. Seek out facilities that allow the RN to attend conferences
   D. All of the above are correct

4. A new nurse is attending the new employee orientation at the facility. She is not sure about the National Patient Safety Goals. When she questioned the nurse manager regarding the safety goals she was informed that they are used to:
   A. Focus performance in areas of patient safety
   B. Complete the employee assessment review
   C. Complete incident reports properly
   D. Determine whether or not the employee will receive additional pay

5. The vice president of human resources in a hospital setting is usually the designated risk manager. You will most likely meet the risk manager at new employee orientation. Your understanding of the program is to:
   A. Prevent the incidence of preventable accidents, injuries, and errors
   B. Only use the program when there is a sentinel event
   C. Evaluate the incident reports daily
   D. Reprimand nurses who do not follow the risk management program

6. You have decided to work in the operating room as your first nursing position. You will have a long nursing orientation because this is a specialty. You have witnessed the surgeon begin operating on the wrong leg. This is considered a:
   A. Sentinel event
   B. Incident report
   C. Firing of the surgeon
   D. Firing of the RN

7. Health care organizations were challenged to ensure that services were:
   A. Safe, effective, patient-centered, timely, efficient, and equitable
   B. Safe, effective, patient-centered, timely, efficient
   C. Patient-centered, timely, efficient, and equitable
   D. Safe, effective, efficient, and equitable

8. Which of the following is not a focus of PI?
   A. Meeting and exceeding the needs of the customer/stakeholder
   B. Building organizational learning into each work process
   C. Being data driven
   D. Evaluating the work process one time

9. When using the FOCUS method of quality the nurse should be aware of this method. F = focus on an opportunity for improvement, O = organize a team involved with the process, C = clarify the current process, U = understand the causes of variation in the process, and S = based on evidence, select the improvement. Your unit has had an increase in the number of falls on the 7 p.m. to 7 a.m. shift. Which of the following does this refer to?
   A. F = focus on an opportunity for improvement
   B. O = organize a team involved with the process
   C. C = clarify the current process
   D. U = understand the causes of variation in the process
   E. S = search for evidence

Answers: 1. B   2. D   3. D   4. A   5. A   6. A   7. A   8. D   9. A

REFERENCES

Advisory Commission of Consumer Protection and Quality in the Health Care Industry. (1998). *Better Health Care for all Americans. Quality First. Quality First.* Retrieved August 1, 2019, from www.hcqualitycommission.gov/final/.

American Nurses Credentialing Center. (2013). *Magnet Application Manual.* Silver Spring, MD: ANCC.

American Nurses Credentialing Center. (2019). *Magnet Application Manual.* Silver Spring, MD: ANCC.

Baldrige National Quality Program. (2014). *Health care criteria for performance excellence.* Gaithersburg: MD: National Institute of Standards.

Bronson Methodist Hospital. (2007). Baldrige application. Retrieved August 1, 2019, from baldrige.nist.gov/PDF_files/Bronson_Methodist_Hospital_Application_Summary.pdf.

Clinical Dashboard Metrics. (n.d.). www.dashboardzone.com/hospital-dahsboard-clinical-dashboard-metrics.

Deming, W. E. (2000a). *Out of the crisis.* Cambridge, MA: Massachusetts Institute of Technology.

Deming, W. E. (2000b). *The new economics: for industry, government, education* (2nd ed.). Cambridge, MA: MIT Press.

Donabedian, A. (1992). The role of outcomes in quality assessment and assurance. *Quality Review Bulletin, 18,* 356–360.

GE. (2014). GE's DMAIC Approach. Retrieved August 1, 2019, from www.ge.com/capital/vendor/dmaic.htm.

Institute for Healthcare Improvement. (2015). *The Triple Aim.* Retrieved August 1, 2019, from www.ihi.org/Engage/Initiatives/TripleAim/pages/default.aspx.

Institute for Medicine. (1998). *Crossing the quality chasm: a new health system for the 21st century.* Washington, DC: National Academies Press.

Joosten, T., Bongers, I., & Janssen, R. (2009). Application of lean thinking to health care: issues and observations. *International Journal of Health Care Quality, 21,* 341–347.

Juran, J. M. (1989). *Juran on leadership for quality: An executive handbook.* New York: Free Press.

Kavaler, F., & Spiegel, A. (2003). *Risk management in health care institutions: A strategic approach* (2nd ed.). Boston: Jones & Bartlett.

Miller, D. B. (Ed.), (2005). *Going lean in health care.* [IHI Innovation Series white paper.] Cambridge, MA: 2005 Institute for Healthcare Improvement. Retrieved August 1, 2019, from www.ihi.org/IHI/Results/WhitePapers/GoingLeaninHealthCare.htm.

Naik, G. (2006). *Hospital races to learn lessons of Ferrari crew.* November 14, 2006 The Wall Street Journal. November 14, 2006.

Nielsen D. M., Merry M. D., Schyve P. M., & Bisognano, M. (2004). *Can the gurus' concepts cure health care?* [September 25–34] Quality Progress.

Phelps, C. E. (1997). *Health economics* (2nd ed.). Reading, MA: Addison-Wesley.

North Mississippi Health System. (2012). *Baldrige Application* [Fig. 7.2-7]. Retrieved January 4, 2022, from <https://www.nist.gov/baldrige/north-mississippi-health-services>, p. 45.

Press Ganey. (2021). Lets reshape healthcare. Retreived January 4, 2022, from www.pressganey.com.

Sackett, D., Strauss, S., Richardson, W., Rosenberg, W., & Haynes, R. (2000). *Evidence-based medicine: How to practice and teach EBM* (2nd ed.). Edinburgh: Churchill Livingstone.

The Joint Commission. (2007). *Sentinel event policies and procedures*. Retrieved August 1, 2019, from www.joint-commission.org/SentinelEvents/PolicyandProcedures/.

The Joint Commission. (2014). *National patient safety goals*. Oak Brook, IL: Author.

The Joint Commission. (2015). *National Patient Safety Goals 2015*. Oak Brook, IL. Retrieved August 1, 2019, from www.jointcommission.org/assets/1/6/2015_HAP_NPSG_ER.pdf.

Womack, J., & Jones, D. (2003). *Lean thinking: Banish waste and create wealth in your corporation*. New York: Free Press.

Yoder-Wise, P. (2011). *Leading and managing in nursing*. St. Louis: Mosby.

Evidence-Based Practice

OBJECTIVES

- Differentiate among research, evidence-based practice (EBP), and performance improvement.
- Review the nurse's role in the implementation of evidence-based practice.
- Identify the various models of EBP.
- Identify the hierarchy of evidence.

- Discuss the critical appraisal process in evaluating evidence.
- Identify the PICOT (population, intervention, comparison, outcome, time) format of identifying a question.

KEY TERMS

correlational study a study examining the relationship between or among two or more variables in a single group; it does not examine cause and effect

descriptive study used to identify and describe variables and examine relationships that exist in a situation; provides an accurate portrayal of the phenomenon of interest

evidence-based practice conscientious use of current best practice or research evidence in making clinical decisions

nonrandomized clinical trial same as a randomized clinical trial, but patient placement in treatment or nontreatment group depends on study variables, with not every individual having an opportunity for selection

observational study use of structured and unstructured observations to measure study variables

randomized clinical trial effects of an intervention are examined by comparing the treatment group with the nontreatment group; patients are placed in treatment or nontreatment group through random sampling

research generation of new knowledge through the rigorous study of variables

research use findings from a single study or a set of studies for the development of patient care

TREATMENT MYTHS AND TRUTHS

Two sentinel publications by the Institute of Medicine (IOM), *To Err Is Human* and *Crossing the Quality Chasm* (Institute of Medicine [IOM], 2000, 2001), drew attention to quality issues in U.S. health care. A major theme of both reports is that although the technology of health care has advanced at lightning speed, the delivery system has not advanced, causing potentially lethal situations in health care. One of the most common situations seen is the increased rate of hospital-acquired infections, and one of the proposed solutions to the improvement of care is the use of evidence-based decision making in health care.

The vision for the future of nursing in *The Future of Nursing* report (Institute of Medicine IOM, 2011) focuses on the convergence of knowledge, quality, and new functions in nursing. The recommendation that nurses lead interprofessional teams to improve delivery systems and care brings to the fore the necessity for new competencies, beyond evidence-based practice, that are requisite as nurses transform health care. These competencies focus on using knowledge in clinical decision making and producing research evidence on interventions that promote uptake and use by individual providers and groups of providers (Stevens, 2013).

Evidence-based practice (EBP) requires a shift from the traditional paradigm of clinical practice grounded in pathophysiology and clinical experience to one of the integration of best practice and scientific evidence. This paradigm shift allows for the continuous improvement of practice and a creation of environments that stimulate innovation.

A recent survey of the state of EBP in nurses indicated that although nurses had positive attitudes toward EBP and wished to gain more knowledge and skills, they still faced significant barriers in employing it in practice (Melnyk, Fineout-Overholt, Gallagher-Ford, & Kaplan, 2012). This will prove to be a challenge if we are to meet the IOM goal of 90% of practice being informed by evidence by 2020.

As a new nurse, there will be many times that you will ask yourself the following: "Why do we do it this way?" or "Is there a better way to do this?" For answers to these questions you must look to the evidence. What is the best practice, or what is the best way to do this? Some of our standard practices are "sacred cows," meaning they represent the way it has always been done. For instance, does every patient admitted to your unit need their temperature taken at 7 a.m.? Perhaps not, but that is just the way we do it, or perhaps that was the "best practice" when the policy was implemented. But what does the evidence (scientific data) tell us today? As nurses, we should remain current within our practice area because the evidence is always changing and growing. Estabrooks (1998) and Pravikoff, Tanner, and Pierce (2005) found that knowledge sources most frequently used by nurses were school experiences and colleague experience. Assuming this is the case, a nurse with 15 years of experience may be using "evidence" that is 15 years out of date, and this experienced nurse who is mentoring new nurses may be fostering practice that is 15 years out of date. A colleague of this author once said that "health care was a long history of tradition unimpeded by progress"—the move to EBP is changing this.

EXAMPLES OF SOME TRADITIONAL PRACTICES NOT SUPPORTED BY EVIDENCE

Use of Oxygen in Patients with Chronic Obstructive Pulmonary Disease

The use of oxygen at levels that potentially may eliminate "hypoxic drive" in patients with chronic obstructive pulmonary disease (COPD) has long been a clinical concern (Makic, Martin, Burns, Philbrick, & Rauen, 2013). Statements such as "if you give oxygen, you will wipe out their drive to breathe and their carbon dioxide will increase," and "it is OK for the COPD patient to have a high $Paco_2$ and a low Pao_2, they live there" are often repeated in clinical practice settings, in academic classrooms, and even in textbooks (Table 18.1).

TABLE 18.1   Debunking "Hypoxic Drive" and Support for Providing Oxygen to Patients With Chronic Obstructive Pulmonary Disease (COPD)

Evidence-Based Literature (Author, year)	Provide Oxygen for Acute on Chronic Respiratory Failure	Provide Oxygen for Chronic Respiratory Failure	Main Points
Rudolf, Banks, & Semple,[38] 1977	NA	NA	Hypercapnia during oxygen therapy in acute exacerbations of chronic respiratory failure not due to "hypoxic drive" but other mechanisms
Easton, Slykerman, & Anthonisen,[36] 1986	NA	NA	Minute ventilation may decrease in some patients in acute respiratory failure who are given oxygen; $Paco_2$ subsequently increases
Crossley, McGuire, Barrow, & Houston,[40] 1997	Yes	NA	Described response of COPD patients to high fractions of inspired oxygen after a period of rest on mechanical ventilation; provision of oxygen did not result in hypercarbia or respiratory muscle failure
Dick, Liu, Sassoon, Berry, & Mahutte,[35] 1997	NA	NA	Described the oxygen-induced change in ventilation and ventilatory drive in COPD; was not due to "hypoxic drive"; although hypoxic drive is a real phenomenon, it is responsible for only ~10% of the total drive to breathe
Pierson,[28] 2000	NA	Yes	Dangerous to withhold oxygen. Effects of chronic hypoxia include organ failure and a shortened life span
Singapore Ministry of Health SMOH, 2006	Yes	Yes	Evidence-based recommendations for the use of oxygen in both chronic and acute on chronic COPD
West,[34] 2008	NA	NA	Describes Haldane effect and hypoxic vasoconstriction as mechanisms of increased carbon dioxide with provision of oxygen in COPD
Global Initiative for Chronic Obstructive Lung Disease GOLD, 2009	Yes	Yes	Evidence-based recommendations for the use of oxygen in both chronic and acute on chronic COPD

NA, Not applicable.

Use of Large-Bore IV Needles for Blood Administration

Administration of packed red blood cells (PRBCs) is often a life-sustaining measure for patients to replace lost blood or treat symptomatic anemia (Makic et al., 2013). The size of the intravenous catheter traditionally was believed to influence the delivery of PRBCs; it was thought that smaller-bore catheters (e.g., 22-gauge needle or smaller) result in slower infusion rates and cell hemolysis. The common misperception, or sacred cow, is the belief that it is necessary to insert the largest-bore intravenous catheter possible to administer PRBCs to avoid destruction of cells through the administration process (Table 18.2).

TABLE 18.2   Catheter Gauge Recommendations and Blood Product Infusion Based on American Association of Blood Banks Practice Guidelines

Gauge of Intravenous Catheter	Description
22–14	Acceptable for transfusion of cellular blood components in adults (catheter size may need to be adjusted for rate of infusion)
24°22	Acceptable for transfusion of cellular blood components in infants and toddlers (may require infusion through pump or syringe)

(Based on information from Roback, J.M.D., Combs, M.K., Grossman B., Hillyer, C. (2008). The AABB technical manual: Chapter 21 (p. 615). Hoboken, NJ: Blackwell Publishing.)

Changing Peripheral IV Catheter Sites Every 72 to 96 Hours

The most common, minimally invasive hospital procedure performed worldwide is the insertion of peripheral IV catheters (Wu & Casella, 2013). Over 200 million peripheral IVs are inserted each year in the United States (Hadaway, 2012). Routine institutional policy requires replacement of peripheral IV sites every 72 to 96 hours. In a critical appraisal of the evidence, compared with routine replacement, replacing PIV sites when clinically indicated resulted in no greater rates of PIV complications including phlebitis, infiltration, catheter-related bloodstream infections, occlusion, accidental removal, infusion failure, or in-hospital mortality (Gilton, Seymour, & Baker, 2019; Morrison & Holt, 2015). In addition to not being harmful, changing PIV sites only when clinically indicated resulted in decreased costs, reduction in resource utilization, and happier patients (Bolton, 2015).

Evaluating practice and continually questioning "why" should become a norm in every nurse's practice.

DECISION-MAKING MODEL

EBP is a decision-making model based on the "conscientious, explicit and judicious use of current best practice in making decisions about the care of individual or groups of patients" (Sackett, Rosenberg, Gray, Haynes, & Richardson, 1996). "This practice requires the integration of individual clinical expertise with the best available external clinical evidence from systematic research, available resources, and our patient's unique values and circumstances" (Sackett et al. 1996). This definition requires nurses to carefully and thoroughly integrate evidence into their practice.

This new paradigm of EBP requires the development of a clinical inquiry approach. Nurses must ask ourselves the following questions and not blindly accept standard practice (Salmon, 2007):

- Why are we doing it this way?
- Is there a better way to do this?
- What is the evidence to support what we are doing?
- What practice guidelines support this practice?
- Would doing this be as effective as doing that?
- What constitutes best practice?

MODELS OF EVIDENCE-BASED PRACTICE

There are numerous models of EBP. These models are the following:

- The Iowa Model of Evidence-Based Practice to Promote Quality Care
- Johns Hopkins Nursing Evidence-Based Practice Model
- Stetler Model of Research Utilization
- ACE Star Model of Knowledge Transformation
- ARCC Model: Advancing Research and Clinical Practice Through Close Collaboration Model

The ACE Star Model of Knowledge Transformation is depicted as a five-point star defining the following forms of knowledge:

Point 1: Discovery, representing primary research studies;

Point 2: Evidence Summary, which is the synthesis of all available knowledge compiled into a single harmonious statement, such as a systematic review;

Point 3: Translation into action, often referred to as evidence-based clinical practice guidelines, combining the evidential base and expertise to extend recommendations;

Point 4: Integration into practice is evidence-in-action, in which practice is aligned to reflect best evidence; and

Point 5: Evaluation, which is an inclusive view of the impact of EBP on patient health outcomes, satisfaction, efficacy and efficiency of care, and health policy (Stevens, 2013).

EVIDENCE-BASED PRACTICE

EBP consists of five steps (Strauss, 2005):
1. Ask a searchable clinical question
2. Find the best evidence to answer the question
3. Appraise the evidence
4. Apply the evidence with clinical expertise, taking the patient's wants/needs into consideration
5. Evaluate the effectiveness and efficiency of the process

Question Formulation

The first thing you will need to do is to formulate the question. Defining and narrowing down the problem is very important. As nurses, we often decide on an intervention before we adequately define the problem. The first step in EBP is to identify either a problem-focused trigger or a knowledge-focused trigger that will initiate the need for change. A problem-focused trigger could be a clinical problem or a risk management issue; knowledge triggers might be new research findings or a new practice guideline (Dontje, 2007). Patient outcomes are a perfect starting point.

As nurses, we make numerous decisions when caring for our patients. As we make these decisions we are influenced by a number of factors (Craig & Smyth, 2002):

- Clinical expertise
- Beliefs, attitudes
- Routine (tradition)
- Organizational factors
- State and federal policies
- Regulatory factors
- Funding
- Time
- Factors related to the patient
- Clinical circumstances
- Preferences, beliefs, attitudes, and needs

Up-to-date, valid evidence needs to be integrated with these factors to maximize the likelihood of what we want to happen (the outcome). The more explicit the question, the easier it is to run searches through the multiple electronic databases available to nurses (CINAHL, MEDLINE, and Cochrane). For example, you are interested in determining best practice for end-of-shift reports. If you enter "end-of-shift report" into the search line, you will receive 56 references. If you narrow the search to within the past 5 years, the number of references is cut to 32. A focused question makes your search strategy much easier. It is helpful for any nurse working in a hospital to develop a good relationship

with the hospital librarian, who will assist you in the gathering of research evidence (Table 18.3).

Reliable Evidence

Once you have focused your question, you need to select the best evidence. Just because something has been published either in print or on the Internet, it does not mean it is a valid source of evidence. You must first determine the reliability of the source. Your librarian will assist you in this. A research study on urinary catheters funded by the company that makes urinary catheters may not be

TABLE 18.3	Resources for Forms of Knowledge in the Star Model
Form of Knowledge	**Description of Resources**
Point 1: Discovery	Bibliographic databases such as CINAHL—provide single research reports, in most cases, multiple reports.
Point 2: Evidence Summary	Cochrane Collaboration Database of Systematic Reviews—provides reports of rigorous systematic reviews on clinical topics. See www.cochrane.org/
Point 3: Translation into Guidelines	National Guidelines Clearinghouse—sponsored by the Agency for Healthcare Research and Quality (AHRQ), provides online access to evidence-based clinical practice guidelines. See www.guideline.gov
Point 4: Integration into Practice	AHRQ health care innovations exchange—sponsored by AHRQ, provides profiles of innovations, and tools for improving care processes, including adoption guidelines and information to contact the innovator. See http://innovations.ahrq.gov/
Point 5: Evaluation of Process and Outcome	National quality measures clearinghouse—sponsored by AHRQ, provides detailed information on quality measures and measure sets. See http://qualitymeasures.ahrq.gov/

(From Stevens, K. (2013). The impact of evidence-based practice in nursing and the next big ideas. *OJIN: The Online Journal of Issues in Nursing*, 18(2).)

the most reliable source of evidence; a study supporting their catheter is in the company's best interest. The first question in your critical appraisal of the evidence is whether or not this study is good enough to use the findings. You will be attempting to determine whether the quality of the study is good enough for you to use the results in the design of a nursing protocol. You would need to look at the research design, the sample, and the sample size. Obviously, results from a study directed at children may not be appropriate in the design of a protocol addressed to adults. Also, a study with a sample size of four will not carry as much strength as will a study with a sample size of 1000. Some research designs are more powerful than others. The fact that some studies are more powerful than others has given rise to the hierarchy of evidence (Peto, 1993). The hierarchy of evidence for questions about effectiveness of an intervention follows (Polit & Beck, 2013):

Level 1
   a. Systematic review of randomized controlled trials
   b. Systematic review of **nonrandomized trials**
Level 2
   a. Single randomized controlled trial
   b. **Single nonrandomized trial**
Level 3: Systematic review of **correlational/observational studies**
Level 4: Single correlational/observational study
Level 5: Systematic review of descriptive/qualitative/physiologic studies
Level 6: Single **descriptive**/qualitative/physiologic **study**
Level 7: Opinions of authorities, expert committees

Fig. 18.1 shows an example of an evidence-based pyramid.

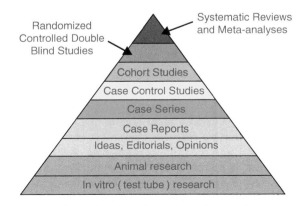

Fig. 18.1 Example of evidence-based pyramid.

There will be differences in the actual numbers associated with the varying levels of evidence depending on the model used. You need to become knowledgeable about the model used in your institution.

Critical Appraisal

The next question to ask in your critical appraisal is whether or not the findings are applicable to your setting. The patients used in a study will never be identical to yours, but there may be similarities. The following questions can be asked to determine applicability of the study to your practice area:

- Is it clear what the study is about?
- Is the sample/context adequately described?
- Are my patients/contexts so different that the results will not apply?
- Is the intervention available, or is the change possible in my setting?
- Do the benefits of the change for my patient/context outweigh the costs?
- Are the patients' values and preferences satisfied by change?

Part of this question will be to ask what these results mean for your patients.

POPULATION, INTERVENTION, COMPARISON INTERVENTION, OUTCOME

A framework for formulating evidence-based questions is PICOT (**p**opulation, **i**ntervention, **c**omparison intervention, **o**utcome, time). Box 18.1 describes the focus of the **p**opulation, **i**ntervention, **c**omparison intervention, **o**utcome (PICO) question.

The last step in the implementation of any change is the monitoring of outcomes. Was the EBP change successful? And are the outcomes sustained over time?

In health care organizations, there may be many triggers that initiate the need for change. They can be data-driven, resulting from performance review data, risk management data, benchmarking data, and financial data, or they can be knowledge-driven, resulting from new research findings, change in regulatory guidelines and standards, or questions from practitioners.

As a nurse manager, your role will be in the promotion and implementation of EBP in your organization. The algorithm of the Iowa Model of Evidence-Based

BOX 18.1   Focus of the PICOT (Population, Intervention, Comparison Intervention, Outcome, Time) Question

Patient or **P**opulation	Define who or what the question is about. Tip: Describe a group of patients similar to yours.
Intervention	Describe the intervention, test, or exposure that you are interested in. An intervention is a planned course of action. An exposure is something that happens such as a fall, anxiety, exposure to house mites, etc. Tip: Describe what it is that you are considering doing or what has happened to the patient.
Comparison intervention (if any)	Describe the alternate intervention. Tip: Describe the alternative that can be compared with the intervention.
Outcomes	Define the important outcomes, beneficial or harmful. Tip: Define what you are hoping to achieve or avoid.
Time	Over what period of time will this happen?

(Adapted from Craig, J., & Smyth, R. (2002). *The evidence-based manual practice manual for nurses* (p. 30). Edinburgh: Churchill Livingstone.)

Practice provides a visual representation of the development of EBP in a clinical facility (Fig. 18.2).

As a summary, EBP can be used as a guide for implementing a research-based protocol. The steps in this model are to do the following:
- Synthesize relevant research
- Determine the sufficiency of the research base for use in practice
- Pilot the change in practice
- Institute the change in practice
- Monitor outcomes (Chapter 18)

RESEARCH USE

EBP differs from research use. **Research use** is the process of using research-generated knowledge to make an impact on or a change in existing practices (Burns, Grove, & Gray, 2018). EBP requires synthesizing research study findings to determine best research evidence. Research evidence is a synthesis of high-quality, relevant studies to form a body of empirical knowledge for the selected area of practice. The best research evidence is then integrated with clinical expertise and patient values and needs to deliver quality, cost-effective care (Sackett, Straus, Richardson, Rosenberg, & Haynes, 2000).

RESEARCH

Research is the systematic investigation, testing, and evaluation designed to generate new knowledge or to contribute to generalizable knowledge (adapted from U.S. Department of Health and Human Services, 2009). There is now a focus on patient-centered outcomes research (PCOR). As evidence mounted on standard medical metrics (mortality and morbidity), it was noted that metrics and outcomes of particular interest to patients and families (such as quality of life) were understudied. Thus attention is now drawn to the need to produce evidence on patient-centered outcomes from the perspective of the patient.

Research is critical to the growth of any profession, and in nursing it is mandatory for the continued improvements in patient care. The Iowa Model offers a visualization of how a clinical inquiry brought by a nurse may develop into a research project. In reviewing and appraising the evidence, the nurse may find that there is little or no published information about the clinical inquiry. This will then lead to the development of research. Health care institutions that are centers of excellence will have infrastructures and resources available for nurses interested in pursuing research.

A first step for any nurse interested in research is to join the nursing research committee at the institution. Such research committees are part of the shared governance structures within the nursing departments (see Chapter 6). A novice nurse may assist in an ongoing research project as step one and gradually increase research responsibilities as he or she matures in

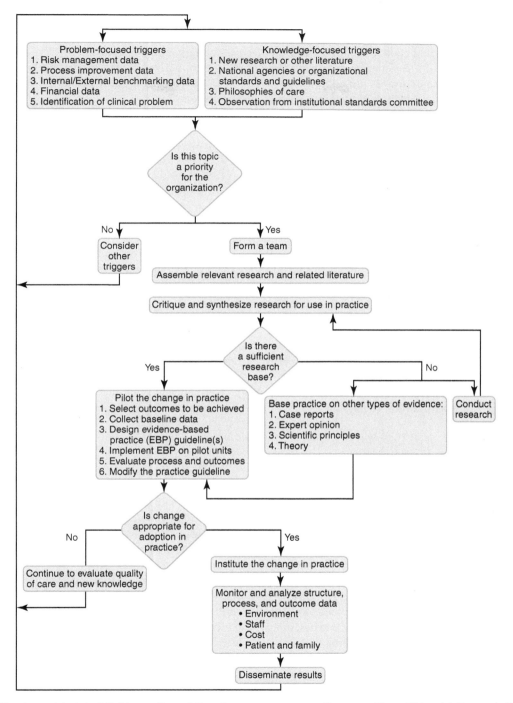

Fig. 18.2 The Iowa Model of Evidence-Based Practice to promote quality care. (From Titler, M.G., et al. [2001]. The Iowa Model of Evidence-Based Practice to promote quality care. *Crit Care Nurs Clin of North Am, 13*[4], 497–509; reprinted from Burns, N., & Grove, S. K. [2007]. *Understanding nursing research: Building an evidence-based practice*, (p. 514). St. Louis: Saunders Elsevier.)

professional responsibilities. Another important step is to continually ask those clinical questions that come to mind. This constant spirit of clinical inquiry is what differentiates the nurse with a passion for improving care from the nurse who sees nursing as "just a job."

The following is the Magnet (American Nurses Credentialing Center ANCC, 2019, pp. 61–63) template for the communication of research across the institution.

Study Overview
- Title of study
- IRB approval date and type of review (i.e., full board, exempt, expedited)
- Study start date
- Study completion date

Research Team
- Nurses at the organization who are the principal investigators (PI), co-PI, or the site PI involved in the conduct of the study
- Other key personnel on research team

Study Aims
- Study purpose, what new knowledge will be generated, or both

Significance of the Literature Review (two pages maximum)
- Key references to support the significance
- Why the study is important to nursing

- What is currently known about the topic, if an intervention study, what evidence supports the intervention or innovation
- Summarize the gap in current knowledge about the topic being addressed by the study

Innovation
- How the study will produce actionable information for nursing

Sample Description
- Type of sample (convenience, cohort, random)
- Inclusion and exclusion criteria
- Sample size

Location of Study (within the applicant organization)
- Hospital unit(s), ambulatory care area

Study Procedures
- Procedures from initial screening through end of contact with subjects
- Data collection methods

Results
- Results of data analysis (description of sample characteristics and analysis for research question or hypotheses)

Discussion
- Discussion and interpretation of the findings
- Implications of the findings and recommendations to the organization

SUMMARY

As a new nurse entering the profession, it is imperative that you maintain currency within your profession. Here are some strategies for using research evidence in your own practice:

- Read widely and critically: Professionally accountable nurses keep abreast of their practice by reading journals relating to their practice.
- Join a professional organization related to your specialty: Many innovations in practice and best practices are shared through professional organizations.
- Attend professional conferences and continuing education seminars.

- Participate in evidence-based projects.
- Participate in nursing research.
- Always assume that it can be done better.
- Focus on the triple aim: delivery of effective, efficient, and patient-centered care.

The IOM report (Institute of Medicine IOM, 2003) stated that as a core competency nurses must employ EBP, integrate best research with clinical expertise and patient values for optimum care, and participate in learning and research activities to the extent feasible.

CLINICAL CORNER

What Works: Innovation Tip Sheet

Innovation is a term that we hear constantly in all fields from health care to business to technology. But what does innovation *really* mean?

Innovation Defined

Innovation can be defined as the intentional introduction and application within a role, group, or organization of ideas, processes, products, or procedures new to the relevant unit of adoption, designed to significantly benefit the individual, the group, or wider society.

This definition is largely accepted because it captures the most important characteristics of innovation:
a. novelty
b. an application component
c. an intended benefit

More generally, innovation can be defined as a new method and/or practice device. It is an idea, practice, or object that is perceived as new by an individual or other unit of adoption.

Innovation in Nursing

It is no surprise that the founder of modern nursing, Florence Nightingale, was also an adept innovator. We all know that nurses are creative and get the job done no matter what. The American Nurses Association Scope and Standards of Practice (2015) reinforced innovation as essential to nursing's history and future, calling on all nurses to be leaders within the profession by working to influence policies and encourage innovation.

Although innovation, as a concept, is not new to the nursing profession, the term "nursing innovation" does not seem to be universally defined. A proposed working definition of nursing innovation is nursing professionals utilizing their acquired knowledge and skills to creatively develop new ways of working, drawing on technologies, systems, theories, and associated partners/stakeholders to further enhance and evaluate nursing practice.

Innovation in Practice

Nursing innovation is a fundamental driver of progress for health care systems around the world. Nurses work in a variety of settings with all types of patients, families, communities, and our interprofessional partners. This global perspective enables nurses to provide innovative solutions to the challenges and demands of health care delivery. Innovation in nursing care continues to be an accelerating force seeking to balance cost containment and health care quality. It is considered a critical component of business productivity and competitive survival.

Innovation in Nursing Leadership

Navigating Innovation: Acting as Validators
Leaders at the Helm: Acting as Influencers
Leading in Disruption: Acting as Strategic Advisors

Tips to Innovation: Questions to Consider

1. Does the innovation fit?
   - What is the innovation?
   - Does it further our goals?
   - Is it compatible with our organization?
2. Should we do it here?
   - What are the potential benefits? Costs?
   - Can we build a business case?
   - What are the risks?
3. Can we do it here?
   - Are we ready for this change?
   - What changes will we have to make?
   - Do we have the ingredients for success?
4. How will we do it here?
   - How will we measure the impact of the innovation?
   - Can we try the innovation first?
   - How will we implement the innovation?

(AHRQ, 2011)

TIPS for Selection of an Innovation

1. Select a concept (interesting, relevant, important, useful)
2. Determine the aims or purpose of the analysis (to distinguish between ordinary and scientific usage of the same concept, to clarify meaning of an existing concept, to develop an operational definition, to develop on operational definition, to add to existing theory, etc.)
3. Identify all uses of concept (sources, all uses of the term, in all fields)
4. Determine the definitional attitudes
5. Identify
   a. A model case
   b. Borderline cases, related cases, contrary cases, invented cases, illegitimate cases
   c. Antecedents, consequences
6. Define empirical reference

Examples from Practice

Role of the Registered Nurse	Practice
Admission nurse	Sepsis bundle
Nurse navigator	Cauti bundle
Discharge nurse	VAP bundle

CLINICAL CORNER—cont'd

Role of the Registered Nurse	Practice	Role of the Registered Nurse	Practice
Patient safety investigators	TCAB initiatives	Mobilization nurse	Mentorship program
Resource nurse	Hourly rounding	Nurse scribe	Leadership rounds
Pivot nurse	Antibiotic stewardship	Clinical leadership (DNP)	Nurse residency program

Agency for Healthcare Research and Quality. (n.d.). AHRQ health care innovations exchange. Retrieved from https://innovations.ahrq.gov/.
(From Agency for Healthcare Research and Quality [AHRQ]. (2011). Will it work here? A decisionmaker's guide to adopting innovations. Retrieved from https://innovations.ahrq.gov/qualitytools/will-it-work-here-decisionmakers-guide-adopting-innovations.
American Nurses Association. (2015). Nursing: Scope and standards of practice (3rd ed.). Silver Spring, MD. ANCC.
American Nurses Credentialing Center. (2017). 2019 Magnet® application manual. Silver Spring, MD. ANCC.
Centers for Disease Control and Prevention. (2009). Guidelines for prevention of catheter-associated urinary tract infections. Retrieved from https://www.cdc.gov/infectioncontrol/pdf/guidelines/cauti-guidelines-H.pdf.

EVIDENCE-BASED PRACTICE

Nearly 20 years ago, it was determined that the average time for scientific evidence to be translated into practice is 17 years. These observations have led to the development of translation and implementation science, which aims to reduce delays and understand what factors facilitate the successful adoption and implementation of new knowledge into practice.

There are various EBP implementation models, frameworks, and theories that have been developed in implementation science to advance EBP and expedite uptake of evidence into real-world settings. The approaches were categorized as models that guide the process and steps of moving research into practice, frameworks for understanding and exploring factors that influence implementation, classic theories explain change processes, specific implementation models, and evaluation frameworks.

Process Models

Process models take an action or application approach. Example: The *Iowa EBP Model* was developed and originally implemented at the Iowa Hospitals and Clinics to serve as a guide to help nurses identify methods appropriate in the improvement of patient care. The *Advancing Research and Clinical Practice through Close Collaboration* developed by Melynk begins with an organizational assessment of EBP readiness, emphasizes EBP mentors, and promotes changing beliefs and skills about EBP.

Determinants and Evaluation Frameworks

These frameworks emphasize specific factors or characteristics that will improve the uptake of evidence into practice. They aim to improve adherence to guidelines or EBPs by leveraging enabling factors and minimizing barriers. Example: *The Promoting Action on Research Implementation in Health Services* emphasizes the characteristics of the evidence, the context for the adoption of the evidence, and the facilitation that promotes the EBP initiative and implementation strategies. Another example: *The Consolidated Framework for Implementation Research* addresses the gap between what research trails have shown to work and what actually occurs in real practice settings.

Implementation and Classic Theories

Implementation theories were developed to advance knowledge about best strategies and processes for promoting evidence uptake. They build on classic (social cognitive theory, diffusion of innovation) and change theories from other fields. Example: *The Transtheoretical Model (TTM)*, also known as *Stages of Change Model*, proposes that people move through a series of stages when modifying behavior. The stages identified are precontemplation (not ready), contemplation (getting ready), preparation with plan (ready), action (moving forward), maintenance (managing and preventing drift), and termination (when appropriate).

Implementation is a major step in the EBP process, but it is often overlooked and not fully evaluated post implementation. The sustaining of the action plans and outcomes are necessary to determine adherence to the practice change and to prevent practice drift back to less than required outcomes.

(From Tucker, S. (2019). Implementation: The linchpin of evidence-based changes. Take a strategic approach to translating research into practice. *American Nurse Today, 14*(3), 8–13.)

NCLEX® EXAMINATION QUESTIONS

1. Quality issues in patient care came to the forefront when there were two sentinel publications by the Institute of Medicine (IOM), *To Err Is Human* and *Crossing the Quality Chasm* (Institute of Medicine [IOM], 2000, 2001). Which of the following occurred?
   A. A shift from traditional paradigm of clinical practice and pathophysiology
   B. A shift to best practices and scientific evidence
   C. The use of evidence-based practice only
   D. The use of research only

2. Evidence-based practice can be used as a guide for implementing a research-based protocol. The steps in this model are to synthesize relevant research, determine the sufficiency of the research base for use in practice, pilot the change in practice, institute the change in practice, and monitor outcomes. What will the nurse need to know when implementing the process?
   A. That change will meet resistance
   B. That change will be easy
   C. That change is always welcome in the best practice as a nurse
   D. That change is the first step in the process

3. The vision for the future of nursing in *The Future of Nursing* report (Institute of Medicine IOM, 2011) focuses on the convergence of knowledge, quality, and new functions in nursing. The recommendation is that nurses:
   A. Lead interprofessional teams in improving delivery systems and care
   B. Bring to the forefront the necessity for new competencies
   C. Use knowledge in clinical decision making and producing research evidence on interventions that promote uptake and use by individual providers and groups of providers
   D. All of the above

4. Evidence-based practice consists of five steps (Strauss, 2005): ask a searchable clinical question, find the best evidence to answer the question, appraise the evidence, apply the evidence with clinical expertise, take the patient's wants/needs into consideration, evaluate the effectiveness and efficiency of the process. Although each step is important, which step is key?
   A. Ask a searchable clinical question
   B. Take the patient's wants/needs into consideration

C. Appraise the evidence
D. Evaluate the effectiveness

5. As a new nurse you may find resistance from "seasoned" nurses regarding patient care. If this should occur, what would you do?
   A. Explain evidence-based practice regarding patient care
   B. Report the nurse to the charge nurse immediately
   C. Do it the way the "seasoned" nurse does it
   D. Say you will do it your way and she can do it her way

6. When the new nurse is attending new employee orientation, he or she will be in an all-inclusive orientation with other new hires. Nurses then have an orientation of nursing. At this time the nurse is informed of policies, protocols, and procedures and is with a preceptor on the unit. If a patient needs insertion of a foley catheter, for example, the nurse should:
   A. Have the preceptor observe you doing the procedure
   B. Review the protocol for foley insertion
   C. Explain the procedure to the patient
   D. All of the above

7. Health care institutions that are centers of excellence will have infrastructures and resources available for nurses interested in pursuing research. One can join the nursing research committee. A novice nurse may assist in an ongoing research project. Barriers for the new nurse would be:
   A. Being overwhelmed in first nursing position
   B. Being hired at an institution that is not a "Magnet" facility
   C. Feeling insecure
   D. All of the above

8. The National Patient Safety Goals:
   A. Form the basis of all process improvement activities
   B. Are a nationwide initiative
   C. Are mandated by the Institute of Medicine (IOM)
   D. Will improve patient safety

9. One model of quality is FOCUS PDCA (Plan-Do-Check-Act). The U stands for:
   A. Understand the causes of variance in the process
   B. Underlying causes for assessment
   C. Unlikely reason for a variance
   D. Understand the end result of the process improvement

10. Nurses need to know the outcomes that directly affect their unit. Common outcomes for all units are:
    A. Infection rates
    B. Patient satisfaction
    C. Performance on The Joint Commission Core Measures
    D. All of the above

11. Two of the common vendor satisfaction measures are:
    A. Press Ganey and Gallup
    B. Press Ganey and The Joint Commission
    C. Gallup and Occupational Safety and Health Administration (OSHA)
    D. Gallup and National Institute of Occupational Safety and Health (NIOSH)

12. Organizations that recognize "best practice" are:
    A. American Nurses Association
    B. American Nurses Credentialing Center Magnet Status
    C. Malcolm Baldrige National Quality Award
    D. Press-Ganey Questionnaire

13. Which of the following is not one of W. Edwards Deming's 14-point management philosophy?
    A. Institute training on the job
    B. Cease dependence on inspection to achieve quality
    C. Adopt the new philosophy
    D. Begin the practice of awarding business on the basis of price tag

14. A goal of organizational learning is to make learning:
    A. The end product of all data collection
    B. Part of all activities within the organization
    C. Required of all employees in clinical positions
    D. Match the goals of The Joint Commission (TJC)

15. "Lean" refers to:
    A. The attempt to make do with the smallest amount possible
    B. A type of financial arrangement in which dollars are saved
    C. Getting rid of waste in all work processes
    D. The streamlining of all patient processes for cost saving

16. A root-cause analysis:
    A. Focuses on risk management
    B. Is a Six Sigma model
    C. Determines process variation
    D. Is a prospective review

17. Six Sigma is a model of quality focusing on:
    A. Process development
    B. Improving performance
    C. Decreasing the process variation
    D. Statistical analysis

Answers: 1. B   2. A   3. D   4. A   5. D   6. D
7. B   8. C   9. C   10. C

REFERENCES

American Nurses Credentialing Center [ANCC]. (2019). *The 2019 Magnet application manual.* Silver Spring, MD: ANCC.

American Nurses Credentialing Center [ANCC] (2019). *Magnet application manual (pp. 61–63).* Silver Spring, MD: ANCC.

Bolton, D. (2015). Clinically indicated replacement of peripheral cannulas. *MA Healthcare Limited, 2015 Therapy Supplement, 24,* S4–12.

Burns, N., & Grove, S. K. (2007). *Understanding nursing research: building an evidence-based practice* (pp. 515–517) (4th ed.). St. Louis: Saunders Elsevier.

Burns, N., Grove, S., & Gray, J. (2018). *The practice of nursing research* (8th ed.). St. Louis: Saunders Elsevier.

Craig, J., & Smyth, R. (2002). *The evidence-based manual practice manual for nurses.* Edinburgh: Churchill Livingstone.

Crossley, D. J., McGuire, G. P., Barrow, P. M., & Houston, P. L. (1997). Influence of inspired oxygen concentration on dead space, respiratory drive, and $Paco_2$ in intubated patients with chronic obstructive pulmonary disease. *Critical Care Medicine, 25*(9), 1522–1526.

Dick, C. R., Liu, Z., Sassoon, C. S., Berry, R. B., & Mahutte, C. K. (1997). O_2-induced change in ventilation and ventilatory drive in COPD. *American Journal of Respiratory Critical Care Medicine, 155*(2), 609–614.

Dontje, K. (2007). Evidence-based practice: Understanding the process. *Topics in Advanced Practice Nursing, 7*(4).

Easton, P. A., Slykerman, L. J., & Anthonisen, N. R. (1986). Ventilatory response to sustained hypoxia in normal adults. *Journal of Applied Physiology, 61,* 906–911.

Estabrooks, C. (1998). Will evidence-based nursing practice make practice perfect? *Canadian Journal of Nursing Research, 30*(1), 15–36.

Gilton, L., Seymour, A., & Baker, R. (2019). Changing peripheral intravenous sites when clinically indicated:

An evidence-based practice journey. *Worldviews on Evidence-Based Nursing, 16*(5). https://doi.org/10.1111/wvn.12385.

Global Initiative for Chronic Obstructive Lung Disease (GOLD). (2009). *Global strategy for the diagnosis, management, and prevention of chronic obstructive pulmonary disease*. Bethesda, MD: Global Initiative for Chronic Obstructive Lung Disease (GOLD).

Hadaway, L. (2012). Short, peripheral intravenous catheters and infections. Infusion Nursing *(Jul-Aug 2012), 35*(4), 230–240.

Institute of Medicine [IOM]. (2000). *To Err is Human: Building a safer health care system*. Washington, DC: National Academy Press.

Institute of Medicine [IOM]. (2001). *Crossing the quality chasm: A new health system for the 21st century*. Washington, DC: National Academy Press.

Institute of Medicine [IOM]. (2003). In A. C. Greiner & E. Knebel (Eds.), *Health professions education: A bridge to quality*. Washington, DC: National Academies Press.

Institute of Medicine [IOM]. (2011). *The future of nursing: Leading change, advancing health [prepared by Robert Wood Johnson Foundation Committee Initiative on the Future of Nursing]*. Washington, DC: National Academies Press.

Makic, M., Martin, S., Burns, S., Philbrick, D., & Rauen, C. (2013). Putting Evidence into Nursing Practice: four traditional practices not supported by the evidence. *Critical Care Nurse, 33*(2), 28–42.

Melnyk, B., & Fineout-Overholt, E. (2011). *Evidence based practice in nursing and health care: A guide to best practice* (2nd. ed). Philadelphia, PA: Lippincott, Williams & Wilkins.

Melnyk, B. M., Fineout-Overholt, E., Gallagher-Ford, L., & Kaplan, L. (2012). The state of evidence-based practice in US nurses: Critical implications for nurse leaders and educators. *Journal of Nursing Administration, 42*(9), 410–417.

Morrison, K., & Holt, K. (2015). The effectiveness of clinically indicated replacement of peripheral intravenous catheters: An evidence review with implications for clinical practice. *Worldviews on Evidence-Based Nursing, 12*(4), 187–198. https://doi.org/10.1111/wvn.12102.

Wu, M., & Casella, F. (2013). . Is clinically indicated replacement of peripheral catheters as safe as routine replacement in preventing phlebitis and other complications? *(April 2013). Internal and Emergency Medicine, 8*(5).

Patient-Centered Outcomes Research Institute (PCORI). (2013). Mission and vision. www.pcori.org/about/mission-and-vision/.

Peto, R. (1993). Large scale randomized evidence; large sample trials and overview trials. *Annals of the New York Academy of Science, 703*, 314–340.

Pierson, D. J. (2000). Pathophysiology and clinical effects of chronic hypoxia. *Respiratory Care, 45*, 39–51.

Polit, D., & Beck, C. (2013). *Essentials of nursing research: Appraising evidence for nursing practice* (9th ed.). Philadelphia: Lippincott Williams & Wilkins.

Pravikoff, D., Tanner, A., & Pierce, S. (2005). Readiness of US nurses for evidence-based practice. *American Journal of Nursing, 105*(9), 40–51.

Roback, J. M. D., Combs, M. K., Grossman, B., & Hillyer, C. (2008). *The AABB technical manual (chapter 21)* (16th ed, p. 615) Hoboken, NJ: Blackwell Publishing.

Rudolf, M., Banks, R. A., & Semple, S. J. (1977). Hypercapnia during oxygen therapy in acute exacerbations of chronic respiratory failure: Hypothesis revisited. *Lancet, 2*, 483.

Sackett, D., Rosenberg, W., Gray, J., Haynes, R., & Richardson, W. (1996). Evidence-based medicine: what it is and what it is not. *British Medical Journal, 312*, 71–72.

Sackett, D. L., Straus, S. E., Richardson, W. C., Rosenberg, W., & Haynes, R. M. (2000). *Evidence-based medicine: How to practice and teach EBM* (2nd ed.). New York: Churchill Livingstone.

Salmon. S. (2007). Advancing evidence-based practice. *Orthopaedic Nursing, 26*(2), 118.

Singapore Ministry of Health [SMOH]. (2006). *Chronic obstructive pulmonary disease*. Singapore: Singapore Ministry of Health.

Stevens, K. (2013). The Impact of evidence-based practice in nursing and the next big ideas. *OJIN: The Online Journal of Issues in Nursing, 18*(2). Manuscript 4.

Strauss, S. E. (2005). *Evidence-based medicine: How to practice and teach EBM*. New York: Churchill Livingstone.

SUNY Downstate. (2014). Evidence-Based Medicine Tutorial. http://library.downstate.edu/EBM2/2100.htm.

U.S. Department of Health and Human Services. (2009). *Code of Federal Regulations Title 45: Public Welfare Part 46: Protection of Human Subjects, Title 21 Food and Drugs Part 50: Protection of Human Subjects*. Washington, D.C.: HHS.

West, J. B. (2008). *Respiratory physiology: The essentials* (8th ed). Philadelphia, PA: Lippincott Williams & Wilkins.

19

Monitoring Outcomes and the Use of Data for Improvement

OBJECTIVES

- Discuss the importance in using data to drive decisions.
- Interpret visual representations of performance outcomes.

- Compare levels of performance to benchmark.
- Identify the requirements for presenting improvement initiatives.

KEY TERMS

benchmark comparison information that allows an organization to evaluate its own performance in relation to others

dashboard visual representation of performance using colors to represent levels, usually green (on target) or red (below target)

graph visual representation of levels of performance

trend three data points moving in same direction

In Chapter 17 the improvement of patient care was discussed, and in the Chapter 18 the use of evidence-based practice (EBP) was reviewed. One final and very important step in each of these processes is the continued monitoring of outcomes. To evaluate the success of an EBP practice change, we need to know the levels of performance before the implementation of the changes and after the changes. As nurses we need to be cognizant of the outcomes of our professional practice at all times.

The Institute of Medicine (IOM, 2003) suggested a core competency of nurses should be able to apply quality improvement; identify errors and hazards in care; understand and implement basic safety design principles, such as standardization and simplification; continually understand and measure quality of care in terms of structure, process, and outcomes in relation to patient and community needs; and design and test interventions to change processes and systems of care, with the objective of improving quality. It is the continual measuring and monitoring of quality outcomes that this chapter will address.

NURSING-SENSITIVE INDICATORS

As stated in Chapter 17, nursing-sensitive indicators reflect the structure, process, and outcomes of nursing care. The structure of nursing care is indicated by the supply of nursing staff, the skill level of the nursing staff, and the education/certification of nursing staff. Process indicators measure aspects of nursing care such as assessment, intervention, and registered nurse (RN) job satisfaction. Patient outcomes that are determined to be nursing sensitive are those that improve if there is a greater quantity or quality of nursing care (e.g., pressure ulcers, falls, infections and intravenous infiltrations). Some patient outcomes are more highly related to other aspects of institutional care, such as medical decisions and institutional policies (e.g., frequency of primary C-sections, cardiac failure, readmissions), and are not considered "nursing sensitive." Performance is usually represented in dashboards or graphs.

Some of the nursing-sensitive indicators are as follows:
- Nursing hours per patient day RN hours per patient day (Structure)
  - Licensed practical/vocational nurse (LPN/LVN) hours per patient day
  - Unlicensed assistive personnel (UAP) hours per patient day
- Staffing based on acuity (Structure)
- Nursing turnover (Structure)
- Nosocomial infections (Outcome)
- Ventilator-associated pneumonia (VAP) (Process and Outcome)
- Central line–associated bloodstream infection (CLABSI) (Outcome)
- Catheter-associated urinary tract infection (CAUTI) (Outcome)
- Patient falls with injury (Process and Outcome)
- Hospital-acquired pressure ulcer rate (stage II and greater) (Process and Outcome)
- Device-related hospital-acquired pressure injury (Process and Outcome)
- Pediatric pain assessment, intervention, reassessment (AIR) cycle
- Pediatric peripheral intravenous infiltration (Outcome)
- Psychiatric physical/sexual assault (Outcome)
- RN education/certification (Structure)
- RN survey (Process and Outcome)
  - Job satisfaction scales
- Staff mix (Structure)
  - RN
  - LPN/LVN
  - UAP
  - Percentage of agency staff

Additional data elements collected:
- Patient population (e.g., adult or pediatric)
- Hospital category (e.g. teaching, nonteaching, etc.)
- Type of unit (critical care, step-down, medical, surgical, combined medical-surgical, rehab, and psychiatric)
- Number of staffed beds designated by the hospital

NATIONAL COMPARISON GROUPS AND REPORTS

The data for these nursing sensitive indicators are collected at the institution and uploaded to the National Database of Nursing Quality Indicators (NDNQI) (American Nurses Credentialing Center [ANCC], 2019). There are approximately 2500 U.S. hospitals participating in this database. The hospitals provide unit level performance data to NDNQI. The large number of participating hospitals allows for comparisons of performance across institutions, divisions, and units. A critical care unit at a large teaching hospital on the East Coast can evaluate their performance with all other critical care units in teaching hospitals. National comparison data for the indicators are grouped based on patient (adult/pediatric), and unit type: critical care, step-down, medical, surgical, combined med-surgical, rehab, psychiatric, and staffed bed size. Teaching and Magnet status is identified as it relates to participating hospitals. The quarterly reports provide the national comparison along with unit performance data trended over eight quarters. The Magnet goal is that hospitals outperform the selected benchmark for a majority of the reporting quarters. This comparison is called benchmarking or comparing performance to other like institutions. Such comparisons also allow hospitals to evaluate their performance in relation to the competition, and to the best performers.

Some of the definitions of the data sets within NDNQI are as follows:
- *Patient falls:* All documented falls, with or without injury, experienced by patients on a unit in a calendar month
- *Patient falls with injury:* All documented patient falls with an injury level of minor or greater
- *Pressure ulcer prevalence:* The total number of patients that have nosocomial (hospital-acquired) stage II or greater pressure ulcers
- *Pressure ulcer incidence*: The total number of patients that have stage II or greater pressure ulcers
- *Skill mix:* Percentage of hours worked by RN, LPN, UAP, and contract staff with patient care responsibilities, by type of unit
- *Nursing care hours per patient day:* The number of productive hours worked by RN nursing staff per patient day, and the number of productive hours worked by nursing staff (RN, LVN, LPN, and UAP) per patient day.

(From https://nursingandndnqi.weebly.com/ndnqi-indicators.html)

Let us look at)

Let us look at pressure ulcers. Pressure ulcers cost $9.1 to $11.6 billion per year in the United States. Cost of individual patient care ranges from $20,900 to $151,700 per pressure ulcer. Medicare estimated in 2007 that each pressure ulcer added $43,180 in costs to a hospital stay. (Agency for Healthcare Research and Quality [AHRQ], 2015). Pressure ulcers occur in up to 23% of patients in long-term and rehabilitation facilities and at an incidence of 10% to 41% in intensive care unit patients. AHRQ reported that nearly 2.5 million individuals are affected by pressure ulcers, and more than 60,000 patients in the United States die each year as a direct result of pressure ulcers. Rates are calculated as follows:

- Prevalence measures the number of patients with pressure ulcers at a certain point or period in time:
  - The numerator will be the number of patients with any pressure ulcer (count for both any ulcer and stage II or greater).
  - Just count patients, not the number of ulcers. Even if a patient has four stage II ulcers, they are only counted once.
  - The denominator is the number of patients on your unit or in your facility during that month.
  - Divide the numerator by the denominator and multiply by 100 to get the percentage.

Example: 17 patients with any pressure ulcer ÷ 183 patients = .093 × 100 = 9.3%

- Incidence measures the number of patients developing new pressure ulcers during a period in time:
  - The numerator will be the number of patients who develop a new pressure ulcer (count all ulcers and those stage II or greater) after admission.
  - Just count patients, not the number of ulcers. Even if a patient has four stage II ulcers, they are only counted once.
  - The denominator is the number of all patients admitted during that time period.
  - Sometimes in calculating incidence rates, studies have excluded patients with an existing pressure ulcer on admission. Neither approach is necessarily better; just be consistent.
  - Divide the numerator by the denominator and multiply by 100 to get the percentage.

Example: 21 patients with a new pressure ulcer ÷ 227 patients = .093 × 100 = 9.3%

(From AHRQ, 2015.)

As stated previously, two types of measures can be monitored: incidence and prevalence rates. Incidence rates provide the most direct evidence of the quality of your care. Therefore, your quality improvement efforts should focus on incidence rates. Prevalence may reflect a single point in time, such as on the first day of each month. This is known as point prevalence. However, it can also reflect a prolonged period of time, such as an entire hospital stay. This is known as period prevalence. Both types of prevalence rates (point and period) include pressure ulcers present on admission, in addition to new ulcers that developed while in your facility or on your unit. Therefore, they can provide a useful snapshot of the pressure ulcer burden of care on the staff, but they say less about your quality of preventive care than do incidence rates (AHRQ, 2015).

The majority of this information is presented to the staff in graph format. The frequency of reporting varies according to the information, the monitoring timeline of the organization, and the frequency of assessment. Most institutions look at financial outcomes on a daily or weekly basis. Patient satisfaction may be monitored weekly, monthly, or quarterly. The NDNQI unit-based outcomes are reported on a quarterly basis, with the nurse satisfaction data reported annually.

In reviewing graphs that represent performance, the nurse needs to be able to:

1. Recognize the current level of performance,
2. Determine the relationship of the current level to the strategic goal of the organization/department,
3. Compare performance to professional comparisons, and
4. Determine whether an improvement is required.

This representation of outcomes demonstrates eight quarters of performance. (Insert graph from ANCC Manual, 2019 p 53). The benchmark is listed at the bottom of the graph. With pressure ulcers, the goal is fewer than the benchmark. With outcomes such as patient satisfaction, the goal is to be above the benchmark. The nurses will need to identify the concerns and necessary process or evidence-based changes. If this graph was representing pressure injuries, Unit A was below the benchmark for four of eight quarters. Unit B was below the benchmark for only four of eight quarters.

The challenge with such dashboards is that the performance levels are made available to staff quarterly, and not in "real time." This may preclude rapid process improvement. Many institutions prioritize items such as infections, patient satisfaction, and falls, and review performance on a daily level. It is not uncommon to see units bragging about levels of performance with signs such as "200 days without an infection," or "125 days without a fall" posted on the performance board. On such units, when an event occurs, a "huddle" is called, usually within 15 minutes, to review the event and to determine actions that need to be implemented immediately so that future occurrences can be prevented. However, it is important that lessons learned from the huddle are shared with the performance-improvement representatives on the unit.

A sample of a postfall huddle.

Post-Fall Huddle Guidelines

Date: _____ Time of fall: _____ Time of huddle: _____ Room #: _____ SHIFT *(circle one)*: D/PM/NOC

Diagnosis: _____ Pertinent medical Hx: _____

LOCATION of FALL:

☐ Bed/ Bedside Commode   ☐ Chair   ☐ Gurney   ☐ Hallway   ☐ Room   ☐ Restroom

☐ Other: _____

BACKGROUND: Fall risk factors / risk for injury *(check all that apply)*:

☐ Altered mental status	☐ Pain or discomfort: Location	☐ Age (>85)
☐ Dizziness/lightheadedness	☐ Diagnosis r/t *(Hypoglycemia/ Seizure/Hypotension/Parkinson/Dementia)*	☐ Prior fall history
☐ Change in vital signs	☐ Bones*(Osteoporosis)*	☐ Impaired communication
☐ Medications *(Benzodiazipines, Pain meds, B/P meds, hypnotics)*	☐ Surgery*(recent/Fracture/amputee)*	☐ New infection or illness
☐ SOB	☐ Physical condition *(poor balance, weakness)(equipment)*	☐ Environmental factors
☐ Anticoagulation	☐ Sensory or neural deficit	☐ Other: _____
☐ s/p OD or intoxication	☐ ETOH use	

Information Related to Fall Event	FINDINGS
1. Was patient on fall precaution?	_____ YES _____ NO
2. Most recent fall-risk assessment score?	
3. Was patient alone at the time of fall?	_____ YES _____ NO
4. Describe in patient's own words what they were dong prior to fall.	
5. Elimination problems : (_____ urgency; _____ diarrhea, _____ incontinence)	_____ YES _____ NO

TYPE of FALL	DESCRIPTION
A. _____ Accidental fall	_____ Slip _____ Trip
B. _____ Anticipated physiological fall related to: _____ loss of balance _____ impaired gait or mobility _____ impaired cognition/confusion _____ impaired vision _____ functional deficits _____ disease process _____ unrealistic assessment of their ability	
C. _____ Unanticipated physiological fall *(created by condition that cannot be predicted, e.g., unexpected orthostasis, extreme hypoglycemia, stroke or heart attack)*.	
D. _____ Intentional fall: *(Patient who voluntarily alters body position to lower level)*.	

NURSING OBSERVATION/ASSESSMENT	FINDINGS
Neuro checks: Glasgow Coma Scale: _____	_____ Changes in MS *(Mental Status)* _____ Headache _____ Vomiting _____ Bleeding
Did patient hit his/her head?	_____ YES _____ NO
Fall witnessed?	_____ YES _____ NO
What were the provider's findings and orders?	__ Injury __ Pain __ Functional change __ Other:

ACTION/RECOMMENDATION/PREVENTATIVE MEASURES

_____ Assistive device *(e.g., walker, cane)*   _____ Hip protectors   _____ PT/OT evaluation

_____ Bed alarm   _____ Non-skid socks   _____ Removed clutter/ equipment

_____ Close observation   _____ Moved patient *(higher visibility)*   _____ Toileting plan

_____ Behavioral management plan   _____ Pain management assessment

Follow–up Plan: *(Free text new interventions or family to prevent further falls).*

Print and signature (RN/LVN): _____

*(www.visn8.va.gov/visn8/.../**falls**team/**postfallhuddle**_guideline.docx)*

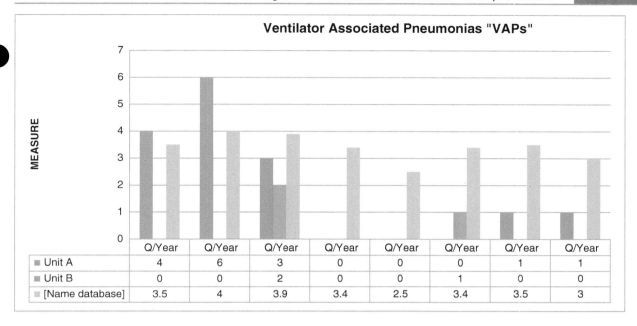

Ventilator Associated Pneumonias "VAPs"

	Q/Year	Q/Year	Q/Year	Q/Year	Q/Year	Q/Year	Q/Year	Q/Year
Unit A	4	6	3	0	0	0	1	1
Unit B	0	0	2	0	0	1	0	0
[Name database]	3.5	4	3.9	3.4	2.5	3.4	3.5	3

The NDNQI benchmark for ventilator associated pneumonias is compared with the actual performance of two critical units over eight quarters. Unit A outperformed the benchmark for six of eight quarters, whereas Unit B unperformed the benchmark for five of eight quarters.

The next graph represents performance on one of the CORE measures.

This graph represents a sustained level of performance that exceeds the benchmark comparison. The hospital was above The Joint Commission national

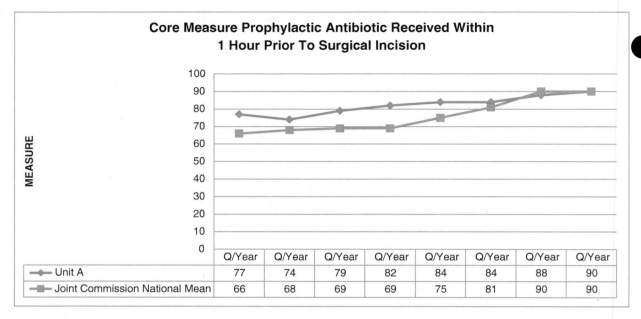

Core Measure Prophylactic Antibiotic Received Within 1 Hour Prior To Surgical Incision

	Q/Year	Q/Year	Q/Year	Q/Year	Q/Year	Q/Year	Q/Year	Q/Year
Unit A	77	74	79	82	84	84	88	90
Joint Commission National Mean	66	68	69	69	75	81	90	90

The graph demonstrates that Unit A outperformed the benchmark six of eight quarters.
When the unit results are the xsame as the benchmark, it is not considered outperforming.

mean (the benchmark) for six of eight quarters. When the unit results are the same as the benchmark, it is not considered outperforming.

The Hospital Consumer Assessment of Healthcare Providers and Systems (HCAHPS) survey is the first national, standardized, publicly reported survey of patients' perspectives of hospital care.

Three broad goals have shaped HCAHPS. First, the survey is designed to produce data about patients' perspectives of care that allow objective and meaningful comparisons of hospitals on topics that are important to consumers. Second, public reporting of the survey results creates new incentives for hospitals to improve quality of care. Third, public reporting serves to enhance accountability in health care by increasing transparency of the quality of hospital care (Centers for Medicare & Medicaid Services [CMS], 2015)

HCAHPS Survey

SURVEY INSTRUCTIONS

◆ You should only fill out this survey if you were the patient during the hospital stay named in the cover letter. Do not fill out this survey if you were not the patient.

◆ Answer <u>all</u> the questions by checking the box to the left of your answer.

◆ You are sometimes told to skip over some questions in this survey. When this happens you will see an arrow with a note that tells you what question to answer next, like this:

☐ Yes
☑ No ➔ *If No, Go to Question 1*

> *You may notice a number on the survey. This number is used to let us know if you returned your survey so we don't have to send you reminders.*
> *Please note: Questions 1-25 in this survey are part of a national initiative to measure the quality of care in hospitals. OMB #0938-0981*

Please answer the questions in this survey about your stay at the hospital named on the cover letter. Do not include any other hospital stays in your answers.

YOUR CARE FROM NURSES

1. **During this hospital stay, how often did nurses treat you with <u>courtesy and respect</u>?**

   ^{1}☐ Never
   ^{2}☐ Sometimes
   ^{3}☐ Usually
   ^{4}☐ Always

2. **During this hospital stay, how often did nurses <u>listen carefully to you</u>?**

   ^{1}☐ Never
   ^{2}☐ Sometimes
   ^{3}☐ Usually
   ^{4}☐ Always

3. **During this hospital stay, how often did nurses <u>explain things</u> in a way you could understand?**

   ^{1}☐ Never
   ^{2}☐ Sometimes
   ^{3}☐ Usually
   ^{4}☐ Always

4. **During this hospital stay, after you pressed the call button, how often did you get help as soon as you wanted it?**

   ^{1}☐ Never
   ^{2}☐ Sometimes
   ^{3}☐ Usually
   ^{4}☐ Always
   ^{9}☐ I never pressed the call button

YOUR CARE FROM DOCTORS

5. **During this hospital stay, how often did doctors treat you with <u>courtesy and respect</u>?**

   ^{1}☐ Never
   ^{2}☐ Sometimes
   ^{3}☐ Usually
   ^{4}☐ Always

6. **During this hospital stay, how often did doctors <u>listen carefully to you</u>?**

   ^{1}☐ Never
   ^{2}☐ Sometimes
   ^{3}☐ Usually
   ^{4}☐ Always

7. **During this hospital stay, how often did doctors <u>explain things</u> in a way you could understand?**

   ^{1}☐ Never
   ^{2}☐ Sometimes
   ^{3}☐ Usually
   ^{4}☐ Always

THE HOSPITAL ENVIRONMENT

8. **During this hospital stay, how often were your room and bathroom kept clean?**

   1 ☐ Never
   2 ☐ Sometimes
   3 ☐ Usually
   4 ☐ Always

9. **During this hospital stay, how often was the area around your room quiet at night?**

   1 ☐ Never
   2 ☐ Sometimes
   3 ☐ Usually
   4 ☐ Always

YOUR EXPERIENCES IN THIS HOSPITAL

10. **During this hospital stay, did you need help from nurses or other hospital staff in getting to the bathroom or in using a bedpan?**

    1 ☐ Yes
    2 ☐ No ➜ If No, Go to Question 12

11. **How often did you get help in getting to the bathroom or in using a bedpan as soon as you wanted?**

    1 ☐ Never
    2 ☐ Sometimes
    3 ☐ Usually
    4 ☐ Always

12. **During this hospital stay, did you need medicine for pain?**

    1 ☐ Yes
    2 ☐ No ➜ If No, Go to Question 15

13. **During this hospital stay, how often was your pain well controlled?**

    1 ☐ Never
    2 ☐ Sometimes
    3 ☐ Usually
    4 ☐ Always

14. **During this hospital stay, how often did the hospital staff do everything they could to help you with your pain?**

    1 ☐ Never
    2 ☐ Sometimes
    3 ☐ Usually
    4 ☐ Always

15. **During this hospital stay, were you given any medicine that you had not taken before?**

    1 ☐ Yes
    2 ☐ No ➜ If No, Go to Question 18

16. **Before giving you any new medicine, how often did hospital staff tell you what the medicine was for?**

    1 ☐ Never
    2 ☐ Sometimes
    3 ☐ Usually
    4 ☐ Always

17. **Before giving you any new medicine, how often did hospital staff describe possible side effects in a way you could understand?**

    1 ☐ Never
    2 ☐ Sometimes
    3 ☐ Usually
    4 ☐ Always

WHEN YOU LEFT THE HOSPITAL

18. **After you left the hospital, did you go directly to your own home, to someone else's home, or to another health facility?**

    1 ☐ Own home
    2 ☐ Someone else's home
    3 ☐ Another health facility ➜ If Another, Go to Question 21

19. **During this hospital stay, did doctors, nurses or other hospital staff talk with you about whether you would have the help you needed when you left the hospital?**

    1 ☐ Yes
    2 ☐ No

Continued

20. During this hospital stay, did you get information in writing about what symptoms or health problems to look out for after you left the hospital?

    ^{1}☐ Yes
    ^{2}☐ No

OVERALL RATING OF HOSPITAL

Please answer the following questions about your stay at the hospital named on the cover letter. Do not include any other hospital stays in your answers.

21. Using any number from 0 to 10, where 0 is the worst hospital possible and 10 is the best hospital possible, what number would you use to rate this hospital during your stay?

    ^{0}☐ 0   Worst hospital possible
    ^{1}☐ 1
    ^{2}☐ 2
    ^{3}☐ 3
    ^{4}☐ 4
    ^{5}☐ 5
    ^{6}☐ 6
    ^{7}☐ 7
    ^{8}☐ 8
    ^{9}☐ 9
    ^{10}☐ 10   Best hospital possible

22. Would you recommend this hospital to your friends and family?

    ^{1}☐ Definitely no
    ^{2}☐ Probably no
    ^{3}☐ Probably yes
    ^{4}☐ Definitely yes

UNDERSTANDING YOUR CARE WHEN YOU LEFT THE HOSPITAL

23. During this hospital stay, staff took my preferences and those of my family or caregiver into account in deciding what my health care needs would be when I left.

    ^{1}☐ Strongly disagree
    ^{2}☐ Disagree
    ^{3}☐ Agree
    ^{4}☐ Strongly agree

24. When I left the hospital, I had a good understanding of the things I was responsible for in managing my health.

    ^{1}☐ Strongly disagree
    ^{2}☐ Disagree
    ^{3}☐ Agree
    ^{4}☐ Strongly agree

25. When I left the hospital, I clearly understood the purpose for taking each of my medications.

    ^{1}☐ Strongly disagree
    ^{2}☐ Disagree
    ^{3}☐ Agree
    ^{4}☐ Strongly agree
    ^{5}☐ I was not given any medication when I left the hospital

ABOUT YOU

There are only a few remaining items left.

26. During this hospital stay, were you admitted to this hospital through the Emergency Room?

    ^{1}☐ Yes
    ^{2}☐ No

27. In general, how would you rate your overall health?

    ^{1}☐ Excellent
    ^{2}☐ Very good
    ^{3}☐ Good
    ^{4}☐ Fair
    ^{5}☐ Poor

28. In general, how would you rate your overall <u>mental or emotional health</u>?

    ^{1}☐ Excellent
    ^{2}☐ Very good
    ^{3}☐ Good
    ^{4}☐ Fair
    ^{5}☐ Poor

29. **What is the highest grade or level of school that you have <u>completed</u>?**

   ¹☐ 8th grade or less
   ²☐ Some high school, but did not graduate
   ³☐ High school graduate or GED
   ⁴☐ Some college or 2-year degree
   ⁵☐ 4-year college graduate
   ⁶☐ More than 4-year college degree

30. **Are you of Spanish, Hispanic or Latino origin or descent?**

   ¹☐ No, not Spanish/Hispanic/Latino
   ²☐ Yes, Puerto Rican
   ³☐ Yes, Mexican, Mexican American, Chicano
   ⁴☐ Yes, Cuban
   ⁵☐ Yes, other Spanish/Hispanic/Latino

31. **What is your race? Please choose one or more.**

   ¹☐ White
   ²☐ Black or African American
   ³☐ Asian
   ⁴☐ Native Hawaiian or other Pacific Islander
   ⁵☐ American Indian or Alaska Native

32. **What language do you <u>mainly</u> speak at home?**

   ¹☐ English
   ²☐ Spanish
   ³☐ Chinese
   ⁴☐ Russian
   ⁵☐ Vietnamese
   ⁶☐ Portuguese
   ⁹☐ Some other language (please print): _____

THANK YOU

Please return the completed survey in the postage-paid envelope.

[NAME OF SURVEY VENDOR OR SELF-ADMINISTERING HOSPITAL]

[RETURN ADDRESS OF SURVEY VENDOR OR SELF-ADMINISTERING HOSPITAL]

Questions 1-22 and 26-32 are part of the HCAHPS Survey and are works of the U.S. Government. These HCAHPS questions are in the public domain and therefore are NOT subject to U.S. copyright laws. The three Care Transitions Measure® questions (Questions 23-25) are copyright of The Care Transitions Program® (www.caretransitions.org).

Continued

Sample Initial Cover Letter for the HCAHPS Survey

[HOSPITAL LETTERHEAD]

[SAMPLED PATIENT NAME]
[ADDRESS]
[CITY, STATE ZIP]

Dear [SAMPLED PATIENT NAME]:

Our records show that you were recently a patient at [NAME OF HOSPITAL] and discharged on [DATE OF DISCHARGE]. Because you had a recent hospital stay, we are asking for your help. This survey is part of an ongoing national effort to understand how patients view their hospital experience. Hospital results will be publicly reported and made available on the Internet at www.medicare.gov/hospitalcompare. These results will help consumers make important choices about their hospital care, and will help hospitals improve the care they provide.

Questions 1-25 in the enclosed survey are part of a national initiative sponsored by the United States Department of Health and Human Services to measure the quality of care in hospitals. Your participation is voluntary and will not affect your health benefits.

We hope that you will take the time to complete the survey. Your participation is greatly appreciated. After you have completed the survey, please return it in the pre-paid envelope. Your answers may be shared with the hospital for purposes of quality improvement. [*OPTIONAL*: You may notice a number on the survey. This number is used to let us know if you returned your survey so we don't have to send you reminders.]

If you have any questions about the enclosed survey, please call the toll-free number 1-800-xxx-xxxx. Thank you for helping to improve health care for all consumers.

Sincerely,

[HOSPITAL ADMINISTRATOR]
[HOSPITAL NAME]

Note: The OMB Paperwork Reduction Act language must be included in the mailing. This language can be either on the front or back of the cover letter or questionnaire, but cannot be a separate mailing. The exact OMB Paperwork Reduction Act language is included in this appendix. Please refer to the Mail Only, and Mixed Mode sections, for specific letter guidelines.

Sample Follow-up Cover Letter for the HCAHPS Survey

[HOSPITAL LETTERHEAD]

[SAMPLED PATIENT NAME]
[ADDRESS]
[CITY, STATE ZIP]

Dear [SAMPLED PATIENT NAME]:

Our records show that you were recently a patient at [NAME OF HOSPITAL] and discharged on [DATE OF DISCHARGE]. Approximately three weeks ago we sent you a survey regarding your hospitalization. If you have already returned the survey to us, please accept our thanks and disregard this letter. However, if you have not yet completed the survey, please take a few minutes and complete it now.

Because you had a recent hospital stay, we are asking for your help. This survey is part of an ongoing national effort to understand how patients view their hospital experience. Hospital results will be publicly reported and made available on the Internet at www.medicare.gov/hospitalcompare. These results will help consumers make important choices about their hospital care, and will help hospitals improve the care they provide.

Questions 1-25 in the enclosed survey are part of a national initiative sponsored by the United States Department of Health and Human Services to measure the quality of care in hospitals. Your participation is voluntary and will not affect your health benefits. Please take a few minutes and complete the enclosed survey. After you have completed the survey, please return it in the pre-paid envelope. Your answers may be shared with the hospital for purposes of quality improvement. [*OPTIONAL*: You may notice a number on the survey. This number is used to let us know if you returned your survey so we don't have to send you reminders.]

If you have any questions about the enclosed survey, please call the toll-free number 1-800-xxx-xxxx. Thank you again for helping to improve health care for all consumers.

Sincerely,

[HOSPITAL ADMINISTRATOR]
[HOSPITAL NAME]

Note: The OMB Paperwork Reduction Act language must be included in the mailing. This language can be either on the front or back of the cover letter or questionnaire, but cannot be a separate mailing. The exact OMB Paperwork Reduction Act language is included in this appendix. Please refer to the Mail Only, and Mixed Mode sections, for specific letter guidelines.

Continued

OMB Paperwork Reduction Act Language

The OMB Paperwork Reduction Act language must be included in the survey mailing. This language can be either on the front or back of the cover letter or questionnaire, but cannot be a separate mailing. The following is the language that must be used:

English Version

"According to the Paperwork Reduction Act of 1995, no persons are required to respond to a collection of information unless it displays a valid OMB control number. The valid OMB control number for this information collection is 0938-0981. The time required to complete this information collected is estimated to average 8 minutes for questions 1-25 on the survey, including the time to review instructions, search existing data resources, gather the data needed, and complete and review the information collection. If you have any comments concerning the accuracy of the time estimate(s) or suggestions for improving this form, please write to: Centers for Medicare & Medicaid Services, 7500 Security Boulevard, C1-25-05, Baltimore, MD 21244-1850."

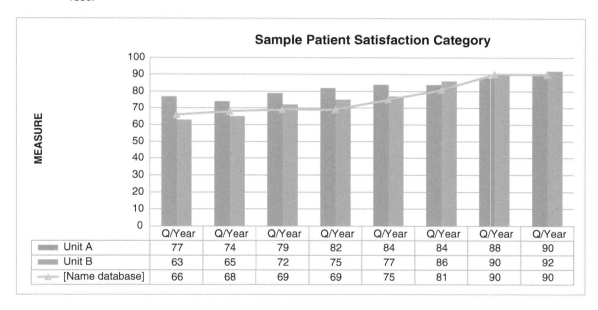

Sample Patient Satisfaction Category

	Q/Year	Q/Year	Q/Year	Q/Year	Q/Year	Q/Year	Q/Year	Q/Year
Unit A	77	74	79	82	84	84	88	90
Unit B	63	65	72	75	77	86	90	92
[Name database]	66	68	69	69	75	81	90	90

The graph demonstrates that Unit A outperformed the benchmark in six of eight quarters and that Unit B outperformed the benchmark in five of eight quarters. When the unit results are the same as the benchmark, it is not considered outperforming.

With regard to this measure of patient satisfaction, Unit A outperformed the benchmark in six of eight quarters. Unit B outperformed the benchmark for five of eight quarters.

These types of graphic representation of performance allow the staff to view trends, to be accountable for patient outcomes, and to continually drive performance improvement. Behind each of the previously mentioned performance metrics, there are processes developed that identify targets for improvement, develop and implement plans for change, and develop and implement plans for change and sustained high levels of performance. Still, there is further documentation that is needed to ascertain what actions, evidence, and research has led to the sustained improvements.

In Magnet-recognized institutions, there is a template that summarizes the reporting and communication of improvements. This tool is a good template for the summarization of such efforts (ANCC, 2013, p. 60) as follows:

- Background/problem
  - Provide relevant background information
  - Describe the problem that exists in the organization
- Goal statement
  - State the goal that is the desired improvement/change/result
  - Identify the measure selected to demonstrate the improvement/change/result (i.e., errors, incidents, indicators, satisfaction)
- Description of the intervention/initiative/activity
  - Describe the action that had an effect on the problem and resulted in the achievement of the goal
    - Include where the intervention/initiative occurred (unit, department)
    - Include the date when the intervention/initiative occurred
- Participants
  - List the participants involved
  - Include name, discipline, title, and department
- Outcomes
  - Demonstrate the achievement of the desired improvement/change/result with data displayed in a clearly labeled graph with a data table:
    - Trended data must be displayed to show change/improvement/result.
    - The selected measure must correlate with desired goal.
    - Preintervention/initiative data and postintervention/initiative data must:
      - Use the same measure to demonstrate the effect of the intervention/initiative and
      - Be clearly identified with dates.
    - The intervention time frame/dates must be clearly identified on the graph.

The Clinical Corner gives an example of an evidence-based improvement with the resultant graph demonstrating improvement.

SUMMARY

The continual monitoring of performance is integral to the continued excellence in the delivery of patient care. Nurses need to play an active role in the constant evaluation of the delivery of care and assume accountability for the outcomes within the organization.

CLINICAL CORNER

Role of Leaders in the Implementation of Therapeutic Activities Such as Dementia Care Best Practice

Sometimes solutions to substantial problems, like agitation behaviors associated with dementia, can be fun and lighthearted for patients and bedside caregivers. Sustaining dementia patients' independence and current level of function is a daily challenge in the acute care setting. Diversional activities, like listening to music and interacting with a baby doll, are cognitively stimulating interventions that divert attention away from agitation behaviors associated with dementia. Nurses and other health care providers must shift the way they think about dementia patients and agitation behaviors. Caregivers must view these patients holistically, assess them for unmet needs, and avoid reaching for sedation and restraints when behaviors begin. Organizational leaders, leader-managers, and frontline leaders can improve care outcomes for hospitalized dementia patients by advocating for nonpharmacologic interventions, like diversional activities, as first-line treatment for agitation behaviors associated with dementia.

Agitation Behaviors Associated With Dementia

The older adult population is increasing and will continue to use the health care system for acute and chronic conditions. The prevalence of dementia is increasing, as well. The Alzheimer's Association (2019) estimates that by 2050, the number of people aged 65 and older with Alzheimer's disease will grow to nearly 14 million people. Dementia is characterized by progressive and irreversible

Continued

cognitive decline. These patients lose their short-term memory, their ability to perform basic tasks, and their ability to communicate. Agitation behaviors associated with dementia are often an expression of unmet physical, cognitive, or psychosocial needs or a manifestation of frustration when patients cannot communicate effectively (Cohen-Mansfield, Dakheel-Ali, Marx, Thein, & Regier, 2015; Dimitriou et al., 2018). Wandering, calling out, repetitive motions, and other behaviors are common for dementia patients when they feel frustrated, anxious, lonely, or pain (Conedera & Kingston, 2013). These behaviors can worsen in the acute care setting where the patient is out of his or her usual element and at risk for delirium (Cohen-Mansfield et al., 2015). Dementia patients are also at risk for falls, removing critical medical equipment like central venous catheters, and other iatrogenic events because of their agitation behaviors.

Frontline caregivers often find that the daily difficulties of communication barriers and agitation behaviors make caring for dementia patients challenging. Caregivers face higher patient-care hours, heavier workloads, and more stressful environments when dementia patients are climbing out of bed, hitting, or repeatedly crying out. In these situations, leaders must gently remind caregivers to look past the agitation behaviors to seek safe solutions for the person in front of them. Dementia patients are adults with rich life stories who deserve to be treated with dignity.

Current Treatment of Agitation Behaviors Associated With Dementia
Unfortunately, physical restraints and sedation are often used to address agitation behaviors associated with dementia in the acute care setting. These treatment methods can harm dementia patients further. Many medications have historically caused exacerbation of behaviors and decline in patients' baseline cognitive status. According to the Beers Criteria, benzodiazepines and anticholinergics, like lorazepam and diphenhydramine, among others should be avoided in older adults because of risk for delirium, somnolence, and increased agitation (American Geriatrics Society, 2015). Physical restraints can also cause delirium, soft tissue limb injuries, broken bones, and death (Mccabe, Alvarez, Mcnulty, & Fitzpatrick, 2011; American Geriatrics Society, 2015). Delirium increases patients' length of stay and risk for further iatrogenic events, including falls, which add up to high human and financial costs.

Lack of Health Care Providers Trained in Older Adult-Specific Best Practices
Even though older adults are the most extensive and fastest growing population in acute care settings, most health care providers lack sufficient older adult-specific training and expertise (Gillis, MacDonald, & MacIssaac, 2008). Leaders must advocate for this vulnerable population by encouraging geriatric-specific training and dissemination of older adult best practices to nursing staff.

Therapeutic Activities as First-Line Treatment for Behaviors
Therapeutic activities are interventions that divert the patient's attention away from agitation behaviors while providing cognitive and psychosocial stimulation to address patients' needs (Ricker & Mulligan, 2017). Patient-centered, nonpharmacologic interventions should be the first-line treatment for older adult patients exhibiting behaviors associated with dementia (Conedera & Kingston, 2013). Whereas physical restraints and sedation can cause physical harm and threaten the dignity and personhood of dementia patients, therapeutic activities are low risk for harm and promote the patients' well-being. By implementing therapeutic activities into nursing practice, leaders provide caregivers with patient-centered tools to deal with these behaviors in safe and humane ways.

Review of Literature and Highlight on Activities
Diversional activities are patient-centered, noninvasive, and fun interventions that patients can refuse, but generally, do not raise patient objections. Listening to music and interaction with a baby doll are two types of therapeutic, diversional activities.

Music: Good for Patients and Caregivers
Music, in various forms, is a commonly discussed nonpharmacologic intervention for agitation. Music interventions improve the dementia patient's overall well-being and reduce agitation behaviors associated with dementia (Livingston et al., 2014; de Oliviera et al., 2015; Shibazaki & Marshall, 2015; Dimitriou et al., 2018). Nonpharmacologic interventions that are based on the patient's interests or needs are the most effective and long-acting in positive behavioral effects (Livingston et al., 2014; de Oliviera et al., 2015). Listening to preferred age-appropriate music taps into patients' long-term memories and can increase enthusiasm and enjoyment (Shibazaki & Marshall, 2015). Music can meet patients' needs for cognitive stimulation, which is demonstrated by singing along with songs from memory (Shibazaki & Marshall, 2015). Shibazaki & Marshal (2015) found that dementia patients' family members describe that their loved ones had improved happiness and communicativeness after music concerts. Improved communication skills can assist patients in expressing needs, which can decrease frustration and incidence of agitation behaviors associated with

dementia. Regular implementation of a music intervention can also help meet cognitive and psychosocial needs before behaviors start.

In addition to decreasing patients' agitation behaviors, music interventions help decrease patients' family members' caregiver distress levels (Dimitriou et al., 2018). Shibazaki & Marshall (2015) describe that facility-based music concerts lifted the mood of the entire organization (Shibazaki & Marshall, 2015). Music interventions can improve the overall well-being of people who care for dementia patients.

Baby Doll Provides Comfort and Safety

Interacting with a baby doll is a natural, nonthreatening, and nontoxic intervention that provides comfort to severe-stage dementia patients and decreases agitation behaviors (Green et al., 2011; Braden & Gasper, 2015). The baby doll provides participants with feelings of ownership, purpose, companionship, and bonding (Alander, Prescott, & James, 2015). This intervention reminds patients of their experiences as caregivers to children and loved ones. Dementia patient doll users often increase their communicativeness and socialization as they interact with the doll and with individuals around them (Alander et al., 2015). This intervention provides a calming effect for patients, decreases agitation, and decreases aggressive behaviors (Green et al., 2011; Alander et al., 2015).

Occasionally, a patient's family members will object to the use of the baby doll intervention for their loved one with dementia. These family members have described the baby doll as "childish" and inappropriate for adults. In these cases, staff members must act as leaders to educate and reassure families regarding the benefits of the nonpharmacologic baby doll intervention for agitation behaviors associated with dementia. Doll users must always be given a choice whether to interact with the doll (Alander et al., 2015). Nursing staff members should help families understand that the baby doll provides a vehicle for their loved ones' to feel purpose during their hospitalization and, at times, meets the patients' past attachment needs (Bisiani & Angus, 2015). If the baby doll successfully decreases a patient's agitation, it preserves that individual's dignity (Alander et al., 2015). Most of all, nursing staff members must convey that the baby doll is offered with respect. For clinical nursing staff, the baby provides just the right amount of lightheartedness coupled with evidence-based practice affiliation.

Synthesis of Evidence

Nonpharmacologic activities have a positive effect on agitation in dementia patients and are favorable to pharmacologic treatment (Livingston et al., 2014; de Oliviera et al., 2015, Staedler & Nunez, 2015). Interventions that are supervised and involve staff understanding of patients' needs have a sustained decrease in agitation over months and during treatment (Livingston et al., 2014). These treatments are most effective when they are based on participants' interests (de Oliviera et al., 2015). A holistic, nonpharmacologic approach should be applied to all of dementia care, not just symptom management (Spears, 2018).

Saint Joseph's Health Therapeutic Activity Kit

Saint Joseph's Health (SJH) located in northern New Jersey, implemented the SJH Therapeutic Activity Kit throughout its hospital system as a toolbox of interventions for cognitively impaired older adults who are exhibiting or at risk for agitation behaviors. The SJH Therapeutic Activity Kit includes music and the baby doll as part of its nine therapeutic activities. Every piece of the SJH Therapeutic Activity Kit is evidence based and made for the older adult patient, including large-print materials, large-sized crayons, and age-appropriate music (Ricker & Mulligan, 2017). The activities are easy to use and take minimal time to implement.

Since the rollout of the SJH Therapeutic Activity Kit, interprofessional staff members have recounted countless success stories. Although every inpatient unit in the hospital system has the same kit, the utilization of each therapeutic activity varies based on the care setting. Music is the most common intervention in critical care units, whereas the baby dolls are frequently used in medical-surgical units (Ricker & Mulligan, 2017).

The SJH Therapeutic Activity Kit uses portable CD players, age-appropriate CDs, and an online streaming music program. These supplies are inexpensive, easy to clean, and reusable. Endless types of music can be played on bedside computers or workstations on wheels through free websites like YouTube and Pandora. Depending on the setting, patients are put in cohorts and invited to listen to music together in common areas. Nursing staff members do not need significant training to implement music intervention for patients, but their company and understanding of patients' needs can further decrease agitation behaviors (Livingston et al., 2014). At SJH, it is not uncommon to walk through a patient care unit and to hear multiple types of music floating out of patient's rooms.

The baby doll was a particular catalyst for cultural change in the care of dementia patients at SJH. Severe-stage dementia patients are frequently found sitting in the hallway cuddling a baby doll, or asking staff members to

Continued

CLINICAL CORNER—cont'd

"babysit" the doll while they are at a procedure. The baby doll solidifies the caring engagement between patients and staff. The elevation of patients' agitation behaviors combined with the lightheartedness of the intervention contributes to staff buy-in. Once, a nurse called a "missing baby doll alert" and posted missing signs when she could not find the baby doll on the unit.

To disseminate therapeutic, diversional activities throughout the hospital system, the creators of the SJH Therapeutic Activity Kit had to garner buy-in from hospital administration and bedside nurses. Integrating therapeutic activities into the care of the dementia patient can positively change caregivers' connectedness to patients and improve their experience of providing care (Ricker & Mulligan, 2017). Communication of the importance of this practice must be consistent but engaging. If bedside nurses do not buy into the intervention, they will not follow through with the practice. Nurses should be allowed to ask questions and raise concerns about diversional activity interventions. Leaders should meet opposition with openness, explanation of the intervention, and conviction that the diversional activities will improve patient outcomes.

Conclusion

Nonpharmacologic interventions are patient centered, safe, effective, inexpensive, and without adverse side effects (Staedtler & Nunez, 2015). Nursing staff and organization buy-in is key to the successful implementation of the intervention. However, education for staff members does not need to be extensive, just clear and consistent. Nursing staff will buy into the concept of diversional activities intervention if they understand that these interventions will improve patient outcomes and prevent behaviors that increase care workload. Music and the baby doll add levity that improves the environment for nursing staff and patients. Hospital administration will recognize that the financial cost of music equipment is negligible if in-patient falls and delirium can be prevented in the dementia patient population. Ultimately, diversional activities are nonpharmacologic best practices that can significantly improve the well-being, safety, and dignity of dementia patients.

Jennifer Racine Ricker
Maureen Mulligan
(September 1, 2019, St. Joseph's Health, Patterson, NJ.)

EVIDENCE-BASED PRACTICE

(From Dempsey, C., & Assi, M. J. (2018). The impact of nurse engagement on quality, safety, and the experience of care. What nurse leaders should know. *Nursing Administration Quarterly, 42*(3), 278–283.)

To lead others in achieving stellar outcomes, nurse leaders need to understand the vital and interdependent connection between quality, safety, the patient and nurse experience of care, and registered nurse (RN) engagement. With the many generations present in today's health care environment along with the challenging work, understanding the key drivers of joy and meaning is critically important.

Measures of nurse engagement include autonomy, professional development, leadership access and responsiveness, interprofessional relationships, quality of nursing care, resources and staffing, and nurse-to-nurse teamwork and collaboration. Recent analyses of one engagement database indicate that 15 of every 100 nurses are disengaged and lack commitment and/or satisfaction with their work. This is expensive for an organization. Conservative estimates suggest that a disengaged nurse costs an organization more than $22,000 in lost

revenue caused by lost productivity, but it also exacts a toll on the patient experience. The patient and caregiver experience of care coordination includes the following key Hospital Consumer Assessment of Healthcare Providers and Systems (HCAHPS) measures:

- Communication with nurses
- Communication with hospital staff
- Communication about medicines
- Discharge information

These make up to 25% of the value-based purchasing score for the health care facility. All of these measures are influenced by the experience of the people who care for them as patients. An analysis of the more than 1.5 million responses to inpatient surveys identified teamwork and nurse communication as top drivers of HCHAPS global ratings. Yet the findings from the 2015 National Healthcare Average employee engagement database demonstrate low engagement among direct caregivers, including nurses, which has been linked to poor teamwork and lack of effective communication. Furthermore, loyalty is lowest for those employees aged 25 to 39 years who represent close to 38% of the workforce.

EVIDENCE-BASED PRACTICE—cont'd

To address engagement in an effort to improve both the patient and nurse experience, leaders must understand the perceptions of both groups of stakeholders. Through measuring engagement at the work unit level and identifying the key performance drivers for each unit, leaders can identify the key performance drivers necessary for success in each unit. Celebrating high-performing units and leveraging their success to educate and support less engaged groups are strategies that high performing organizations consistently employ.

Findings from qualitative interviews of top performing nurse managers revealed their behaviors that lead to how they establish a meaningful connection with their staff. Their emphasis is on

• An unwavering focus on quality and safety of care;

• A culture of respect;
• Nurse manager relationships and visibility;
• Promotion of autonomy;
• Support of professional development;
• Interprofessional rounds and team building;
• Huddles to improve communication and teamwork;
• The use of data and evidence to support decisions and practice;
• Safe and appropriate staffing; and
• A bundle that includes bedside report, white boards, pain management, communication, peer review, and auditing.

The connection of nurse engagement to the experience of care and to nurse and patient outcomes is evident throughout all of the evidence-based boxes in this text.

NCLEX® EXAMINATION QUESTIONS

1. You are the nurse in the operating room. The patient was having left eye cataract surgery. Once the procedure began you informed the surgeon that he was operating on the wrong eye. This is considered a(n):
   A. Sentinel event
   B. Risk management
   C. Outcomes
   D. Incident

2. After you have informed the surgeon that he was operating on the right eye, you would then inform:
   A. The medical director
   B. Your immediate supervisor
   C. The nursing unit
   D. The family

3. In 1998 in the quest for improvement in health care, the _____ issued a report, to Err is Human: Building a Safer Health System.
   A. The Advisory Commission on Consumer Protection and Quality
   B. The American Nurses Association
   C. The Institute of Medicine (IOM)
   D. The Board of Physicians

4. Which of the following has been shown to be a powerful tool to help health care organizations become safer, more efficient, and patient centered?
   A. Performance improvement (PI)
   B. Total quality management (TQM)
   C. Quality improvement (QI)
   D. All of the above

5. The focus on outcomes uses a(n) _____ _____ model. Examples of organizations that recognize this are the American Nurses Association and its Magnet Award for Nursing, the Malcolm Baldrige National Quality Award for performance excellence.
   A. High-reliability
   B. Best practice
   C. Improvement
   D. Accommodation

6. A majority of health care organizations across the United States measure patient satisfaction. Two of the common vendor satisfaction measures are:
   A. Press Ganey and Gallup
   B. Press Ganey and The Joint Commission
   C. Gallup and The Joint Commission
   D. Gallup and Six Sigma

7. Common outcomes for most units are infection rates, patient satisfaction, and performance scales. These are the:
   A. Core measures
   B. Unit-specific measures
   C. Measures of The Joint Commission
   D. Infection measures

8. Outcomes that are used by hospitals include financial measures, human resource measures, and ethical measures and are referred to as the:
   A. Management plan
   B. Strategic plan

C. Administrative plan

D. Nursing plan

9. The FOCUS method is:

A. F: focus on an opportunity for improvement, O: organize a team involved with the process, C: clarify the current process, U: understand the causes of variation in the process, S: Select the improvement

B. F: find an opportunity for improvement, O: organize a team involved with the process, C: clarify the current process, U: understand the causes of variation in the process, S: select the improvement

C. F: focus on an opportunity for improvement, O: organize a team involved with the process, C: communicate, U: understand the causes of variation in the process, S: select the improvement

D. F: focus on an opportunity for improvement, O: organize a team involved with the process, C: clarify the current process, U: understand the causes of variation in the process, S: solve the problem

10. The next step is the Plan–Do–Study–Act (PDSA) cycle. Which of the following is NOT part of the plan?

A. Plan: plan a change, with activity aimed at improvement

B. Do: carry it out

C. Check/study: Study the results. What happened? What did you learn? Did the change work?

D. Assess the outcomes

Answers: 1. A   2. B   3. D   4. D   5. B   6. A
7. A   8. B   9. A   10. D

REFERENCES

Alander, H., Prescott, T., & James, I. (2015). Older adult's views and experiences of doll therapy in residential care homes. *Dementia*, 14(5), 574–588.

Alzheimer's Association. (2015). *2019 Alzheimers disease facts and figures*. <https://www.alz.org/media/Documents/alzheimers-facts-and-figures-infographic-2019.pdf>. (Accessed December 21, 2021).

American Geriatrics Society. (2015). American Geriatrics Society 2015 updated Beers Criteria for potentially inappropriate medication use in older adults. *Journal of the American Geriatrics Society*, 63(11), 2227–2246. https://doi.org/10.1111/jgs.13702. (Accessed 21 December 2021).

Bisiani, L., & Angus, J. (2012). Doll therapy: a therapeutic means to meet past attachment needs and diminish behaviors of concern in a person living with dementia–a case study approach. *Dementia*, 12(4), 447–462.

Braden, B., & Gaspar, P. (2015). Implementation of a baby doll therapy protocol for people with dementia: innovative practice. *Dementia*, 14(5), 696–706.

Cohen-Mansfield, J., Dakheel-Ali, M., Marx, M. S., Thein, K., & Regier, N. G. (2015). Which unmet needs contribute to behavior problems in persons with advanced dementia? *Psychiatry Research*, 228(1), 59–64. https://doi.org/10.1016/j.psychres.2015.03.043 (Accessed 21 December 2021).

Conedera, F., & Kingston, L. (2013). Try this: best practices in nursing care to older adults with dementia. *The Hartford Institute for Geriatric Nursing*, (D4). New York University: NY, NY.

de Oliveira, A. M., Radanovic, M., De Mello, P. C., Buchain, P. C., Vizzotto, A. D., Celestino, D. L., & Forlenza, O. V.
(2015). Nonpharmacological interventions to reduce behavioral and psychological symptoms of dementia: a systematic review. *BioMed Research International*, 2015, 1–9. https://doi.org/10.1155/2015/218980. (Accessed 21 December 2021).

Dimitriou, T. D., Verykouki, E., Papatriantafyllou, J., Konsta, A., Kazis, D., & Tsolaki, M. (2018). Non-pharmacological interventions for agitation/aggressive behavior in patients with dementia: a randomized controlled crossover trial. *Functional Neurology*, 33(3), 143–147.

Gillis, A., MacDonald, B., & MacIssaac, A. (2008). Nurses' knowledge, attitudes, and confidence regarding preventing and treating deconditioning in older adults. *Journal of Continuing Education in Nursing*, 39(12), 547–554. https://doi.org/10.3928/00220124-20081201-07. (Accessed 21 December 2021).

Green, L., Matos, P., Murillo, I., Neushotz, L., Popeo, D., Aloysi, A., & Fitzpatrick, J. (2011). Use of dolls as a therapeutic intervention: relationship to previous negative behaviors and pro re nata (prn) Haldol use among geropsychiatric inpatients. *Archives of Psychiatric Nursing*, 25, 388–389.

Livingston, G., Kelly, L., Lewis-Holmes, E., Baio, G., Morris, S., Patel, N., & Cooper, C. (2014). Non-pharmacological interventions for agitation in dementia: systematic review of randomised controlled trials. *British Journal of Psychiatry*, 205(6), 436–442. https://doi.org/10.1192/bjp.bp.113.141119

Mccabe, D. E., Alvarez, C. D., Mcnulty, S. R., & Fitzpatrick, J. J. (2011). Perceptions of physical restraints use in the elderly among registered nurses and nurse assistants in a single acute care hospital. *Geriatric Nursing, 32*(1), 39–45. https://doi.org/10.1016/j.gerinurse.2010.10.010

NDNQI. (2021). NDNQI Nursing-Sensitive Indicators. NDNQI. https://nursingandndnqi.weebly.com/ndnqi-indicators.html. (Accessed 21 December 2021).

Ricker, J. R., & Mulligan, M. (2017). Activity kits as a first line intervention to care for individuals with dementia. *Geriatric Nursing, 38*(6), 604–605. https://doi.org/10.1016/j.gerinurse.2017.10.003. (Accessed 21 December 2021).

Shibazaki, K., & Marshall, N. A. (2015). Exploring the impact of music concerts in promoting well-being in dementia

care. *Aging & Mental Health, 21*(5), 468–476. https://doi.org/10.1080/13607863.2015.1114589. (Accessed 21 December 2021).

Spears, M. M. (2018). *Nonpharmacological behavioral interventions for patients with dementia: an integrative literature review, unpublished doctoral dissertation. Minneapolis, MN*: Walden University.

Staedtler, A., & Nunez, D. (2015). Nonpharmacological therapy for the management of neuropsychiatric symptoms of Alzheimer's disease: linking evidence to practice. *Worldviews on Evidence-Based Nursing, 12*(2), 108–115.

BIBILOGRAPHY

Agency for Healthcare Research and Quality [AHRQ]. (2015). Pressure Ulcer Resources. < www.ahrq.gov/professionals/systems/long-term-care/resources/pressure-ulcers/pressureulcertoolkit/putool5.html>. (Accessed January 26, 2015).

American Nurses Association [ANA]. (2014) Nursing Sensitive Indicators. www.nursingworld.org/MainMenu Categories/ThePracticeofProfessionalNursing/Patient SafetyQuality/Research-Measurement/The-National-Database/Nursing-Sensitive-Indicators_1. (Accessed December 21, 2021).

American Nurses Credentialing Center [ANCC]. (2013). *2014 Magnet Application Manual.* Silver Spring, MD: author.

American Nurses Credentialing Center [ANCC]. (2019). *2019 Magnet Application Manual.* Silver Spring, MD: Author.

Centers for Medicare and Medicaid Services [CMS]. (2015) HCHAPS—The Patient Perception of Care Survey. www.cms.gov/Medicare/Quality-Initiatives-Patient-

Assessment-Instruments/HospitalQualityInits/HospitalHCAHPS.html. (Accessed December 21, 2021).

Cramer, E., Staggs, V., & Dunton, N. (2014). Improving the nursing work environment. *American Nurse Today, 9*(1), 55–57.

Hall, J., & Kelly, C. (2014). A partnership to enhance outcomes through quality dashboards and action planning. *American Nurse Today, 9*(1), 57–58.

Institute of Medicine (2003). Keeping pateints safe: transforming the work environment of nurses. Washington, D.C.: The National Academies Press.

Montalvo. I. (2007). The National Database of Nursing Quality Indicators™ (NDNQI®). Manuscript 2. *OJIN: The Online Journal of Issues in Nursing, 12*(3).

NDNQI Nursing-Sensitive Indicators. (Accessed 21 December 2021).

VISN. Post Falls Huddle, Palo Alto Veterans Administration Hospital. www.visn8.va.gov/visn8/.../fallsteam/postfall-huddle_guideline.docx. (Accessed December 21, 2021).

Case Scenario: An advanced practice nurse (APN) in pediatrics at a Magnet-recognized institution is proud of the way evidence-based practice and research are integrated into her unit's clinical and operational processes. This integration has enabled her unit's nurses to not only explore safest and best practices but contribute to generating new knowledge among the team.

Now she is taking on a new role. After a resurgence of measles in the city and surrounding communities, the hospital's on-site clinic for low-income children and families is looking for ways to improve the organization's performance in outreach specifically aimed at overcoming barriers to immunization among the institution's immediate, low-income community. As someone practiced in evidence-based research, the APN is tasked with leading the investigation. She has defined the problem, welcoming input from her pediatric team. As a result of their input, she is now compiling her literature review. The first question in her critical appraisal of the evidence is determining the quality of each study before she can begin to apply their results to the design of her unit's nursing protocol for immunizations.

ITEM TYPE: CLOZE

1. Out of 618 children in the immediate community's elementary school, (1) 23 children contracted measles last year, (2) 11 new cases developing in the month of April alone. What are the incidence and prevalence rates? **Choose the *most likely* options to complete the statement below** (Chapter 19).
   The incidence rate for last year was _____1_____, while last prevalence rate for April was _____2_____.

Options for 1	Options for 2
A. 0.037%	D. 0.018%
B. 3.7%	E. 0.18%
C. 0.37%	F. 1.8%

Answers: The incidence rate for the year was (B) 3.7% while the prevalence rate for April was (F) 1.8%.

Objective: Calculate incidence and prevalence rates of an outbreak.

Rationale: Two types of measures can be monitored: incidence and prevalence rates. Incidence rates provide the most direct evidence. Incidence measures the number of children/patients who contract measles during a period in time—in this case, last year. (A) Incidence rates are calculated as follows: The numerator will be the number of children at our school who developed measles over the last year. So 23 is our numerator. The denominator is the total number of children in our school, so 618 is our denominator. Divide the numerator by the denominator and then multiply by 100 to get the percentage: 23 divided by 618 equals 0.03721. When we multiply this by 100, we get 3.721. Rounded to the nearest whole number, we get 3.7%. The other choices—(A) 0.037% and (C) 0.37%—represent errors in decimal placement. (B) Prevalence may reflect a single point in time, such as on the first day of each month. Prevalence rates are calculated as follows: The numerator will be the number of patients who contract measles in the month of April. So 11 is our numerator. The denominator is the number of children in the school. So 618 is the denominato. Divide the numerator by the denominator: 11 new cases in April divided by 618 children. Then multiply the result by 100 to get the percentage: 1.779. Round this up to 1.8%. The other choices—(D) 0.018% and (E) 0.18%—represent errors in decimal placement.

Source: Motacki, K., Burke, K. (2021). *Nursing delegation and management of patient care* (3rd ed., ch. 19). Philadelphia: Elsevier.

ITEM TYPE: EXTENDED MULTIPLE RESPONSE

2. Using an evidence-based practice model, the APN prepares graphs to help visualize areas of performance. **Place a check mark next to each data point that will be relevant in graphing the problem. Check all that apply** (Chapter 19).

_____A. Current level of success in helping families take advantage of scaled-fee or sometimes free immunizations at the clinic

_____B. Relationship between the current percentage of eligible children and the ultimate strategic goal of the clinic's outreach

_____C. Comparison of each staff member's performance

_____D. Comparison of clinic's overall performance to that of other free or scaled-fee children's and family clinics

_____E. Mix of staff members' education and skill levels

_____F. Indicators of whether there's a better way to reach these families

Answers: A, B, D, F

Objective: Interpret or plan visual representations of performance outcomes.

Rationale: Data points relevant to graphing the problem areas of performance include: current level of performance—in this case, the current level of success in helping families take advantage of services; relationship of the current level to the strategic goal; comparison of performance to other parallel professional entities—in this case comparing the clinic's performance to that of similar scaled-fee or free family clinics, and indicators of whether an improvement is required—that is, ways to improve outreach to this group of families. Comparing each staff member's performance is not a relevant data point to graphing the problem of performance using an evidence-based practice model. Finally, visually representing the mix of staff members' education and skill levels is not a relevant data point to include in this graph, as it is instead an example of a nursing-sensitive indicator, reflecting the structure, process, and outcomes of nursing care.

Source: Motacki, K., Burke, K. (2021). _Nursing delegation and management of patient care_ (3rd ed., ch. 19). Philadelphia: Elsevier.

ITEM TYPE: CLOZE

3. The APN and her team conclude from data analyses that they will (1) expand their hours of availability to working families; (2) apply for new grants to fund more vaccines for those who are uninsured; and (3) improve their family education programming. **Choose the _most likely_ options to complete the statement below** (Chapters 18 and 19).

Research   use   is   _____1_____,   while evidence-based practice is _____2_____.

Options for 1	Options for 2
Generation of new knowledge through the rigorous study of variables	Utilization of structured and unstructured observations to measure study variables
Process of applying findings from a single study or a set of studies for the development of patient care	Process of applying findings from a single study or a set of studies for the development of patient care
Utilization of structured and unstructured observations to measure study variables	Conscientious use of current best practice or research findings in making clinical decisions

Answers: Research use is the process of applying findings from a single study or a set of studies for the development of patient care, while evidence-based practice is the conscientious use of current best practice or research findings in making clinical decisions.

Objective: Differentiate among research, evidence-based practice, and performance improvement.

Rationale: Evidence-based practice differs from research use in that, for one thing, research use is the process of using research-generated knowledge to make an impact on or a change in existing practices (Burns et al., 2012) and applies findings from a single study or a set of studies for the development of patient care. Evidence-based practice, however, is the conscientious use of current best practice or research findings in making clinical decisions; it requires synthesizing research study findings to determine best research evidence to integrate into practice. Research evidence is a synthesis of high-quality, relevant studies to form a body of empirical knowledge for the selected area of practice. The best research evidence is then integrated with clinical expertise and patient values and needs to deliver quality, cost-effective care (Sackett et al., 2000). As for the other definition choices, the generation of new knowledge through the rigorous study of variables describes research and the utilization of structured and unstructured observations to measure study variables refers to an observational study.

Source: Motacki, K., Burke, K. (2021). _Nursing delegation and management of patient care_ (3rd ed., ch. 18). Philadelphia: Elsevier.

Congratulations

SECTION OUTLINE

To those readers who are students, this chapter is about progression after graduation. First of all, congratulations! It is not yet time to relax, however. There is much work to be done on entry to the new role of a professional nurse. This chapter will review the process for registering and taking the licensure exam, getting your first job, the means to continue professional growth, and continuation of your nursing education.

20

New Graduates: The Immediate Future: Job Interviewing, NCLEX® and Continuing Education

OBJECTIVES

- Review the recruitment process for patient care staff.
- Identify the steps in the employment process.
- Review the importance of a résumé in the employment process.
- Differentiate between the various types of interviewing techniques used in health care.
- Differentiate between various types of questions used in the employment interview.
- Identify the role of the nurse manager in the hiring process.

- Review the process for registering for the licensing examination.
- Identify states participating in the Nurse Licensure Compact.
- Elaborate on the decision making surrounding selection of the first job.
- Identify specialty organizations in nursing.
- Review the types of certification examinations available to the nurse.
- Discuss the importance of continued education in nursing.

KEY TERMS

ANCC American Nurses Credentialing Center

home state the nurse's primary state of residence

interview formal consultation to evaluate qualifications of a potential employee

NCLEX National Council Licensure Examination

NCSBN National Council of State Boards of Nursing

Nursing Licensure Compact states recognizing the license regulation of other states

party state any state that has adopted this compact

Pearson VUE company under contract with NCSBN to administer NCLEX® examination

recruitment process of obtaining individuals for employment

remote state any party state other than the home state

résumé summary of an individual's past employment, education, and honors

retention preservation or maintenance of staff

specialty certification examination credential specifying the candidate's knowledge level within a specialty

THE EMPLOYMENT PROCESS

It is the responsibility of the organization to provide staffing adequate to deliver safe and competent care. The number of staff required will depend on the acuity of the patients, the requirements of the job, mandatory staffing law (if applicable), health department regulations, and organization policies. As positions become vacant or new ones created, the first step in the employment process is to determine the competencies required for the position. This will require a job description.

All organizations will have a template for the job description. You need to familiarize yourself with the format in your organization. An effective job description needs to minimally include: (1) title, (2) job objectives, and (3) a list of duties. The job description also includes nursing competencies and expected behaviors, and competencies as they relate to the strategic objectives of the organization. As the job description is finalized, the job is "posted" according to the organization's policies. The process of "posting" is the initial stage in the nine-stage process of recruitment (Huber, 2018) that include:

1. Position posting
2. Advertising
3. Screening
4. Interviewing
5. Selecting
6. Orienting
7. Counseling/coaching/mentoring
8. Performance evaluation
9. Staff development

As a nurse manager you will play a role in each stage of this recruitment process. Your actual role in each stage of the process will depend on the organization's hierarchical structure. As a new nurse you need to be aware of the process, which you will be exposed to in your first hire.

Position Posting

Once a position becomes vacant within an organization, the facility posts the position internally for staff review and selection. Then the position is posted externally in the local newspapers and with staffing and recruiting agencies.

Advertising

Health care organizations may place ads in professional nursing journals or magazines, and/or on professional organization websites. This encourages a broad range of individuals to be exposed to the position posting.

Screening

Health care organizations use this process by reviewing applications and then determining whether or not the nurse meets the position criteria. Facilities that are equal opportunity employers must meet all federal government guidelines during the screening process. Screening for nursing positions may include criminal background checks, drug and alcohol screens, and nursing grade point averages (GPAs). Many institutions also use proficiency examinations, such as pharmacology or critical thinking examinations to screen candidates. Some organizations are testing potential new hires via simulations.

Other institutions are now also using examinations that attempt to match the personality of the potential employee with the organizational culture.

Interviewing

Interviews are usually done in person, but they may also be conducted via telephone or teleconference. The interview may be one-on-one with the human resources representative and then with the nurse manager, or the interview may be conducted with multiple personnel at the same time.

Selecting

The nurse manager or clinical director usually makes the selection for a nursing position. If the position is a management position, the nurse manager and clinical director, and other members of the management team may select the candidate together.

THE INTERVIEW PROCESS

The most challenging aspect of the hiring process is to find the right person for the job. The job interview is the best way of determining the "fit" of the individual for the job and for your unit and organization. Remember, matching the job qualifications with the individual is only one aspect of the "right fit"; the personality and values of the individual also play a role in determination of the "right person for the job."

Before the interview process, a professional résumé is shared with individuals in the recruitment process. A résumé is a summary of professional and personal experiences (education, clinical experience, employment, skills, and interests) designed to introduce the candidate to potential employers. Often the résumé is the employer's first impression of the candidate. As a new nurse manager, you will need to evaluate the résumé for the right fit.

For a résumé to be effective, it must be targeted to the job being applied for. A single "catch-all" résumé that a candidate expects to use in looking for various types of jobs is much less effective than several well-focused résumés that highlight pertinent experience or expertise. For example, if a candidate is planning to apply to both hospital-based and community-health-center–based positions, they might be better served by having two résumés, one focusing on hospital experience and the other focusing on their community-health

background. Remember, for a nurse looking for a job, the purpose of a résumé is to obtain an interview, so it must make a strong argument to the reader that you have something to offer. The purpose of the résumé to the nurse manager is for evaluation of a potential candidate's education, skills, and experience related to the open position. A résumé is different from a curriculum vitae (CV) in that a résumé is a summary of your academic and work history, whereas a CV is a more detailed document of work history, academic experience, publications, and so on. A CV is usually used in the academic world. All nurses need to keep their résumé current; it is very frustrating to attempt to write a résumé after 5 years and try to remember everything you have accomplished! Update your résumé at least every 6 months.

RÉSUMÉ WRITING

New nurses and nurse managers and leaders all need to pay attention to their résumé. Tips for résumé writing are listed in Box 20.1.

Name and Address Section

- The name and address may be centered on the page or split on each margin.
- The name should be in a slightly larger type-size than the rest of the résumé.
- The name should be in bold font.

BOX 20.1   Tips for Résumé Writing and Printing

- Résumés should be one page long, unless you have extensive experience in the position for which you are applying.
- Print on light blue, ivory, white, or beige paper (if you mail your résumé, the envelope must be the same color).
- Use Times Roman or similar font; do not use fancy fonts, underlining, or italics because they do not scan correctly.
- Margins should be 1 inch top, bottom, and sides.
- Use 12-point type size if possible; no smaller than 10-point type size.
- Do not use pronouns.

- List a telephone number where you can be reached; list a home and/or a cell phone number, and make sure you have an answering machine or message capability so a message can be left for you (ensure that the greeting on the answering machine is appropriate for a potential employer to hear). Check your message box frequently to make sure that the box is not "full."
- Use an email address that is professional and appropriate; avoid "cutesy" email addresses such as Cutesypie@....
- Check email and telephone messages several times a day.

Objective

Be very specific, even if you have to list more than one job title. If you cannot be specific, omit this section. Make sure that this objective matches the facility to which you are applying.

Education

- List your college name, city, and state (not street address), and the years attended.
- List most recent degree first.
- List the graduation date or anticipated graduation date.
- List the degree and major or program.
- Give your GPA (if your overall GPA is not good, give your nursing GPA [e.g., Nursing GPA 3.5]).
- Once you have graduated, you can list your degree first and then the school and date.
- If you have graduated from a college or university, you do not need to list your high school.

Relevant Skills and Experience or Accomplishments

Use bullet format for clinical rotations, volunteer experiences, accomplishments at other jobs if relevant, computer skills, and so on. Special qualifications such as bilingual ability is important here.

Certifications

List any professional certification that may be significant here. If you are CPR certified through the American Heart Association (AHA), list it along with expiration date. Have you been certified in electrocardiogram (ECG) interpretation? If so, list the organization certifying you, and the date of the course. As you progress in your professional career, you will add your professional certifications here, including the name of certification, certifying agency, and date of expiration.

Job History

- List jobs starting with the most recent and work back from there.
- List name of company, city, state (not street address), and years you worked (not months).
- Give your job title.
- Use bullets to state your accomplishments.
- Begin each bullet statement with an action verb. Use present tense for current job only; use past tense for all previous jobs,
- Do not use "responsible for" or "duties include"; list accomplishments in each job.
- If you have had jobs in the health care field or experience relevant to the job you are now seeking, give it more space on your résumé; jobs that are unrelated to what you are seeking can be given minimal space.

Professional Affiliation and Honors

- List any organizations that you were a member of as a student and/or other jobs you have had; list all honors and membership in honor societies.
- Do not put "References available on request" at the bottom of the résumé. References are always listed on a separate page that you can take with you to an interview.
- Do not list personal information (age, marital status, height, weight, social security number, etc.).

Proofread! Proofread! And Proofread Again!

Have someone else proofread your résumé. Do not rely on computer software spell check and grammar check to proofread for you. Box 20.2 provides a sample résumé for a graduate nurse.

As a nurse manager evaluating this résumé, you would realize that this new nurse has computer skills, has demonstrated leadership qualities within her nursing education, and meets the basic needs of a new staff nurse. If you were looking for a nurse with extensive experience in the cardiac setting, this candidate does not meet that need.

As a new nurse developing a first professional nursing résumé, you need to access the resources available at your school of nursing. Most schools have resources to assist you in the development of a professional résumé; it is in your best interest to use these services.

BOX 20.2 Sample Résumé for a Nurse

Jane Doe

1111 South Green Street, Anywhere, USA 00222

222-555-1212 (cell) 555-212-3333 (home)

Job Target: Long-term association with an acute care hospital acknowledged for nursing excellence

Skills

- Registered nurse highly skilled in care of the critically ill patient
- Strong ability to rapidly prioritize patient care and manage complex patient care
- Bilingual Spanish

Education and Certifications

University of State, Anywhere, USA

Bachelor of Science Degree, Nursing. GPA 3.76, 2003

Outstanding Student Award: attained for excellence in clinical area

American Association of Critical-Care Nurses: CCRN certification current to 2015

Basic Life Support Certificate and Advanced Cardiac Life Support Certificate

Professional Experience

Surgical Intensive Care Staff Nurse: June 2007 to present

Mercy Medical Center, Somewhere, NY

Level II trauma center with 678 beds. 20-bed adult surgical intensive care unit

Postcardiac, renal, and gastrointestinal surgery patient population

Cardiac Intensive Care Staff Nurse: March 2005 to June 2007, Hammondton Medical Center, Somewhere, NY

Community hospital with 320 beds. 10-bed cardiac intensive care unit. Postcardiac intervention unit

Staff Nurse, Telemetry: July 2003 to March 2005

Hammondton Medical Center, Somewhere, NY

40-bed telemetry unit

License

State of Anywhere, USA Registered Professional Nurse

Awards

Staff Nurse of the Year Hammondton Medical Center, 2006

Sigma Theta Tau, International Honor Society of Nursing. Chapter, inducted 2003

EFFECTIVE COVER LETTERS

All résumés need to be accompanied by a cover letter to the institution to which you are applying. The cover letter needs to be written in a professional tone. As a new nurse, this letter will set the tone for the individual reading the cover letter. For the nurse manager, this letter will let you know if this individual is someone who may be appropriate for the position. The qualities of an effective cover letter follow (Jones, 2007, p. 383):

- Brief, neat, and without errors.
- In business format.
- Name and title of person to whom the letter is addressed.
- Why you are interested, and what position you would like to apply for.
- Appointed time for taking NCLEX®-RN (for a new nurse).
- Certifications that match the posted job (for an experienced nurse).
- Express appreciation for consideration and eagerness to be part of team.
- How you can be reached (telephone number).

- Use 9- × 12-inch envelope to send résumé and cover letter (first-class mail).
- Expect response to letter in 2 weeks.
- If not, call after 3 weeks; check with the human resources department.
- Box 20.3 provides an example of an effective cover letter.

THE INTERVIEW

Credentials are often reviewed before or during the interview. These credentials usually consist of the following:

- Copy of the complete résumé.
- Copy of nursing license or a copy of notice of passing board scores.
- Two copies of a complete typed list of all references and previous managers (one copy for the human resources department, and one for the hiring manager). Be sure to include the references' complete names and titles, and current addresses and telephone numbers.

BOX 20.3 Example of an Effective Cover Letter

May 1, 2014
Elizabeth B. Wise, PhD, RN
Director of Nurse Recruitment and Hiring
Caring Hospital, USA
Joy City, LA 70777
RE: Nursing Position on Medical-Surgical Unit
Dear Dr. Wise:

I have just graduated from Caring College and would like to apply for a new graduate nurse position on the Medical-Surgical Unit II at Caring Hospital. I served there as a nurse technician while attending nursing school. I plan to take the NCLEX®-RN examination in early June 2014, and will be available to start work by July 1, 2014.

Having worked as a nurse technician on the Medical-Surgical Unit II for 3 years, I developed positive interpersonal and professional relationships with the team. Furthermore, I am well organized, have effective time-management skills, and am enthusiastic about the prospect of returning to the unit. I am proud to have worked at Caring Hospital for 3 years in light of its high rating and Magnet status. The mission of Caring Hospital is congruent with my values.

Thank you very much for your consideration. You may reach me any time on my cell phone at (999) 709-2525. I look forward to hearing from you to schedule an interview at your convenience.

Sincerely,
Scelitta Source

(Adapted from Jones, R. A. (2007). *Nursing leadership and management: Theories, processes, and practice*. Philadelphia: F. A. Davis.)

- Permission for a criminal background check. Be sure to have a list of your addresses from the previous 5 to 7 years.
- Permission for a drug and alcohol screen.
- For a new nurse, a copy of a recent cumulative grade report to show that you are a graduation candidate, and that you are not at risk for failing the licensing examination.

In many institutions, the initial interview is with the nurse recruiter. During this interview the employment process is reviewed, the salary and benefits are reviewed in a cursory manner, and the potential employee is evaluated as to what position in the organization might be appropriate. The individual is then interviewed by the nurse manager of the particular area of interest. Some nurse managers will also include staff in the interviewing process. This is a reflection of the culture of the organization.

It is important that you have prepared for the interview and do not try to "wing it." This is important for both the job candidate and the nurse manager. As the candidate, before the interview you will need to make a self-assessment of your abilities, your strong points, and your challenges. You also need to do a thorough review of the organization: What is their mission, vision, values? What is the philosophy of nursing? What is the care delivery model? Much of this information is available on the organization website. Remember you need to be able to put your best foot forward, and your self-awareness and organization awareness will greatly assist you in this endeavor. As the nurse manager, this is when the candidate assesses your abilities and judges whether or not they would like to work with you.

Styles of Interviewing

As you move forward to the interview process, you will need to have an idea of what you will ask or be asked. There are various styles of interviewing for the nurse manager, but you need to remember that the goal of the interview is to determine the capabilities of the individual, and to determine whether this individual would be an asset to the unit.

The more traditional styles of interviewing ask questions that elicit standard answers from the prospective employee. Samples of such questions include:

- How would you describe yourself?
- What specific goals have you established for your career?
- What will it take to attain your goals, and what steps have you taken toward attaining them?
- How would you describe the ideal job for you?
- How would you describe yourself in terms of your ability to work as a member of a team?
- What short-term goals and objectives have you established for yourself?
- How would you evaluate your ability to deal with conflict?
- Describe what you have accomplished toward reaching a recent goal for yourself.
- Can you describe your long-range goals and objectives?
- What plans do you have for continued study? An advanced degree?

- Can you describe your long-range goals and objectives?
- Why have your chosen this health care organization?

Many institutions are moving toward a behavior-based interviewing technique. This technique allows the manager to more critically evaluate a person's capabilities based on the following questions:

- Describe a situation in which you were able to use persuasion to successfully convince someone to see things your way.
- Describe a time when you were faced with a stressful situation that demonstrated your coping skills.
- Give me a specific example of a time when you used good judgment and logic in solving a problem.
- Give me an example of a time when you set a goal, and were able to meet or achieve it.
- Give me a specific example of a time when you had to conform to a policy with which you did not agree.
- Tell me about a time when you had to go above and beyond the call of duty to get a job done.
- Tell me about a time when you had too many things to do, and you were required to prioritize your tasks.
- Give me an example of a time when you had to make a split-second decision.
- What is your typical way of dealing with conflict? Give me an example.

- Tell me about a time you were able to successfully deal with another person even when that individual may not have personally liked you (or vice versa).
- Tell me about a difficult decision you have made in the last year.
- Give me an example of a time when you tried to accomplish something and failed.
- Give me an example of when you showed initiative and took the lead.
- Tell me about a recent situation in which you had to deal with a very upset patient or coworker.

These questions can also be customized to deal with specific patient situations.

Lawful and Unlawful Inquiries

As the manager, there are also some rules for things to avoid in the interviewing process that include the following:

- Do not make promises that you cannot keep.
- Do not ask about anything that the law prohibits you from considering, in making your decision. For example, do not ask about an applicant's race or religion because you are not allowed to consider these factors in making your decision. Table 20.1 provides some ideas about how to get relevant information while staying within the bounds of the law. And do not panic if an applicant raises a delicate subject (such as disability

TABLE 20.1	Interview Questions That May and May Not Be Asked	
Subject	Lawful Inquiry/Areas You Can Inquire About	Unlawful Inquiry/Areas You Cannot Inquire About
Age	Are you 18 years of age or older? (to determine whether the applicant is legally old enough to perform the job) If applicant is over age 21 (if job related, e.g., bartender)	How old are you? Date of birth Date of high school graduation Age
Citizenship; national origin or ancestry	Are you legally authorized to work in the United States on a full-time basis? Ability to speak/write English fluently (if job related) Other languages spoken (if job related)	Are you a native-born citizen of the United States? Where are you from? Ethnic association of a surname Birthplace of applicant or applicant's parents Nationality, lineage, national origin Nationality of applicant's spouse Whether applicant is citizen of another country Applicant's native tongue/English proficiency

Continued

TABLE 20.1	Interview Questions That May and May Not Be Asked—cont'd	
Subject	Lawful Inquiry/Areas You Can Inquire About	Unlawful Inquiry/Areas You Cannot Inquire About
Disability	These [provide applicant with list of job functions] are the essential functions of the job. How would you perform them?	Do you have any physical disabilities that would prevent you from doing this job? If applicant has a disability Nature or severity of a disability Whether applicant has ever filed a workers' compensation claim Recent or past surgeries and dates Past medical problems
Drug and alcohol use	Do you currently use illegal drugs?	Have you ever been addicted to drugs?
Sex and family arrangements	If applicant has relatives already employed by the organization	Sex of applicant Number of children Marital status Spouse's occupation Childcare arrangements Health care coverage through spouse
Race	No questions acceptable	Applicant's race or color of skin Photograph to be affixed to application form
Religion	No questions acceptable	Maiden name (of married woman) Religious affiliation/availability for weekend work Religious holidays observed
Other	Convictions, if job related Academic, vocational, or professional schooling Training received in the military Membership in any trade or professional association Job references	Number and kinds of arrests Height or weight, except if a bona fide occupational qualification Veteran status, discharge status, branch of service Contact in case of an emergency (at application or interview stage)

or national origin) without any prompting from you. You cannot raise such subjects, but the applicant can.

- Respect the applicant's privacy. Although federal law does not require you to do so, many state laws and rules of etiquette do.

It is also a good strategy to ask the candidate if they have any questions of you, the interviewer. The interview is a time for both the candidate and interviewer to find the answers to any potential questions they have regarding the candidate and the organization. Box 20.4 provides guidelines for the interview process for the nurse manager.

RECRUITMENT STRATEGIES

The final stage in the recruitment process, the selection and acceptance of the candidate, often relies on many of the various recruitment activities of the organization. Many of these strategies reflect compensation, benefits, or work alternatives that are important to the nurses whom the organization is trying to recruit. Some recruitment strategies are listed in Box 20.5.

If you are the individual being interviewed, you need to know in advance, which of these recruitment strategies are important to you. If you are the nurse manager, you need to be aware of the recruitment strategies that are made available to members of your unit. Some questions that may be asked include the following:

- What are the specific duties of the position?
- What are the strategic objectives for this unit?
- What is the nurse-to-patient ratio?
- Is there support staff on the unit to assist nurses?
- In what ways are nurses held accountable for high qualities of practice?

BOX 20.4 Important Guidelines for the Nurse Manager Interview Process

- Prepare questions in advance on an interview guide.
- Take accurate and complete notes, without writing on the résumé or application.
- Save interview notes of all the candidates interviewed, in case of potential legal challenges.
- Use behavioral interviewing techniques in addition to skills assessments. When feasible, include an additional person in the interview process.
- Confirm that human resources will conduct thorough reference and background checking.
- Collaborate with human resources before extending an offer, promising compensation, and scheduling orientation planning.
- Human resources will prepare an offer letter of employment for the Chief Nursing Officer's (CNO's) signature.

(From Yoder-Wise, P. S., & Kowalski, K. E. (2006). *Beyond leading and managing: Nursing administration for the future* (p. 319). St. Louis, MO: Elsevier.)

BOX 20.5 Recruitment/Retention Strategies

- Transition to practice program
- Flexible hours
- Competitive salaries
- Bonus pay
- Relocation pay
- Fixed shifts
- Weekend option program
- Part-time pay with bonus hours
- Flexible benefits packages
- Scholarships for Bachelor of Science in Nursing (BSN) or graduate studies
- Tuition benefit plan
- Educational loan repayment
- Registered nurse (RN) specialty internships
- Professional development opportunities
- Career opportunities
- Specialty certification reimbursement
- Low nurse-to-patient ratios (workload staffing)
- Shared governance/leadership models
- Care delivery model that promotes professional care at the bedside
- Clinical ladder/career ladder
- Free parking
- Magnet recognition
- Culture of safety: zero tolerance for incivility
- Research/evidence-based practice
- Qualified managerial support
- Clinical support; staff educators, clinical nurse specialists
- Workforce diversity
- Interdisciplinary collaboration opportunities

(From Huber, D. (2018). *Leadership and nursing care management*. St Louis, MO: Elsevier.)

- How much input do nurses have regarding systems, equipment, and the care environment? As a new nurse, what opportunities will I have to participate in shared governance?
- What particular opportunities/challenges presently exist on this unit?
- What professional development opportunities are available to nurses?
- Tell me about your culture of patient safety in this institution.
- Can you tell me how the nurses at this institution strive for excellence?
- Tell me about your commitment to the educational advancement of your nurses.

As a new nurse, you should determine the qualities of a work environment that are important to you before the interview. Review the organization's mission, philosophy, and vision to determine whether it is congruent with your professional values. As a nurse manager, realize which qualities of the work environment are important to members of your staff. Although pay is an important issue, it is generally not an acceptable first or early question to ask of an interviewer. Pay information is usually available on the job posting site.

Many of these strategies play an important role in the satisfaction of the nurses and serve to assist with the retention of nurses. With the nursing shortage, the competition for qualified staff members is at an all-time high, and the environment created with the emphasis on some of these strategies plays a vital role in the recruitment and retention of staff. Salaries vary according to locale, type of institution, professional credentials, and past experience of the staff member.

Once the employee is hired, it is the responsibility of the organization to provide orientation, performance evaluation, training, and professional development and a professional work environment.

When the nurse has entered the professional work environment, there are policies and programs that support a safe work environment (Chapter 9). The autonomous work environment, supported by a shared governance was discussed in Chapter 6.

YOUR FIRST JOB AS A NURSE

This is a very exciting time, and the decision about the first professional position is a challenging one. John (2006) has suggested the following tips to help the new graduate get through this decision and survive the first year as a nurse:

- *Go on several interviews*. Try to find a job that feels "right." This is important in making the decision. The culture of the institution; its mission, vision, and values; and the work environment are all important variables in determining whether the institution is a good fit. Evaluate your own strengths and challenges, and determine what type of work environment is important for your success.
- *Get to know the new job*. Gather all of the materials that you were given during the interview process. Read them and look at your job description; do they match what you want to do?
- *Find out how long your orientation will be*. Will you have a mentor? The first year of work is a period of tremendous learning, and it is important that you will be supported through this process. You need to realize that you are a novice nurse, with lots to learn and experience. Be realistic about your abilities and choose a workplace based on these abilities and expectations.
- *Take some time off before you begin work*. You have just finished an arduous journey through your nursing education. Take some time for yourself to recover and to prepare for the next challenge in your nursing life.
- *Take care of yourself*. One of the major challenges in the first work year has been found to revolve around balancing work and life. Watch your diet, sleep, and exercise. Try to maintain a balance. Also, find someone you can speak to about work outside of the workplace. Have you ever noticed that when nurses get together, they all talk "shop"? You will need to talk about your experiences with someone who will understand. Keep in touch with the support group that you formed at school.
- *Stay positive and motivated*. Be positive every day, and avoid negative energy and negative people who will drain you.

New Nurse Residency Programs (Transition to Practice)

The first year of nursing has been demonstrated, in multiple studies, to be a period of high stress, with many new nurses opting out of nursing after less than a year of practice Halfer & Graf, 2006; PricewaterhouseCoopers' Health Research Institute, 2007; (Spector, Blegen, Silvestre, Barnsteiner, & Lynn, 2015). To address this concern, new nurse residency/transition to practice programs have been developed to support the new nurse in the critical first year of practice. Such programs have been demonstrated to decrease the turnover of new nurses, and to increase their feelings of confidence in the first year of employment (Williams, Goode, Krsek, Bednash, & Lynn, 2007; Fink, Krugman, Casey, & Goode, 2008; (Spector, Blegen, Silvestre, Barnsteiner, & Lynn, 2015). Registered nurse (RN) residency/transition to practice programs are designed to provide new nurse graduates with new learning opportunities through mentorships within a framework that supports the advancement from beginner nurse to advanced-beginner nurse role, while promoting increased competency in the RN role (Benner, Sutphen, Leonard, & Day, 2010; (Spector, Blegen, Silvestre, Barnsteiner, & Lynn, 2015). They consist of a curriculum, guidance from a preceptor, support groups, and access to a facilitator (usually an experienced nurse who has advanced through a clinical ladder), who guides the residents in professional role development. Residency/transition to practice programs vary in length of time, pay benefits, and guarantee of employment, so it is important to know the expectations of a residency program. The outcomes of transition programs for new graduates had significantly better outcomes when the programs had the following characteristics:

- A formalized program that is integrated into the institution, with support from higher administration
- A preceptorship, with a preceptor trained for the role
- A program 9 to 12 months in length
- Content includes patient safety, clinical reasoning, communication and teamwork, patient-centered care, evidence-based practice, quality improvement, informatics
- Time for new graduates to learn and apply the content and obtain feedback and share their reflections
- Customization so that the new graduates learn specialty content in the areas where they are working (Adapted from Spector, Blegen, Silvestre, Barnsteiner, & Lynn, 2015 <https://www.ncsbn.org/6889.htm> Accessed 19.11.8)

YOUR FIRST JOB INTERVIEW

At this time in the career path, it is the new nurse's responsibility to make a concerted effort in the job search. This decision should be made diligently with several factors taken into consideration. Preparation for the interview is key. Begin by listing your strengths and weaknesses. Take into consideration your student clinical evaluations from your professors. Was one of your weaknesses tardiness? If yes, you can list or discuss it as one of your weaknesses, but you can add ways in which you have made corrections to this issue. If one of your strengths was clinical group leadership, play this up during the interview process. Be prepared with a list in hand on the day of the interview. You will be asked for references, both personal and professional. Request a letter of recommendation from one of your clinical professors in a course in which you did exceptionally well that will clearly point out your assets and strengths. Be prepared to answer the question, "Why do you want to work at this facility?" You may know the culture, the mission, and vision of an association if you have worked there, but if you have not, do some investigation. Evaluate the website for information about the organization, including the facility's mission and vision. Note this in answering a question that addresses why you have chosen to interview at this particular facility. If the health care organization holds Magnet status, you may say you would very much like to begin your nursing career at a facility with Magnet status. You may be asked about your short-term goals and long-term goals. For example, you may be interviewed for a 7 p.m. to 7 a.m. nursing position on the pediatric unit. A short-term goal might be that you may want to be working the 7 a.m. to 7 p.m. shift within 1 year. A long-term goal would be that you plan on taking the ANCC Pediatric Nursing Certification when you are eligible. Some institutions will ask you to analyze clinical situations and to present potential solutions.

Where to Look

Where do you look for a nursing position? There are endless ways to search for positions; the Sunday newspaper classified section, nursing journals, online at a facility's website, by word of mouth, and on in-hospital human resources job postings. Job fairs are also an excellent place to job search. The National Student Nurses Association website is one place to evaluate (see https://www.nsna.org/).

Most hospitals have numerous components to the application process. The first contact will be through the application process on the web. That is usually followed by the interview by human resources personnel or the nurse recruiter. This interview is usually used to determine the potential fit between the institution and candidate. Afterward, the candidate is usually interviewed by the nurse manager and perhaps staff. Potential interview topics and questions are listed earlier in this chapter.

After the Interview

Once the interview is complete, it is very professional to send a brief message thanking the interviewer for their time and consideration for the position. The message should be handwritten on professional stationery, not a quick e-mail. If it is the candidate's first choice for a position, they should state interest in further discussion about the position at the interviewer's convenience. This is a perfect way to begin a professional future.

PREPARING FOR LICENSURE EXAMINATION

Entry into the practice of nursing in the United States and its territories is regulated by the licensing authorities within each jurisdiction. To ensure public protection, each jurisdiction requires a candidate for licensure to pass an examination that measures the competencies needed to perform safely and effectively as a newly licensed, entry-level registered nurse. The NCSBN develops two licensure examinations: the National Council Licensure Examination for Registered Nurses and the National Council Licensure Examination for Practical Nurses, which are used by state and territorial boards of nursing to assist in making licensure decisions.

The new nurse needs to decide where they wish to be licensed. Most graduates take the examination in the state where they intend to work. They first contact the state board of nursing in the state where they intend to work. For the current addresses and contact information on the various state boards go to the website of the NCSBN (see https://www.ncsbn.org/contactbon.htm).

Although many states require practicing nurses to take the examination in that state or to apply through the state board for reciprocity, the Nurse Licensure Compact (NLC) of the NCSBN is moving toward mutual recognition of licensure by the states. There are 23 such states, with legislation pending in three others, and legislation enacted and awaiting full implementation in three others as of this writing. Not all state boards have enacted such legislation, but a list of states participating in the Nurse Licensure Compact is given in Table 20.2.

If you move to another state and one of the states has a compact agreement, the process is listed in Fig. 20.1.

After the graduate decides where to take the examination, he or she needs to begin the registration process.

NCSBN maintains a website for all candidates for the NCLEX® examination, which provides answers for most questions that applicants have.

This process needs to begin before graduation. The steps identified by NCSBN are listed in Box 20.6. The examination is administered by Pearson VUE, which is a company contracted by NCSBN to provide test administration services.

An overview of the registration process is as follows.

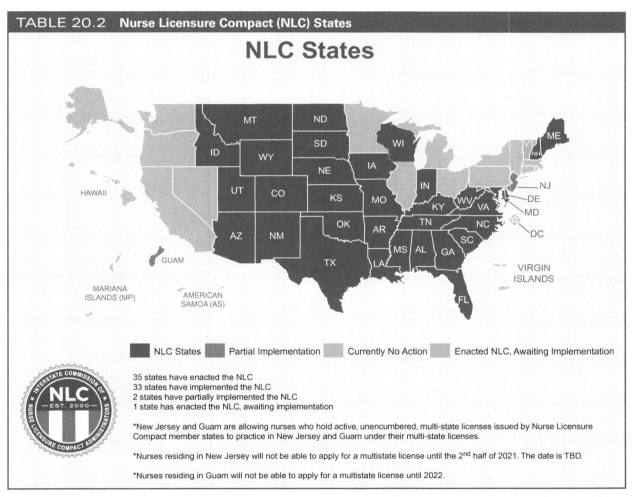

TABLE 20.2 Nurse Licensure Compact (NLC) States

NLC States

Legend: NLC States | Partial Implementation | Currently No Action | Enacted NLC, Awaiting Implementation

35 states have enacted the NLC
33 states have implemented the NLC
2 states have partially implemented the NLC
1 state has enacted the NLC, awaiting implementation

*New Jersey and Guam are allowing nurses who hold active, unencumbered, multi-state licenses issued by Nurse Licensure Compact member states to practice in New Jersey and Guam under their multi-state licenses.

*Nurses residing in New Jersey will not be able to apply for a multistate license until the 2nd half of 2021. The date is TBD.

*Nurses residing in Guam will not be able to apply for a multistate license until 2022.

If you have questions regarding NLC licensure, please contact your state board of nursing in your primary state of residence for specific requirements.
This table indicates which states have enacted the registered nurse (RN) and licensed practical nurse/vocational nurse (LPN/VN) nurse licensure compact (NLC). Please note that Illinois, Massachusetts, Minnesota, New York, and Oklahoma had pending legislation in 2016.
(Modified from Development Dimensions International, Inc. (2003). *Legal considerations in selection [U.S. version]*. Bridgeville, PA: Author.)

Examples of Moving to Different States

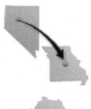

From noncompact to compact:
You must apply for licensure by endorsement in the new state of residency. Your individual state license issued by the noncompact state is not affected and will remain active if you maintain licensure and if so provided by the laws of the nonparty state.

From compact to noncompact:
You must apply for licensure by endorsement in the new state of residency. Your compact license is changed to a single-state license valid only in that state. You must notify the board of nursing that you have moved out of state.

From one compact state to another:
You can practice on the former residency license for up to 30 days. You will be required to:
- Apply for licensure by endorsement (It is recommended that nurses apply 1 to 2 months in advance of a move.).
- Pay any applicable fees.
- Complete a declaration of primary state of residency in the new home state.You will be issued a new multistate license and the former is inactivated. You must notify the board of nursing in the former residency state that you have moved out of state. Proof of residency may be required.

(www.ncsbn.org/nlc.htm)

Fig. 20.1 In the narrative above the fig

Registration Process Overview

1. Submit an application for licensure to the board of nursing where you wish to be licensed.
2. Meet all of the board of nursing's eligibility requirements to take the NCLEX® examination.
3. Register for the NCLEX® examination with Pearson VUE.
4. Receive confirmation of registration from Pearson VUE.
5. The board of nursing makes the candidate eligible to take the NCLEX® examination.
6. Receive authorization to test (ATT) from Pearson VUE.

If you choose to provide an e-mail address at the time you register for the NCLEX® examination (whether by mail, telephone, or via the Internet), please note that all of your correspondence from Pearson VUE will arrive only by e-mail. If you do not provide an e-mail address when you register, your correspondence from Pearson VUE will arrive only through U.S. mail. Remember that all documents need to have identification information that is similar, for example, if your birth certificate reads "Jane Doe" but your transcript reads Jane Allyson Doe," this will cause a delay in your receipt of a permission to test number.

If more than 2 weeks have passed after you have submitted a registration for an NCLEX® examination and received confirmation from Pearson VUE, and you have not received an ATT, please call Pearson VUE at the appropriate number listed on the inside front cover (National Council of State Boards of Nursing, 2019).

Before the Examination

Some schools of nursing administer "readiness examinations" as a requirement for graduation. These examinations are also administered by companies that manage NCLEX® review courses. Many students take such courses on graduation as a preparation for the examination. Most of these courses are valuable preparation tools for examination candidates. They offer large test banks that allow the graduate to constantly practice and review NCLEX®-type questions. Although

BOX 20.6 The Eight Steps of the NCLEX® Examination Process

1. Apply for licensure to the board of nursing in the state or territory where you wish to be licensed. Contact the state board for the requirements.
2. Register for the NCLEX® examination with Pearson VUE by mail, telephone, or via the Internet.
   A. The name with which you register must match exactly with the printed name on the identification you present at the test center
   B. If you provide an email address when registering for the NCLEX® examination, all subsequent correspondence from Pearson VUE will arrive only by email. If you do not provide an email address, all correspondences will arrive only through the U.S. mail.
   C. All NCLEX® examination registrations will remain open for a 365-day time period during which a board of nursing may determine your eligibility to take the NCLEX® examination.
   D. There is no refund of the $200 NCLEX® registration fee for any reason.
3. Receive confirmation of registration from Pearson VUE.
4. Receive eligibility from the state board of nursing you applied for licensure with.
5. Receive the Authorization to Test (ATT) from Pearson VUE.
   If more than 2 weeks have passed after you have submitted a registration for the NCLEX® examination and you received a confirmation from Pearson VUE, and have not received an ATT, please call Pearson VUE.
   A. You must test within the validity dates of your ATT. These validity dates cannot be extended for any reason.
   B. The printed name on your identification must match exactly with the printed name on your ATT. If the name with which you have registered is different from the name on your identification, you must bring legal, name change documentation with you to the test center on the day of your test. The only acceptable forms of legal documentation are marriage licenses, divorce decrees, and/or court action legal name change documents. All documents must be in English, and must be the original documents.
6. Schedule an appointment to test by visiting https://www.pearsonvue.com/nclex or by calling Pearson VUE.
   A. To change your appointment date:
   - For examinations scheduled on Tuesday, Wednesday, Thursday, and Friday, call Pearson VUE at least 24 hours in advance of the day of the appointment.
   - For examinations scheduled on Saturday, Sunday, and Monday, call Pearson VUE no later than the Friday before, at least 1 full business day in advance of your appointment.
7. Present one form of acceptable identification and your ATT on the day of the examination.
   A. The only acceptable forms of identification in test centers in the United States, American Samoa, Guam, Northern Mariana Islands, and the U.S. Virgin Islands are:
   - U.S. driver's license (not a temporary or learner's permit)
   - U.S. state identification
   - Passport
   B. For all other test centers (international), only a passport is acceptable. All identification must be written in English, have a signature in English, be valid (not expired), and include a photograph. Candidates with identification from a country on the U.S.-embargoed countries list will not be admitted to the test.
   C. You will not be admitted to the examination without acceptable identification and your ATT. If you arrive without these materials, you forfeit your test session and must reregister; this includes repayment of the $200 registration fee.
8. Receive your NCLEX® examination results from the board of nursing you applied for licensure with within 1 month from your examination date.
   For more detailed information on the NCLEX® examination and registration process, consult the Candidate Bulletin by visiting https://www.ncsbn.org or https://www.pearsonvue.com/nclex.

(From National Council of State Boards of Nursing [NCSBN]. (2019). Used with permission.)

they are an additional expense for the student, many students believe that the continued exposure to testing situations is worth the expense. Most schools of nursing will assist the student in finding appropriate courses in the area.

PROFESSIONAL GROWTH

As nurses mature in the profession, it is expected that they take a leadership role. How a nurse chooses to do this depends on their practice area. The most important thing is to maintain currency in the profession. Many states require nurses to obtain continuing education (CE) credits to renew the nursing license. Although this is a way to maintain currency, much more work is required to keep up with the rapid changes occurring on a day-to-day basis in the profession. A good way to keep up-to-date is to belong to a professional organization that represents the area of practice and interest. There are numerous organizations representing the various specialties within the profession.

Professional nursing organizations, at both the national and local chapter level, provide opportunities to connect with peers in your specialty; share best practices; and learn about new trends, education, and technical advances. There are many reasons for a nurse to join a professional organization. They include the following:

- *Education:* Science and technology change rapidly and you need to keep up with the changes that affect health care. Some of these boards even offer CE activities to members at reduced prices.
- *Annual conventions:* As a member of a professional organization, you'll get notices announcing major conventions that you may be able to attend at a discount rate. Making professional contacts is a big draw at these conventions, where you'll meet other nurses in your specialty.
- *Networking:* As a member of a professional association, you will have plenty of other networking opportunities along with connecting with other health care professionals at national, state, or local conventions. For example, you will probably have access to online chats or forums at your association's Internet site. Not only can you network with your peers and other professionals, but you can also hear how others are handling some of the same issues you face.
- *Certification:* Many professional organizations offer certification.
- *Targeted products and resources:* When you join a professional organization, you may get discounts to obtain online CE, newsletters, certification review materials, and much more. Some nursing organizations offer members discounts on auto, life, and professional liability insurance, and feature special credit card offers. Many nursing organizations offer members an official journal that may contain peer-reviewed clinical articles and research relevant to the specialty.
- *Career assistance:* When you are searching for a new job, look to your association's career center for openings, advice, and opportunities. In fact, keep an eye

on that information periodically, whether you are job searching or not, to stay in touch with the latest trends in your specialty. Review job openings for salaries and benefits so you know current earning potentials.
- *The Internet:* Practically all nursing associations have Internet sites you can explore. Typically, they offer general information about the association that anyone can access, in addition to member-only areas with restricted access.

(Adapted from Greggs-McQuilkin, 2015.)

A sample listing of professional organizations is given in Chapter 10.

When the nurse has decided on a specialty, it is highly recommended that, when eligible, they sit for the certification examination in the chosen specialty field. Specialties have differing requirements for eligibility for the examination. There are advanced-level examinations for nurse practitioners and clinical nurse specialists. There are also specialty examinations for specific practice areas; the ANCC certifications are listed in Chapter 10.

Other **specialty certification examinations** are given by specialty organizations, such as the Certified Emergency Nurse (CEN) examination, which is administered by the Emergency Nurses Association, and the Adult, Neonatal and Pediatric Acute/Critical Care Nursing Certification (CCRN), and several other certification examinations, which are administered by The Association of Critical Care Nurses Certification Corporation. (American Nurses Credentialing Center [ANCC], 2018).

Some institutions recognize these accomplishments through monetary awards. It is also an accreditation that would provide the nurse with "an edge" if they were to seek an advanced position in nursing.

CONTACT HOURS

Many states have passed legislation that requires a nurse to have obtained a certain number of contact hours of CE to renew a nursing license. When hired it is important to ask about the hospital policy on funding for CE, both within the facility and out of the facility. Ask whether the facility will pay a travel allowance for the nurse to attend a conference out of state. There are also contact hours offered in nursing magazines and online CE contact hours. It is up to the nurse to be aware of the state's licensure requirements for renewal.

RETURNING TO SCHOOL

As a nurse begins to assume a leadership role within the profession, it is time to think about advancing his or her education. Most hospitals have tuition reimbursement for nurses who return to school for an advanced degree. There has been movement in some states (New York and New Jersey) to require nurses to receive the Bachelor of Science in Nursing degree within 10 years of becoming an RN. Some hospitals, especially Magnet-certified hospitals, expect their nurses to continue their education and receive an advanced degree. There are numerous studies that document better patient outcomes in facilities with nurses with advanced education (Aiken, Clarke, Cheung, Sloane, & Silber, 2003, 2004). Remember that although the new nurse has just finished his or her initial education, it is only the first step. Nursing is a profession that demands continued education and growth.

SUMMARY

You have finally done it! You have graduated, but this is only the first step. You will need to prepare for the NCLEX® licensing examination, decide on your first job, and settle into the profession. The profession will demand that you keep up-to-date with changes in patient care, evidence, practice, and professional issues. You will need to join a professional organization, consider taking the certification examination, and return to school for an advanced degree.

CLINICAL CORNER

What I Look For in a Potential Hire

I am going to direct this to you, the potential hire, and I hope that you take this advice, freely given, to make you the hire for the job that you aspired to, and now have the background and experience necessary to apply for the position. This also goes for you, the new registered nurse (RN) graduate, because your first job is extremely important to you. It will be the foundation that you will build your career on.

After 25 years in recruitment, and doing a job that I absolutely love, when I find that fantastic hire, it truly makes my day. Here are some tips for applicants that I hope will help make you that fantastic hire!

- A cover letter is your introduction to the recruiter. Not every recruiter feels as strongly as I do regarding an excellent cover letter, but it sure cannot hurt to do a good one and grab that recruiter's attention. For me, I want to hear your passion about being an RN, and why you would want to work at my institution. Do your homework for this letter and for the interview. It also helps to direct this to the person who will be doing the hiring. Just call the human resources department to find out the name. It shows you have done that little bit extra and that can go a long way.
- Your résumé is going to tell a story of sorts regarding your education, experience, and your other accomplishments. It should begin with your current experience and other experience to follow. Make sure that your dates of employment are correct, and check again when you fill out the application that the dates match with your résumé because background checks are done before the hiring process is complete.
- Make sure a professional message is on your phone or answering machine, for you are a professional seeking employment. When you get to speak use proper grammar (as you have done in your cover letter), and communicate well, as this is a screening process for the recruiter. I cannot even count the times that I have called to set up a possible interview and have not done so because of poor communication skills; after all, an RN is going to communicate with patients, families, physicians, and everyone else connected with patient care. Effective communication is so very important in the life of a nurse or any health care employee. I listen for proper grammar, tone, and attitude in my first contact, and I wish more applicants understood how very important this first voice contact is.
- You have made it to having an interview scheduled. Give yourself enough time to get to the location where the interview will take place. Take a ride there beforehand, at the same time of day your interview is scheduled, so that you have an idea of what traffic is like at that time. If your interview is on a weekday, as most are, do not take that trip on a Sunday when there is a completely different traffic pattern. Take a good look in the mirror before you leave; "dress for success" is not just a tag line. If any recruiter is being honest,

CLINICAL CORNER—cont'd

they will tell you that first impressions set the tone for any interview. "Dress for success" states how you feel about yourself, and how you wish to be viewed. The less skin shown the better; go light on the makeup and the perfume, and for men, the cologne. Suits give a professional appearance and are a good and wise investment.

- Prepare for the interview by coming with questions that you might have. Remember that an interview is a conversation with the recruiter wanting to get to know you and your desire for information about the position. I think that if you keep that in mind and are honest, your interview will go well. Show your passion, why you have chosen nursing, and what you can bring to the institution you are interviewing for. Be prepared to be asked behavioral questions because they show how you have handled situations in the past, and they are a good indicator of how you will handle things in the future. This gives the recruiter excellent insight on how you will probably handle situations in the future. Body language is observed, and I watch facial expressions very closely. I want to see a face light up when talking about a patient or why you have chosen nursing; to me it shows your compassion, and I get a fairly good idea about your commitment to nursing. We can teach clinical aspects of nursing but cannot change one's personality and traits; you will not only be caring for patients, you also will be an ambassador for your institution both at work and in the outside world. No one leaves my office for a second interview without my feeling that I would want them to take care of me or my family. And remember, this is your chance to convince the recruiter that you are the one for this position.

- Follow up with a cover letter to both the recruiter and to anyone else who has interviewed you. An e-mail is acceptable, but a written letter or note shows that little bit extra. This follow-up shows both courtesy and professionalism, and is extremely important. It keeps you in mind. It is perfectly okay to follow up with an e-mail if you have not heard in a few weeks, but stop at one.

- I hope that these pieces of advice have and will help you to be not just the potential hire but that hire. The last thing I will leave you with is to just be yourself. Good Luck!

Joan Orseck
Nurse Recruiter, Holy Name Medical Center,
Teaneck, NJ

EVIDENCE-BASED PRACTICE

(From Needleman, J., Buerhaus, P., Mattke, S., Stewart, M., & Zelevinsky,. (2002). Nurse-staffing levels and the quality of care in hospitals. *New England Journal of Medicine*, 30(22):346; Boyle, D. (2017). Nursing specialty certification and patient care outcomes: What we know in acute care hospitals and future directions. *The Journal of the Association for Vascular Access, 22*(3), 137–142.)

Over the last two decades the Institute of Medicine (IOM) and Magnet have promoted the role of nurses in patient safety. Recently, the IOM promoted individual nurse and nurse organization credentialing as a means to protect the public by improving the quality of care. For individual nurses, credentialing means voluntary specialty certification that "improves access to, and quality of care, particularly in special populations." Further, nurse credentialing may contribute to standardized care quality and promote nurse participation in leadership roles.

Studies have found relationships between higher rates of nursing specialty certification and lower rates of total patient falls, pressure injuries, selected hospital-acquired infections, failure to rescue, and death. Inconsistent or contradictory evidence exists for the association of specialty certified nurses and lower total fall rates, selected hospital-acquired infection rates, and hospital-acquired pressure injuries. Further, many of the significant associations supporting a relationship between specialty certified nurses and better outcomes are weak and may not be clinically meaningful.

These studies all have been based on a linear framework, where the structure and processes of care influence the outcomes of care. For example, structure (i.e., rates of specialty certified nurses) and processes (e.g., risk assessment and prevention measures) can be examined for effect on a particular set of patient outcomes. Needleman et al., 2002 asserted that the factors contributing to outcomes in today's complex health care environment interact in a nonlinear fashion. Needleman modified the research model by specifying three sets (pathways) of nonlinear intervening variables that can directly or indirectly influence how the effects of specialty certification are translated into practice. This new model is the Expanded Conceptual Model for Credentialing Research and the three intervening pathways are invisible architecture, work organization, and nursing performance. Four outcomes were specified: organization, nurse, patient, and population health.

The invisible architecture pathway includes factors such as organizational and unit climate, culture, and leadership. The work organization pathway examines how specialty

Continued

certified nurses provide secondary benefits to their workplace, peers, and patients not in their care. The nurse performance pathway focuses on how specialty certified nurses affect the outcomes of patients directly in their care. When providing illustrations of how the three pathways work, Needleman gives positive examples of how specialty certified nurses influence outcomes. For example, using the invisible architecture pathway, one could posit how the unit culture might suppress the ability of certified nurses to practice to the fullest extent of their education and training.

The following are examples of research formulated with the work organization pathway:

- Is there a threshold dose (rate) of specialty certified nurses needed on units to improve patient outcomes?
- Is the threshold different for different unit types?
- Is there an interaction between threshold dose (rate) and the level of autonomy and decision making on units?

The Expanded Conceptual Model provides a mechanism for driving theory-based research about the association of specialty certification and patient outcomes by providing specific intervening variables: invisible architecture, work organization, and performance.

NCLEX® EXAMINATION QUESTIONS

1. An effective job description includes:
   A. Title, job objectives, list of duties
   B. Title, job opportunity, list of duties
   C. Job objectives, unit, competencies needed
   D. Job objectives, unit, list of duties

2. A nurse manager is legally not allowed to ask the following question during an interview:
   A. When you are available to begin work
   B. Race
   C. Past work history
   D. University attended

3. Regarding position posting, once a position becomes vacant in an organization, the institution posts the position _____ first.
   A. Externally
   B. Internally
   C. In nursing journals
   D. Online

4. Health care institutions that are equal opportunity employers must meet all _____ guidelines
   A. Federal government
   B. State
   C. Government
   D. Cultural

5. Nursing compact states:
   A. Recognize the license regulation of other states
   B. Recognize that the registered nurse (RN) must take the NCLEX® in all states they are working in
   C. Decide what state the RN wants to work in
   D. Be aware that RNs do not have to pay for a license in every state they are working

6. A résumé is different from a curriculum vitae in that:
   A. A résumé is a summary of academic and work history
   B. A curriculum vitae is a summary of academic and work history
   C. A résumé is usually used in academia
   D. A curriculum vitae is education and skills

7. An effective cover letter should be sent with a résumé for all jobs you are applying for. The cover letter should include:
   A. A business format
   B. How to be reached
   C. Addressed to a specific individual
   D. Addressed to the human resource manager

8. Some states have passed legislation that requires a nurse to have obtained a certain number of contact hours of continuing education to renew a nursing license. What question should the RN ask at an interview?
   A. What amount of funds will the hospital pay for continuing education?
   B. Will the hospital pay for internal and external education?
   C. How many contact hours does a nurse need in a particular state?
   D. All of the above are correct

9. What is true regarding returning to college for a Bachelor of Science in Nursing (BSN)?
   A. Some hospitals will pay for the tuition
   B. Most hospitals require the RN to have a BSN

    C. Some hospitals do not require a diploma school graduate to obtain a BSN

    D. Both A and B are correct

10. After a job interview, the RN should:

    A. Write a note to thank the person for the interview

    B. An e-mail is best to send a thank you

    C. Call the nurse manager to say thank you

    D. Call human resources if you have not heard from the hospital in 1 week

Answers: A. A   2. B   3. B   4. A   5. A   6. A   7. C   8. D   9. D   10. A

BIBLIOGRAPHY

Aiken, L. H. (2004). RN education: a matter of degrees. *Nursing, 34*, 50–51.

Aiken, L. H., Clarke, S. P., Cheung, R. B., Sloane, D. M., & Silber, J. H. (2003). Education levels of hospital nurses and patient mortality. *Journal of the American Medical Association, 290*, 1617–1623.

American Nurses Credentialing Center [ANCC]. (2018) National certifications. www.nursecredentialing.org/Magnet/Magnet-CertificationForms. Accessed 18.09.21.

Benner, P., Sutphen, M., Leonard, V., & Day, L. (2010). *Educating nurses: A call for radical transformation*. San Francisco: Jossey-Bass.

Casey K, K., & Goode, C. (2008). The Graduate nurse experience. Journal of Nursing Administration, 38(7/8 July/August).

Fink, R., Krugman, M., Casey, K., & Goode, C. (2008). The graduate nurse: Qualitative residency program outcomes. The graduate nurse: Qualitative residency program outcomes. The graduate nurse: Qualitative residency program outcomes. *Journal of Nursing Administration, 38*(7), 341–348.

Greggs-McQuilkin, D. (2015). Why join a professional organization? *Nursing, 35*, 19.

Huber, D. (2018). *Leadership and nursing care management*. Philadelphia: Elsevier.

Halfer, D., & Graf, E. (2006). Graduate perceptions of the work environment. Nursing Economics, 24(May-June)(3), 150–155, 123.

John, T. (2006). Your first year as a nurse. NSNA Imprint.

Jones, R. A. (2007). *Nursing leadership and management: Theories, processes, and practice*. Philadelphia: F. A. Davis.

Needleman, J., Buerhaus, P., Mattke, S., Stewart, M., & Zelevinsky, K. (2002). Nurse-staffing levels and the quality of care in hospitals. New England Journal of Medicine, 346(May)(22).

National Council of State Boards of Nursing. Nurse Licensure Compact. www.ncsbn.org/nlc.htm. Accessed 18.09.21.

National Council of State Boards of Nursing (2019). Application for licensure flowchart www.ncsbn.org/NCLEX_Flowchart.pdf. NCSBN. Available from www.ncsbn.org/NCLEX_Flowchart.pdf. Accessed 18.09.21.

PricewaterhouseCoopers' Health Research Institute. (2007). What works: Healing the healthcare staffing shortage. http://pwchealth.com/cgilocal/. Accessed 18.09.21.

Spector, N., Blegen, M.A., Silvestre, J., Barnsteiner, J., & Lynn, M.R., et al., & NCSBN. (2015). Transition to practice in hospital settings. Journal of Nursing Regulation, 5(4), 24–38.

Vice Provost for University Life at the University of Pennsylvania. (2008). Resume guide for undergraduates. www.vpul.upenn.edu/careerservices/nursing/resume.html#sample_resume. Accessed 18.09.21.

Williams, C. A., Goode, C. J., Krsek, C., Bednash, G. D., & Lynn, M. R. (2007). Postbaccalaureate nurse residency: 1-year outcomes. *Journal of Nursing Administration, 37*(7/8), 357–365.

Yoder-Wise, P. S., & Kowalski, K. E. (2006). *Beyond leading and managing: Nursing administration for the future*. St. Louis: Elsevier.

Case Scenario: A nursing student has completed his course work to become a registered nurse (RN), but he must still register for and take the NCLEX® licensure exam. In the meantime, he also begins the challenge of looking for and applying for entry-level nursing positions. He is most interested in a residency program within a large hospital setting or health care organization. He says his dream first job would be a residency in either a surgical or orthopedic hospital—with guaranteed employment on completion, of course! He begins by creating his resume.

ITEM TYPE: CLOZE

1. **Choose the *most likely* options to complete the statement below.**

    When creating a resume, this nursing student must be sure to _____1_____ and _____2_____.

Options for 1	Options for 2
A. Provide his overall or nursing GPA—whichever is higher	D. Proofread to ensure that he has included his name (spelled correctly), phone number, address, and Social Security number
B. Include both his college and his high school under "Education"	E. Either identify a specific job title objective or omit an objective statement altogether
C. Omit volunteer experiences since these will make his resume look less professional	F. List job experiences and degrees earned, starting with first job and ending with most recent

ITEM TYPE: ENHANCED HOT SPOTS

2. One of this student's first priorities is to find a nurse residency or transition-to-practice position. Use an X to indicate which features are associated with a nurse residency/transition to practice. **Check all that apply.**
    _____ A. Outsourced support service
    _____ B. Educational curriculum

_____ C. Postlicensure support only
_____ D. Preceptorship
_____ E. 9- to 12-month programmed support
_____ F. Takes the form of continuing education
_____ G. Formal program within the institution
_____ H. Guaranteed employment

ITEM TYPE: DRAG & DROP

3. In planning to take the professional licensing exam, this new graduate realizes the following about the licensing exam. **Place a check mark next to each.**

Credentialing/Licensure Requirements	True
A. The National Council of State Boards of Nursing (NCSBN) provides only one licensure examination for all nurses: the National Council Licensure Examination for Registered Nurses.	
B. The state may require the nurse to attend annual state nursing conventions.	
C. A nurse may acquire CE credits through social magazines.	
D. All states require practicing nurses to take the examination in that same state.	
E. The NCSBN is currently pushing for reciprocity or mutual recognition of licensure between states.	
F. The nurse's state may require continuing education credits to renew the nursing license.	

ANSWERS

1. A, E
2. B, D, E, G
3. A, E, F

INDEX

Note: Page numbers followed by *b, t,* or *f* refer to boxes, tables, or figures, respectively